Pain
SOURCEBOOK
Third Edition

Injury & Trauma Sourcebook

Learning Disabilities Sourcebook, 2nd Edition

Leukemia Sourcebook

Liver Disorders Sourcebook

Lung Disorders Sourcebook

Medical Tests Sourcebook, 3rd Edition

Men's Health Concerns Sourcebook, 2nd Edition

Mental Health Dis⁄ Edition

Mental Retardati

Movement Disor

Multiple Sclerosi

Muscular Dystro

Obesity Sourceb

Osteoporosis Sou

Pain Sourcebook

Pediatric Cancer

Physical & Ment Sourcebook

Podiatry Sourceb

Pregnancy & Bir Edition

Prostate Cancer

Prostate & Urolo

Reconstructive & Sourcebook

Rehabilitation S

Respiratory Di Edition

Sexually Trans 3rd Edition

Sleep Disorder

Smoking Conc

Sports Injuries

Stress-Related Edition

Stroke Source

Surgery Sourc

Thyroid Disor

Transplantatio

Traveler's Health Sourcebook

Urinary Tract & Kidney Diseases & Disorders Sourcebook, 2nd Edition

Vegetarian Sourcebook

Women's Health Concerns Sourcebook, 2nd Edition

Workplace Health & Safety Sourcebook

Worldwide Health Sourcebook

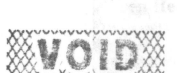

Health Reference Series

Third Edition

Pain
SOURCEBOOK

Basic Consumer Health Information about Acute and Chronic Pain, Including Nerve Pain, Bone Pain, Muscle Pain, Cancer Pain, and Disorders Characterized by Pain, Such as Arthritis, Temporomandibular Muscle and Joint (TMJ) Disorder, Carpal Tunnel Syndrome, Headaches, Heartburn, Sciatica, and Shingles, and Facts about Diagnostic Tests and Treatment Options for Pain, Including Over-the-Counter and Prescription Drugs, Physical Rehabilitation, Injection and Infusion Therapies, Implantable Technologies, and Complementary Medicine

Along with Tips for Living with Pain, a Glossary of Related Terms, and a Directory of Additional Resources

Edited by
Joyce Brennfleck Shannon

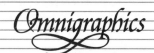

P.O. Box 31-1640, Detroit, MI 48231

Bibliographic Note

Because this page cannot legibly accommodate all the copyright notices, the Bibliographic Note portion of the Preface constitutes an extension of the copyright notice.

Edited by Joyce Brennfleck Shannon

Health Reference Series

Karen Bellenir, *Managing Editor*
David A. Cooke, M.D., *Medical Consultant*
Elizabeth Collins, *Research and Permissions Coordinator*
Cherry Stockdale, *Permissions Assistant*
EdIndex, Services for Publishers, *Indexers*

* * *

Omnigraphics, Inc.

Matthew P. Barbour, *Senior Vice President*
Kevin M. Hayes, *Operations Manager*

* * *

Peter E. Ruffner, *Publisher*

Copyright © 2008 Omnigraphics, Inc.

ISBN 978-0-7808-1006-8

Library of Congress Cataloging-in-Publication Data

Pain sourcebook : basic consumer health information about acute and chronic pain, including nerve pain, bone pain, muscle pain, cancer pain, and disorders characterized by pain, such as arthritis, temporomandibular muscle and joint (tmj) disorder, carpal tunnel syndrome, headaches, heartburn, sciatica, and shingles, and facts about diagnostic tests and treatment options for pain, including over-the-counter and prescription drugs, physical rehabilitation, injection and infusion therapies, implantable technologies, and complementary medicine; along with tips for living with pain, a glossary of related terms, and a directory of additional resources / edited by Joyce Brennfleck Shannon. -- 3rd ed.
    p. cm.
  Includes bibliographical references and index.
  Summary: "Provides basic consumer health information about the causes and treatment of various types of acute and chronic pain, along with prevention and coping strategies. Includes index, glossary of related terms, and other resources"--Provided by publisher.
  ISBN 978-0-7808-1006-8 (hardcover : alk. paper) 1. Pain--Popular works. I. Shannon, Joyce Brennfleck.
  RB127.P346 2008
  616'.0472--dc22

                                                                            2008022070

The information in this publication was compiled from the sources cited and from other sources considered reliable. While every possible effort has been made to ensure reliability, the publisher will not assume liability for damages caused by inaccuracies in the data, and makes no warranty, express or implied, on the accuracy of the information contained herein.

This book is printed on acid-free paper meeting the ANSI Z39.48 Standard. The infinity symbol that appears above indicates that the paper in this book meets that standard.

Printed in the United States

Table of Contents

Visit www.healthreferenceseries.com to view *A Contents Guide to the Health Reference Series*, a listing of more than 14,000 topics and the volumes in which they are covered.

Part III: Diagnosing and Treating Pain

Part V: Additional Help and Information

Preface

About This Book

Virtually everyone has experienced pain—the human nervous system's natural response to injury. For most, it occurs for a specific reason, and then it subsides. For others, however, it lingers long after the cause has been removed. Or, its cause persists. Or, the pain comes even in the absence of an identifiable cause. When all its sources are considered, pain is the number-one reason for unscheduled doctor visits in the United States, and more than 76 million Americans suffer from chronic pain that affects employment, mobility, mood, sleep, concentration, and overall quality of life. Fortunately, new treatment options can minimize and relieve the suffering associated with pain. Furthermore, active personal involvement in pain management offers people the best prognosis for pain relief.

Pain Sourcebook, Third Edition provides updated information about the prevalence and effects of acute and chronic pain. Diagnostic tests and treatment options—including recently approved medications, implantable technologies, and complementary therapies for pain relief—are presented, along with detailed information about specific disorders and conditions associated with pain. Also included is information on coping with chronic pain, a glossary of related terms, and a directory of additional resources for people seeking pain relief.

How to Use This Book

This book is divided into parts and chapters. Parts focus on broad areas of interest. Chapters are devoted to single topics within a part.

Part I: A Universal Disorder summarizes what is currently known about pain and reviews the prevalence and duration of pain. It includes facts about pain management disparities experienced by minority populations, chronic pain's impact on psychological well-being, and current research that may lead to new treatments for pain relief.

Part II: Types of Pain and Disorders Characterized by Pain provides details about specific disorders where pain is a primary symptom. These include arthritis, back pain, cancer pain, carpal tunnel syndrome, fibromyalgia, headache, heartburn, inflammatory bowel disease, kidney stones, nerve pain, shingles and postherpetic neuralgia, temporomandibular muscle and joint (TMJ) disorders, and many others.

Part III: Diagnosing and Treating Pain describes tests and procedures for determining the sources of acute or chronic pain. Guidelines are offered for keeping a pain notebook and effectively communicating pain symptoms to your doctor. The use of over-the-counter and prescription pain medications is described, and facts about the abuse of pain-relieving substances is provided. Physical, surgical, psychosocial, and alternate therapies for pain management, including the use of virtual reality, are also described.

Part IV: Living with Pain offers strategies for managing chronic pain and coping with breakthrough pain, sleep difficulties, and stress. The use of exercise, ergonomics, and positive thinking to prevent and minimize pain conditions is presented, and a separate chapter provides pain management information for caregivers.

Part V: Additional Help and Information provides a glossary of terms related to pain relief and pain conditions and a directory of resources with more information for individuals experiencing acute or chronic pain.

Bibliographic Note

This volume contains documents and excerpts from publications issued by the following U.S. government agencies: Centers for Disease

Control and Prevention (CDC); National Cancer Institute (NCI); National Center for Complementary and Alternative Medicine (NCCAM); National Heart, Lung, and Blood Institute (NHLBI); National Institute of Arthritis and Musculoskeletal and Skin Diseases (NIAMS); National Institute of Biomedical Imaging and Bioengineering (NIBIB); National Institute of Child Health and Human Development (NICHD); National Institute of Dental and Craniofacial Research (NIDCR); National Institute of Diabetes and Digestive and Kidney Disease (NIDDK); National Institute of Neurological Disorders and Stroke (NINDS); National Institute of Mental Health (NIMH); National Institutes of Health (NIH); National Institute on Alcohol Abuse and Alcoholism (NIAAA); National Institute on Drug Abuse (NIDA); U.S. Food and Drug Administration (FDA); and the U.S. Department of Health and Human Services (HHS).

In addition, this volume contains copyrighted documents from the following individuals and organizations: A.D.A.M., Inc.; American Academy of Family Physicians; American Chronic Pain Association; American College of Rheumatology; American Geriatrics Society Foundation for Health in Aging; American Pain Foundation; American Podiatric Medical Association; Cleveland Clinic; Dannemiller Memorial Education Foundation; Christina DiMartino; Joseph S. Dovgan; Elsevier Health Sciences Publications; Harvard Medical School Office of Public Affairs; Long Beach VA Healthcare System; National Sleep Foundation; Nemours Foundation; and the World Health Organization (WHO).

Acknowledgements

In addition to the listed organizations, agencies, and individuals who have contributed to this *Sourcebook*, special thanks go to managing editor Karen Bellenir, research and permissions coordinator Liz Collins, and document engineer Bruce Bellenir for their help and support.

About the Health Reference Series

The *Health Reference Series* is designed to provide basic medical information for patients, families, caregivers, and the general public. Each volume takes a particular topic and provides comprehensive coverage. This is especially important for people who may be dealing with a newly diagnosed disease or a chronic disorder in themselves or in a family member. People looking for preventive guidance, information about disease warning signs, medical statistics, and risk factors for health problems will also find answers to their questions in the *Health Reference Series*. The *Series*, however, is not intended to serve as a tool for diagnosing illness, in prescribing treatments, or as a substitute for the physician/patient relationship. All people concerned about medical symptoms or the possibility of disease are encouraged to seek professional care from an appropriate health care provider.

A Note about Spelling and Style

Health Reference Series editors use *Stedman's Medical Dictionary* as an authority for questions related to the spelling of medical terms and the *Chicago Manual of Style* for questions related to grammatical structures, punctuation, and other editorial concerns. Consistent adherence is not always possible, however, because the individual volumes within the *Series* include many documents from a wide variety of different producers and copyright holders, and the editor's primary goal is to present material from each source as accurately as is possible following the terms specified by each document's producer. This sometimes means that information in different chapters or sections may follow other guidelines and alternate spelling authorities. For example, occasionally a copyright holder may require that eponymous terms be shown in possessive forms (Crohn's disease *vs.* Crohn disease) or that British spelling norms be retained (leukaemia *vs.* leukemia).

Locating Information within the Health Reference Series

The *Health Reference Series* contains a wealth of information about a wide variety of medical topics. Ensuring easy access to all the fact sheets, research reports, in-depth discussions, and other material contained within the individual books of the *Series* remains one of our highest priorities. As the *Series* continues to grow in size and scope, however, locating the precise information needed by a reader may become more challenging.

A Contents Guide to the Health Reference Series was developed to direct readers to the specific volumes that address their concerns. It presents an extensive list of diseases, treatments, and other topics of general interest compiled from the Tables of Contents and major index headings. To access *A Contents Guide to the Health Reference Series*, visit www.healthreferenceseries.com.

Medical Consultant

Medical consultation services are provided to the *Health Reference Series* editors by David A. Cooke, M.D. Dr. Cooke is a graduate of Brandeis University, and he received his M.D. degree from the University of Michigan. He completed residency training at the University of Wisconsin Hospital and Clinics. He is board-certified in Internal Medicine. Dr. Cooke currently works as part of the University of Michigan Health System and practices in Brighton, MI. In his free time, he enjoys writing, science fiction, and spending time with his family.

Our Advisory Board

We would like to thank the following board members for providing guidance to the development of this *Series*:

- Dr. Lynda Baker,
  Associate Professor of Library and Information Science,
  Wayne State University, Detroit, MI

- Nancy Bulgarelli,
  William Beaumont Hospital Library, Royal Oak, MI

- Karen Imarisio,
  Bloomfield Township Public Library, Bloomfield Township, MI

- Karen Morgan,
  Mardigian Library, University of Michigan-Dearborn,
  Dearborn, MI

- Rosemary Orlando,
  St. Clair Shores Public Library, St. Clair Shores, MI

Health Reference Series *Update Policy*

The inaugural book in the *Health Reference Series* was the first edition of *Cancer Sourcebook* published in 1989. Since then, the *Series* has been enthusiastically received by librarians and in the medical community. In order to maintain the standard of providing high-quality health information for the layperson the editorial staff at Omnigraphics felt it was necessary to implement a policy of updating volumes when warranted.

Medical researchers have been making tremendous strides, and it is the purpose of the *Health Reference Series* to stay current with the most recent advances. Each decision to update a volume is made on an individual basis. Some of the considerations include how much new information is available and the feedback we receive from people who use the books. If there is a topic you would like to see added to the update list, or an area of medical concern you feel has not been adequately addressed, please write to:

Editor
Health Reference Series
Omnigraphics, Inc.
P.O. Box 31-1640
Detroit, MI 48231-1640
E-mail: editorial@omnigraphics.com

Part One

A Universal Disorder

Chapter 1

Pain Primer: What Do We Know about Pain?

The Universal Disorder

You know it at once. It may be the fiery sensation of a burn moments after your finger touches the stove. Or it's a dull ache above your brow after a day of stress and tension. Or you may recognize it as a sharp pierce in your back after you lift something heavy.

It is pain. In its most benign form, it warns us that something isn't quite right, that we should take medicine or see a doctor. At its worst, however, pain robs us of our productivity, our well-being, and, for many of us suffering from extended illness, our very lives. Pain is a complex perception that differs enormously among individual patients, even those who appear to have identical injuries or illnesses.

The Two Faces of Pain: Acute and Chronic

What is pain? The International Association for the Study of Pain defines it as: An unpleasant sensory and emotional experience associated with actual or potential tissue damage or described in terms of such damage. It is useful to distinguish between two basic types of pain—acute and chronic.

Excerpts from "Pain: Hope through Research," National Institute of Neurological Disorders and Stroke (NINDS), NIH Publication No. 01–2406, updated January 10, 2008. The full text is available at http://www.ninds.nih.gov/disorders/chronic_pain/detail_chronic_pain.htm.

3

Acute pain, for the most part, results from disease, inflammation, or injury to tissues. This type of pain generally comes on suddenly, for example, after trauma or surgery, and may be accompanied by anxiety or emotional distress. The cause of acute pain can usually be diagnosed and treated, and the pain is self-limiting, that is, it is confined to a given period of time and severity. In some rare instances, it can become chronic.

Chronic pain is widely believed to represent disease itself. It can be made much worse by environmental and psychological factors. Chronic pain persists over a longer period of time than acute pain and is resistant to most medical treatments. It can—and often does—cause severe problems for patients.

Diagnosing Pain

There is no way to tell how much pain a person has. No test can measure the intensity of pain, no imaging device can show pain, and no instrument can locate pain precisely. Sometimes, as in the case of headaches, physicians find that the best aid to diagnosis is the patient's own description of the type, duration, and location of pain. Defining pain as sharp or dull, constant or intermittent, burning or aching may give the best clues to the cause of pain. These descriptions are part of what is called the pain history, taken by the physician during the preliminary examination of a patient with pain. Physicians, however, do have a number of technologies they use to find the cause of pain. Primarily these include electrodiagnostic procedures, imaging, neurological examination, and x-rays.

Gender and Pain

It is now widely believed that pain affects men and women differently. While the sex hormones estrogen and testosterone certainly play a role in this phenomenon, psychology and culture, too, may account at least in part for differences in how men and women receive pain signals. For example, young children may learn to respond to pain based on how they are treated when they experience pain. Some children may be cuddled and comforted, while others may be encouraged to tough it out and to dismiss their pain.

Women, many experts now agree, recover more quickly from pain, seek help more quickly for their pain, and are less likely to allow pain to control their lives. They also are more likely to marshal a variety of resources—coping skills, support, and distraction—with which to deal with their pain.

Research in this area is yielding fascinating results. For example, male experimental animals injected with estrogen, a female sex hormone, appear to have a lower tolerance for pain—that is, the addition of estrogen appears to lower the pain threshold. Similarly, the presence of testosterone, a male hormone, appears to elevate tolerance for pain in female mice: the animals are simply able to withstand pain better. Female mice deprived of estrogen during experiments react to stress similarly to male animals. Estrogen, therefore, may act as a sort of pain switch, turning on the ability to recognize pain.

Investigators know that men and women both have strong natural pain-killing systems, but these systems operate differently. For example, a class of painkillers called kappa-opioids is named after one of several opioid receptors to which they bind. Research suggests that kappa-opioids provide better pain relief in women.

Pain in Aging and Pediatric Populations: Special Needs and Concerns

Pain is the number one complaint of older Americans, and one in five older Americans takes a painkiller regularly. In 1998, the American Geriatrics Society (AGS) issued guidelines for the management of pain in older people. The AGS panel addressed the incorporation of several non-drug approaches in patients' treatment plans, including exercise. AGS panel members recommend that, whenever possible, patients use alternatives to aspirin, ibuprofen, and other non-steroidal anti-inflammatory drugs (NSAIDs) because of the drugs' side effects, including stomach irritation and gastrointestinal bleeding. For older adults, acetaminophen is the first-line treatment for mild-to-moderate pain, according to the guidelines. More serious chronic pain conditions may require opioid drugs (narcotics), including codeine or morphine, for relief of pain.

Pain in younger patients also requires special attention, particularly because young children are not always able to describe the degree of pain they are experiencing. Although treating pain in pediatric patients poses a special challenge to physicians and parents alike, pediatric patients should never be undertreated. Recently, special tools for measuring pain in children have been developed that, when combined with cues used by parents, help physicians select the most effective treatments.

Nonsteroidal agents, and especially acetaminophen, are most often prescribed for control of pain in children. In the case of severe pain or pain following surgery, acetaminophen may be combined with codeine.

A Pain Primer

We may experience pain as a prick, tingle, sting, burn, or ache. Receptors on the skin trigger a series of events, beginning with an electrical impulse that travels from the skin to the spinal cord. The spinal cord acts as a sort of relay center where the pain signal can be blocked, enhanced, or otherwise modified before it is relayed to the brain. One area of the spinal cord in particular, called the dorsal horn is important in the reception of pain signals.

The most common destination in the brain for pain signals is the thalamus and from there to the cortex, the headquarters for complex thoughts. The thalamus also serves as the brain's storage area for images of the body and plays a key role in relaying messages between the brain and various parts of the body. In people who undergo an amputation, the representation of the amputated limb is stored in the thalamus.

Pain is a complicated process that involves an intricate interplay between a number of important chemicals found naturally in the brain and spinal cord. In general, these chemicals, called neurotransmitters, transmit nerve impulses from one cell to another. There are many different neurotransmitters in the human body; some play a role in human disease and, in the case of pain, act in various combinations to produce painful sensations in the body. Some chemicals govern mild pain sensations; others control intense or severe pain.

The body's chemicals act in the transmission of pain messages by stimulating neurotransmitter receptors found on the surface of cells; each receptor has a corresponding neurotransmitter. Receptors function much like gates or ports and enable pain messages to pass through and on to neighboring cells. One brain chemical of special interest to neuroscientists is glutamate. During experiments, mice with blocked glutamate receptors show a reduction in their responses to pain. Other important receptors in pain transmission are opiate-like receptors. Morphine and other opioid drugs work by locking on to these opioid receptors, switching on pain-inhibiting pathways or circuits, and thereby blocking pain.

Another type of receptor that responds to painful stimuli is called a nociceptor. Nociceptors are thin nerve fibers in the skin, muscle, and other body tissues, that, when stimulated, carry pain signals to the spinal cord and brain. Normally, nociceptors only respond to strong stimuli such as a pinch. However, when tissues become injured or inflamed, as with a sunburn or infection, they release chemicals that make nociceptors much more sensitive and cause them to transmit pain signals in response to even gentle stimuli such as breeze or a caress. This condition is called allodynia—a state in which pain is produced by innocuous stimuli.

The body's natural painkillers may yet prove to be the most promising pain relievers, pointing to one of the most important new avenues in drug development. The brain may signal the release of painkillers found in the spinal cord, including serotonin, norepinephrine, and opioid-like chemicals. Many pharmaceutical companies are working to synthesize these substances in laboratories as future medications.

Endorphins and enkephalins are other natural painkillers. Endorphins may be responsible for the "feel good" effects experienced by many people after rigorous exercise; they are also implicated in the pleasurable effects of smoking.

Similarly, peptides—compounds that make up proteins in the body—play a role in pain responses. Mice bred experimentally to lack a gene for two peptides called tachykinins—neurokinin A and substance P—have a reduced response to severe pain. When exposed to mild pain, these mice react in the same way as mice that carry the missing gene. But when exposed to more severe pain, the mice exhibit a reduced pain response. This suggests that the two peptides are involved in the production of pain sensations, especially moderate-to-severe pain. Continued research on tachykinins, conducted with support from the National Institute of Neurological Disorders and Stroke (NINDS), may pave the way for drugs tailored to treat different severities of pain.

Scientists are working to develop potent pain-killing drugs that act on receptors for the chemical acetylcholine. For example, a type of frog native to Ecuador has been found to have a chemical in its skin called epibatidine, derived from the frog's scientific name, *Epipedobates tricolor*. Although highly toxic, epibatidine is a potent analgesic and, surprisingly, resembles the chemical nicotine found in cigarettes. Also under development are other less toxic compounds that act on acetylcholine receptors and may prove to be more potent than morphine but without its addictive properties.

One way to control pain outside of the brain, that is, peripherally, is by inhibiting hormones called prostaglandins. Prostaglandins stimulate nerves at the site of injury and cause inflammation and fever. Certain drugs, including NSAIDs, act against such hormones by blocking the enzyme that is required for their synthesis.

Blood vessel walls stretch or dilate during a migraine attack and it is thought that serotonin plays a complicated role in this process. For example, before a migraine headache, serotonin levels fall. Drugs for migraine include the triptans: sumatriptan (Imitrex®), naratriptan (Amerge®), and zolmitriptan (Zomig®). They are called serotonin agonists because they mimic the action of endogenous (natural) serotonin and bind to specific subtypes of serotonin receptors.

Ongoing pain research, much of it supported by the NINDS, continues to reveal at an unprecedented pace fascinating insights into how genetics, the immune system, and the skin contribute to pain responses. The explosion of knowledge about human genetics is helping scientists who work in the field of drug development. We know, for example, that the pain-killing properties of codeine rely heavily on a liver enzyme, CYP2D6, which helps convert codeine into morphine. A small number of people genetically lack the enzyme CYP2D6; when given codeine, these individuals do not get pain relief. CYP2D6 also helps break down certain other drugs. People who genetically lack CYP2D6 may not be able to cleanse their systems of these drugs and may be vulnerable to drug toxicity. CYP2D6 is currently under investigation for its role in pain.

In his research, the late John C. Liebeskind, a renowned pain expert and a professor of psychology at University of California–Los Angeles (UCLA), found that pain can kill by delaying healing and causing cancer to spread. In his pioneering research on the immune system and pain, Dr. Liebeskind studied the effects of stress—such as surgery—on the immune system and in particular on cells called natural killer or NK cells. These cells are thought to help protect the body against tumors. In one study conducted with rats, Dr. Liebeskind found that following experimental surgery, NK cell activity was suppressed causing the cancer to spread more rapidly. However, when the animals were treated with morphine, they were able to avoid this reaction to stress.

The link between the nervous and immune systems is an important one. Cytokines, a type of protein found in the nervous system, are also part of the body's immune system—the body's shield for fighting off disease. Cytokines can trigger pain by promoting inflammation, even in the absence of injury or damage. Certain types of cytokines have been linked to nervous system injury. After trauma, cytokine levels rise in the brain, spinal cord, and at the site in the peripheral nervous system where the injury occurred. Improvements in our understanding of the precise role of cytokines in producing pain, especially pain resulting from injury, may lead to new classes of drugs that can block the action of these substances.

Hope for the Future

Thousands of years ago, ancient peoples attributed pain to spirits and treated it with mysticism and incantations. Over the centuries, science has provided us with a remarkable ability to understand and control pain with medications, surgery, and other treatments. Today, scientists understand a great deal about the causes and mechanisms of pain, and research has produced dramatic improvements in the diagnosis and treatment of a number of painful disorders. For people who fight every day against the limitations imposed by pain, the work of NINDS-supported scientists holds the promise of an even greater understanding of pain in the coming years. The research offers a powerful weapon in the battle to prolong and improve the lives of people with pain: hope.

Chapter 2

Prevalence and Duration of Pain among U.S. Adults

Prevalence and Duration of Pain among Adults in the Month Prior to Interview

Pain hurts—physically, mentally, emotionally, and at times financially. All persons experience pain at some time during their lives. It affects physical and mental functioning, and can profoundly affect quality of life. Treating it is often expensive, time-consuming, and sometimes extremely frustrating. In addition to the direct costs of treating pain—including medical practitioner and hospital visits for diagnosis and treatment, drugs, therapies, and other medical costs—it causes work-loss time, and loss of productivity and concentration at work or while conducting other activities.

The International Association for the Study of Pain (IASP) defines pain as "an unpleasant sensory and emotional experience associated with actual or potential tissue damage, or described in terms of such damage." Pain is a symptom produced when inflammation or changes to the nervous system due to illness or injury are transmitted to the brain, producing a physical sensation that alerts the brain that damage has occurred. Generally, as the inflammation subsides or the wound heals the pain lessens and eventually goes away, although in

---

Excerpted from "Chartbook on Trends in the Health of Americans," *Health, U.S. 2006*, Centers for Disease Control and Prevention (CDC), 2007. The complete report is available at http://www.cdc.gov/nchs/data/hus/hus06.pdf #chartbookontrends.

some cases it does not. Pain can be constant or episodic, last for a minute or most of a lifetime, and can be dull or sharp, throbbing or piercing, localized or widespread, severe or less severe, and ultimately, tolerable or intolerable. Pain can have an undetectable or a nonphysical cause, making it hard to treat.

Pain is always subjective. Although it is a physical sensation, perceptions of pain are influenced by social, cultural, and psychological factors, producing different sensations in different people. Pain in older adults has been shown to be underreported, possibly because of a reluctance to report pain, resignation to the presence of pain, and skepticism about the beneficial effects of potential treatments. Perceptions of pain differ by the context in which it occurs; expectations about how much pain one should feel; anxiety and feelings about a loss of control that can increase pain; past pain experiences; coexisting physical and mental conditions; and many other factors. Research has shown that distracting patients in severe pain can lessen it, and that focusing on pain can make it worse.

Data from the 1999–2002 *National Health and Nutrition Examination Survey* show that more than one-quarter of Americans (26%) age 20 years and over reported that they had a problem with pain— of any sort—that persisted for more than 24 hours in duration in the month prior to interview. Adults age 45–64 years were the most likely to report pain lasting more than 24 hours (30%). Twenty-five percent of young adults age 20–44 reported pain, and adults age 65 years and over were the least likely to report pain (21%). Women reported pain more often than men, and non-Hispanic white adults reported pain more often than adults of other races and ethnic backgrounds. Adults living in families with income less than twice the poverty level reported pain more often than higher income adults.

Measures of pain prevalence are affected not only by how different people perceive pain, but whether it is reported at all. One factor in whether pain is considered salient enough to report is the duration of the pain that is experienced. Adults 20 years of age and over who reported pain in the month prior to interview were asked a follow-up question about the duration of that pain. Nearly one-third of adults 20 years of age and over who reported pain said that it lasted less than one month, 12% reported pain that lasted 1–3 months, 14% reported pain that lasted three months to one year, and 42% reported pain that lasted more than one year. Although persons age 65 years and over are less likely to report pain lasting 24 hours or more, 57% of older adults who reported pain indicated that the pain lasted for more than one year compared with 37% of adults 20–44 years of age who reported pain. Conversely, adults 20–44 years were considerably more likely to report relatively short-lived pain. Therefore, the duration of pain (long- or short-lived) reported by different age groups may explain, in part, differences in pain reporting and pain prevalence by age.

This chapter provides a general overview of pain experienced by adults in the United States. It focuses on common types of pain using data from several national data sources. Some data were collected during in-person interviews with the participant reporting the location, extent, duration, and severity of selected sites of pain. Because some types of pain persist, while other types recur more or less frequently, pain questions have different recall periods. For example, people are asked about any pain that lasted a day or more in the month prior to interview but about severe headaches and back pain during the 3-month period prior to interview. Prevalence estimates with different recall periods are not directly comparable.

Another way to gather information on pain is to ask respondents about use of medications to control severe pain, such as prescription narcotic drugs. Pain in individuals can be indirectly inferred from measures of health care utilization, for example, use of hospital procedures for pain reduction such as hip and knee replacement. Data is presented on the prevalence and possible effects of pain in terms of health status and health care utilization measures, as well as some economic implications including ambulatory medical care expenditures for headache. The relationships between reported pain and race or ethnicity, gender, age, income level, and health status are complex and raise important issues for individuals, the health care system, and society at large. Focusing on pain prevalence and its effects for population subgroups may provide insight for public health initiatives and policies with the ultimate goal of reducing disparities in quality of life and level of functioning.

Low Back, Migraine or Severe Headache, Neck, and Face Pain

Pain occurs in many different parts of the body, each with its own prevalence and presentation patterns. Low back pain and severe headache are two of the most common sources of pain that interfere with an individual's ability to enjoy social activities and negatively affect quality of life.

In the *National Health Interview Survey*, adults 18 years of age and over were asked a series of questions about whether they had had four types of pain during the three months prior to interview (low back, migraine or severe headache, neck, and facial ache in the jaw or joint in front of the ear). Respondents were instructed to report pain that lasted a whole day or more and not to include minor aches or pains. Respondents could report more than one type of pain and were included in each reported category. Trends in the percentage of Americans reporting each of these types of pain have been stable in recent years.

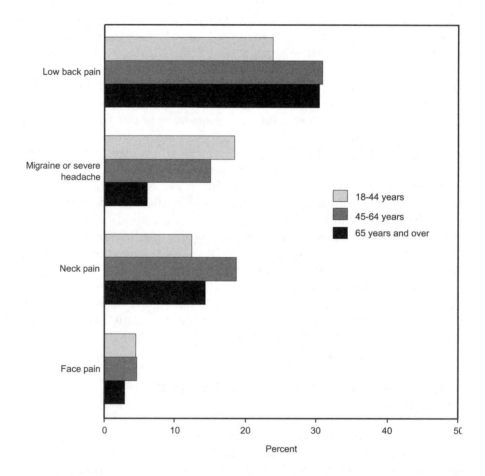

Figure 2.1. *Adults reporting low back pain, migraine, neck, and face pain in the three months prior to interview, by age: United States, 2004. Source: Centers for Disease Control and Prevention (CDC), National Center for Health Statistics (NCHS),* National Health Interview Survey.

Low Back Pain

Low back pain is the second most common neurological ailment in the United States—only headache (when all types and severity levels are considered) is more common. Obesity, smoking, weight gain during pregnancy, stress, poor physical condition, posture inappropriate

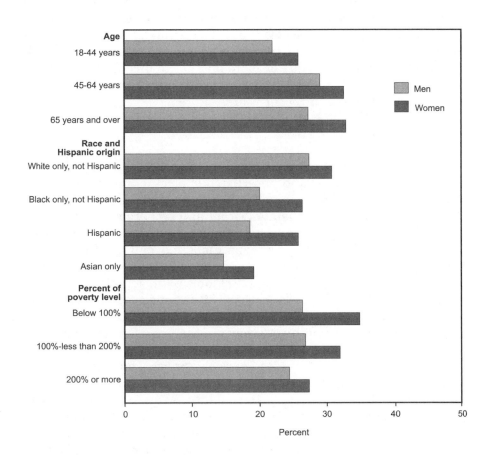

Figure 2.2. *Adults 18 years of age and over reporting low back pain in the three months prior to interview, by selected characteristics: United States, 2004. Note: Asian race includes persons of Hispanic and non-Hispanic origin. Persons of Hispanic origin may be of any race. Percent of poverty level is based on family income and family size and composition using U.S. Census Bureau poverty thresholds. The data table in the full report provides data points graphed and additional notes. Source: CDC, NCHS, National Health Interview Survey.*

for the activity being performed, and poor sleeping position can contribute to low back pain. Low back pain places considerable stress on the health care system in terms of visits and procedures for diagnosis, treatment, and medication management. In addition, there are substantial indirect costs associated with reduced productivity. Low back pain is the most common cause of job-related disability and a leading contributor to missed work, and reduced productivity at work.

In the *National Health Interview Survey*, the presence of pain was measured by asking adult respondents 18 years of age and over about low back pain and other selected types of pain during the three months prior to interview. Respondents were instructed to report low back pain that lasted a whole day or more and not to include minor aches or pains. Trends in the percentage of adults reporting low back pain have remained stable in recent years.

Joint Pain

Severe joint pain is more common among adults age 65 years and over, low-income adults, and non-Hispanic black adults than among adults in other age, income, and racial and ethnic groups. Osteoarthritis is the most common joint disorder and is characterized by joint pain, stiffness, and swelling. Joint pain can also be caused by injury, prolonged abnormal posture, or repetitious movements. In 2003, almost one-third of Americans age 18 years and over and one-half of adults age 65 years and over reported joint pain, aching, or stiffness (excluding the back or neck) during the 30 days prior to interview. The knee was the site of joint pain most commonly reported, followed by the shoulder, fingers, and hips. Trends in the prevalence of joint pain have remained stable in recent years.

In the 2003 *National Health Interview Survey*, only respondents who reported any joint pain, aching, or stiffness in or around a joint during the past 30 days were asked a follow-up question: "During the past 30 days, how bad was your joint pain on average? Please answer on a scale of 0 to 10 where 0 is no pain or aching and 10 is pain or aching as bad as it can be." In this analysis, a reported score of 7–10 was classified as severe pain and 0–6 as lesser pain.

Narcotic Analgesic Drug Visits in Emergency Departments

In one-half of emergency department visits with severe pain recorded, a narcotic analgesic drug was prescribed or received. The presence of pain can be discerned directly by asking people about the presence, type, location, and duration of specific types of pain. In addition, pain can be examined by investigating health care utilization involving pain treatments, such as emergency department (ED) visits during which narcotic analgesic drugs were prescribed. Narcotic analgesic drugs are used primarily to treat severe pain. Physicians' decisions to prescribe narcotic analgesics are highly variable. Some studies conclude that narcotic analgesic drugs are underused in ED visits, particularly among children, older adults, and minority populations.

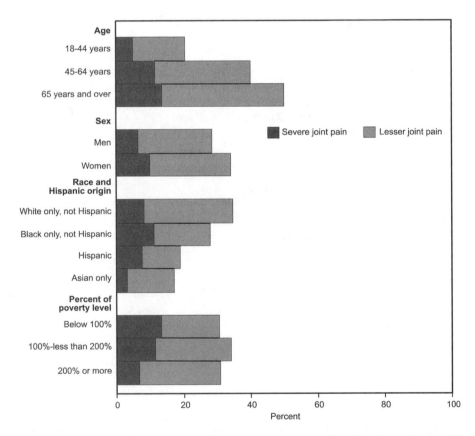

Figure 2.3. *Adults 18 years of age and over reporting joint pain in the 30 days prior to interview, by severity level and selected characteristics: United States, 2003. Note: Percent of poverty level is based on family income and family size and composition using U.S. Census Bureau poverty thresholds. The data table in the full report provides data points graphed, standard errors, and additional notes. Source: CDC, NCHS, National Health Interview Survey.*

In 2003–2004, 23% of all ED visits had a narcotic analgesic drug prescribed or provided during the visit. In the *National Hospital Ambulatory Medical Care Survey, Emergency Room Component*, the presenting level of pain is abstracted from ED records. The presenting level of pain is recorded as none, mild, moderate, severe, unknown, or missing. About 16% of all ED visits in 2003–2004 had a recorded presenting pain level of no pain, 16% mild pain, 21% moderate pain,

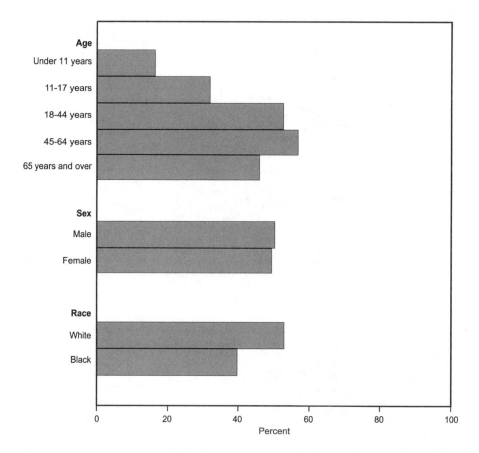

Figure 2.4. *Narcotic analgesic drug visits to the emergency department among visits with a severe pain level recorded, by age, sex, and race: United States, 2003–2004. Notes: Narcotic drug visits are hospital emergency department visits with narcotic drugs prescribed or provided during the visit. The data table in the full report provides data points graphed, standard errors, and additional notes. Source: CDC, NCHS, National Hospital Ambulatory Medical Care Survey, Emergency Department Component.*

14% severe pain, and 33% were unknown or missing on pain level. Children under 11 years of age were more likely to have an unknown or missing presenting pain level, but no difference in the percentage of unknown or missing pain level was noted by gender or by race.

Among ED visits with severe pain recorded, 50% had narcotic analgesic drugs prescribed or provided during the visit. Males and females had similar rates of narcotic drugs for severe pain during ED visits. Children under age 18 were less likely than adults to receive a narcotic drug in the ED, regardless of presenting level of pain. Adults 65 years of age and over with severe pain were less likely to receive a narcotic drug than other adults with severe pain. Black people were less likely than white people to receive narcotic drugs for severe pain in the ED (40% compared with 53%).

Prescription Narcotic Drug Use

The use of narcotic drugs among women has increased from 1988–1994 to 1999–2002, largely due to increased use among non-Hispanic white women and women age 45 years and over. In recent decades, the medical community has increasingly recognized the importance of treating and controlling pain. The goal of pain management is to return patients to a pain level that allows them to function better in their daily lives. Pain may be managed by nonpharmacologic and pharmacologic means. Nonpharmacologic treatments include biofeedback, relaxation techniques, massage, and heat or cold application. These approaches usually supplement pharmacologic treatment. Pharmacologic approaches include a variety of medication options. Minor pain may be controlled by nonnarcotic medications such as aspirin, acetaminophen, or ibuprofen. More severe pain may require the use of narcotic medications, such as codeine and oxycodone.

The *National Health and Nutrition Examination Survey* collects data on the prescription drug use of survey participants living in the community through in-person household interviews. Prescription drug use is determined by examining the prescription labels of the participant's medications.

Between 1988–1994 and 1999–2002, the age-adjusted percentage of women reporting narcotic drug use in the month prior to interview increased by almost one-half from 3.6% to 5.3%. This increase was driven largely by an increase in narcotic drug use among women age 45 years and over. During this period, use of narcotic drugs rose by almost 75% among women 45–64 years of age to 5.7% and by more than 50% among women 65 years and over to 6.8%. This increased use has been primarily among non-Hispanic white women. In contrast, reported narcotic drug use among adult men remained stable from 1988–1994 to 1999–2002 and there were no significant differences in use for men by race or ethnicity. In 1999–2002, women of all ages reported more narcotic drug use than men. Non-Hispanic white women were almost twice as likely to report narcotic use as women of Mexican origin (5.9% compared with 3.2%).

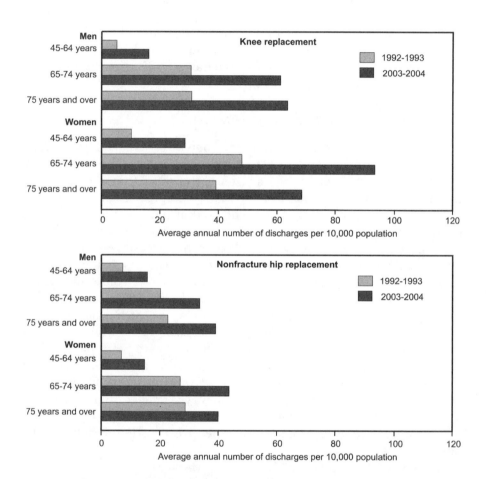

Figure 2.5. Hospital discharges for knee and non-fractured hip replacement surgery among adults 45 years of age and over, by sex and age: United States, 1992–1993 and 2003–2004. Notes: Up to four inpatient hospital procedures were coded for each stay. Hip replacement excludes procedures for hip fracture. The data table in the full report provides data points graphed, standard errors, and additional notes. Source: CDC, NCHS, National Hospital Discharge Survey.

Knee and Hip Replacements

Rates of hospitalizations to replace painful hips and knees have substantially increased since 1992–1993. Knee and hip replacement are two types of surgical procedures for treating significant pain, loss of joint function, and impaired mobility most commonly associated with osteoarthritis. Painful knees and hips are common symptoms among older adults, with about 30% of adults 65 years of age and over reporting knee pain or stiffness in the past 30 days and 15% reporting hip pain or stiffness. In 2003, knee replacement surgery was estimated to cost $11.9 billion and hip replacement $12.2 billion. Aging of the American population and increasing trends in overweight and obesity may further increase the prevalence of joint problems in the future.

Data from the *National Hospital Discharge Survey* provide information on trends in knee and hip replacement surgery. In addition to pain, hip replacement surgery is also performed to treat a fractured hip, often on an emergency basis. Because the focus of this chapter is on pain and its consequences, the analysis of hip replacement surgery excludes hip replacement surgery with a hip fracture diagnosis. Osteoarthritis is the most common diagnosis associated with knee and non-fractured hip replacement procedures—97% of knee replacements and almost 70% of non-fractured hip replacements in 2003–2004 were for patients with a diagnosis of osteoarthritis

Ambulatory Medical Care Expenses Associated with Headaches

Recent statistics on headaches suggest that only a small proportion of adults who experience headaches receive professional medical treatment for their condition, indicating that many people manage their pain themselves using painkillers purchased over the counter, or other self-care. In 2003, 15% of adults reported a migraine or severe headache in the three months prior to interview. However, data from the *Medical Expenditure Panel Surveys* for 2002 and 2003 indicate only 3.5% of adults had ambulatory visits and/or prescribed drug purchases for treatment of headaches over a one-year period. Ambulatory medical care includes care obtained in doctors' offices, hospital outpatient clinics, and emergency rooms, as well as prescribed medicines purchased during the survey year. Ambulatory medical care expenses for headaches averaged about $570 per person with such expenses, although expenses of individuals varied substantially. The

21

median ambulatory medical care headache expense per person with any such expense reported was $212 in 2002–2003.

The percentage of adults who received ambulatory medical care for headaches varied by age and sex. Women were more likely to obtain care than men, reflecting their higher prevalence of headaches. Adults age 45–64 years were most likely to have ambulatory medical care expenses for headaches and those age 65 years or over were least likely to have these expenses.

Average ambulatory medical care expenses for headaches ($566) per adult with such expenses varied little by age and sex. Ambulatory care

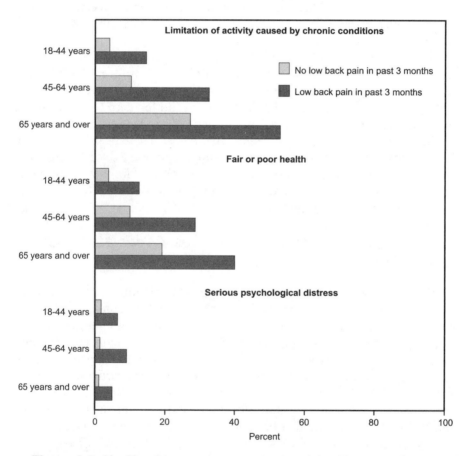

Figure 2.6. *Health status measures among adults 18 years of age and over with and without low back pain, by age: United States, 2004. Note: The full report data table has data points graphed, standard errors, and additional notes. Source: CDC, NCHS, National Health Interview Survey.*

expenses for headache accounted for 15% of total ambulatory expenses for these adults. This percentage decreased with age from 18% among adults age 18–44 years to 10.5% among those 65 years or over. The smaller share of ambulatory care expenses for headaches among adults 65 years and over compared with younger adults resulted in large part from increasing expenses for other medical conditions among older adults.

Health Status Measures among Adults with and without Low Back Pain

People with recent low back pain have worse overall health status as measured by activity limitation, respondent-assessed health status, and serious psychological distress than people without recent low back pain. Pain interferes with an individual's ability to work and engage in many social activities. It may be directly related to health status measures such as activity limitation—for example, people with low back pain may be unable to function in some jobs or to work at all. Moreover, even intermittent pain may affect people's assessments of their physical and mental health. Pain does not necessarily cause serious psychological distress, limitation of activity, or poor health status, but may interact with physical and mental health status to affect perceptions of pain, care-seeking behaviors, speed of recovery, and ability to function.

In the *National Health Interview Survey*, adult respondents were asked about low back pain in the three months prior to interview. Respondents were instructed to report low back pain that lasted a whole day or more and not to include minor aches or pains. Additional questions included respondent-assessed health status, activity limitation due to chronic health conditions, and a series of questions designed to assess serious psychological distress.

Chapter 3

Disparities in Pain Management for Minority Populations

While the undertreatment of pain has been an ongoing problem in the health care setting, this issue has been of particular concern among minority populations. Despite greater general awareness of discriminatory treatment, a recent report by the Institute of Medicine (IOM) states that, "(al)though myriad sources contribute to these disparities, some evidence suggests that bias, prejudice, and stereotyping on the part of health care providers may contribute to differences in care."[1]

Understanding the various forces—explicit and subtle—that contribute to this disparity is indeed complex. To attribute it solely to the failings of health care practitioners is to miss the larger, and more important picture of a systemic failure to address the needs of a substantial part of the population. Beyond human prejudice are issues of a fragmented health care system that provides drastically differing qualities of treatment to different sections of the population, as well as barriers of mistrust between doctor and patient that degrades the quality of care.

And yet there is no turning away from the fact that health care practitioners do discriminate against minorities in a pervasive and surprisingly consistent way. The IOM report, which reviewed well over 100 studies—controlling for such variables as insurance status, patient

Excerpted from "Disparities in Pain Management," *Pain Report, Volume 1, Number 6*, June 2006. © Dannemiller Memorial Educational Foundation. Reprinted with permission.

income, and access to facilities—found an overwhelming majority came to the same conclusion: minorities are less likely to receive needed medical treatment—even clinically necessary treatment—than whites.[1] The area of pain management is no exception to this rule.

A 1997 study comparing different populations of patients with recurrent or metastatic cancer found that 50% of non-minority patients received inadequate analgesic care, while 65% of minorities received inadequate analgesia.[2] This study, typical of its kind, found that in the process of under-medicating, physicians also underestimated the pain of their minority patients at a higher rate. Another study, of Anglo-American and Mexican-American female patients comparing self-reported pain against pain levels assigned by nurses, found a similar discrepancy.[3] A third study found that Hispanics suffering from long-bone fractures were twice as likely to receive no pain medication as their non-Hispanic white counterparts.

In trying to understand how these discrepancies occur, we must first accept the fact that outright prejudice is quite common. Research suggests that more than half, and as much as three-quarters, of white Americans believe that in comparison to themselves minorities—and particularly African-Americans—are less intelligent, more violent, and would prefer to live on welfare.[1] A 2000 study of white doctors found similar views regarding African-Americans, as well as a perception that African-Americans were less likely to comply with medical advice or to have social support.[5] These views were observed even after variables such as income, education, and the personality characteristics of their patients were considered.

Stereotypes of ethnic groups can come into play in a variety of ways. For example, in diagnosing a patient and setting a course of treatment, doctors must weigh the information they gather through observation and interviews with their prior experience and expectations, and the less direct information they are able to gather, the more likely they are to rely on such expectations. If those expectations include preconceived notions about a certain type of patient—whether that type identifies a certain ethnicity, gender, or economic class—an increased risk of misdiagnosis may arise.

Stereotypes, whether they refer to people, experiences, or any other perception of the world, function as a sort of shorthand and may at times be useful to the extent that they don't rely on false or misleading information. Much of diagnostic skill, in fact, depends upon the ability of a physician to recognize symptoms stereotypical of a particular condition. With the serious time constraints put on today's health care practitioner, there is an added pressure to rely on perceptual shortcuts, larger assumptions based on limited information. However, when such shortcuts rely on assumptions about racial and ethnic character traits, the results are likely to be undesirable.[5]

It must be added that along with the physician, the patient may also bring to the table biases counterproductive to a successful medical interaction. If a patient comes in assuming that they will not be properly cared for, there is a higher likelihood that the patient will approach the doctor with mistrust and may be resistant to complying with the doctor's suggested course of treatment. The physician, meanwhile, faced with such resistance, is less likely to be engaged with the patient or with the patient's treatment.

Cultural differences can also play a role in undermining proper treatment, such as when a patient fears the use of certain drugs (for example, opioids) or believes that suffering through pain is a moral requisite. In fact, in the 1997 study mentioned earlier, Hispanic patients were not only more likely to feel they were being undermedicated for their pain, but were also more likely to feel they were being overmedicated.[2] Moreover, limited data suggests that minorities may sometimes be as likely to be undertreated by minority physicians as by white physicians.[6]

The settings of treatment can also play an important role in quality of treatment. Community-based settings, for example, show a significantly better quality of treatment for minority patients compared to clinical settings that treat predominantly minority patient populations.[2] Lack of access to better quality insurance plans or private physicians, regardless of patient income level, is a further impediment to proper treatment. Even where a patient lives can affect their ability to treat their pain: a 2000 study found that while 72% of pharmacies in predominantly white neighborhoods in New York City carried sufficient opioid supplies to treat severe pain, only 25% of pharmacies in non-white neighborhoods did so.[7]

Inevitably, the key to remedying this situation is through education. Cross-cultural education helps health care professionals better understand the cultural and social issues that contribute to inadequate treatment of minority populations. This is not simply sensitivity training for bigots, but is a way of helping even the best intentioned practitioners understand the details that cause such problems, and to teach them the best methods for interacting with their minority patients.

A number of other strategies beyond education need also be applied to remedy the situation, including realigning health plans to better serve all segments of the population. Standardized data collection would further help in getting a clearer picture of disparities in treatment, while promotion of clinical practice guidelines would improve the standardization of health care practice.[6]

References

1. Smedley BD, Stith AY, Nelson AR, eds. *Unequal treatment: confronting racial and ethnic disparities in health care*. Committee on Understanding and Eliminating Racial and Ethnic Disparities in Health Care, Board on Health Sciences Policy, Institute of Medicine. Washington D.C.: The National Academies Press. 2002.

2. Cleeland CS, Gonin R. Pain and treatment of pain in minority patients with cancer: the eastern cooperative oncology group minority outpatient pain study. *Ann Intern Med* 1997; 127: 813–816.

3. Calvillo ER and Flaskerud JH. Evaluation of the pain response by African-American, Mexican-American, and Anglo-American women and their nurses. *Journal of Advanced Nursing* 1993;18: 451–9.

4. Todd KH, Samaroo N, Hoffman JR. Ethnicity as a risk factor for inadequate emergency department analgesia. *JAMA* 1993; 269(12):1537–1539.

5. Van Ryn M, Burke J The effect of patient race and socioeconomic status on physician's perceptions of patients. *Soc Sci and Med* 2000; 50:813–828.

6. Chen J, Rathore SS, Radford MJ, et al. Racial differences in the use of cardiac catheterization after acute myocardial infarction. *N Engl J Med* 2001; 344:1443–1449.

7. Morrison RS, Wallenstein S, et al. "We don't carry that"—failure of pharmacies in predominantly nonwhite neighborhoods to stock opioid analgesic. *N Engl J Med* 2000; 342:1023–1026.

Chapter 4

Chronic Pain and Psychological Well-Being

Mental Disorders Account for Large Percentage of Adult Role Disability

A National Institute of Mental Health (NIMH)-funded study found that more than half of U.S. adults have a mental or physical condition that prevents them from working or conducting their usual duties (role disability) for several days each year, and a large portion of those days can be attributed to mental disorders. The study, published in the October 2007 issue of the *Archives of General Psychiatry*, is based on data from the *National Comorbidity Survey Replication* (NCS-R), a nationwide survey among 9,282 Americans ages 18 and older.

Role disability is increasingly recognized as a major source of the societal costs of illness, but these indirect costs—the result of impaired functioning and lost productivity—are not easily measured, making it difficult to estimate the total costs of illness.

Researchers found that over a one-year period, 53 percent of U.S. adults have one or more mental or physical conditions that result in role disability. Among those adults, each experienced an average of 32 days of disability per year. Nationwide, about 2.4 billion disability days resulted from physical conditions, and about 1.3 billion disability days resulted from mental conditions.

This chapter includes text from "Mental Disorders Account for Large Percentage of Adult Role Disability," National Institute of Mental Health (NIMH), October 1, 2007; and "Depression and Chronic Pain," by Richard W. Hanson, Ph.D., *Self-Management of Chronic Pain Patient Handbook*, April 2007, Chronic Pain Management Program, Long Beach VA Healthcare System. Reprinted with permission.

Estimating the impact of specific diseases on disability is difficult because people tend to have more than one illness or disorder at a time, such as depression and heart disease. By accounting for the likelihood of coexisting disorders, the authors found that musculoskeletal disorders, especially back and neck pain, resulted in the greatest number of disability days (1.2 billion) while major depression resulted in the second greatest number of disability days (387 million). This research documents that the level of disability associated with chronic mental conditions is as large as that associated with many chronic physical conditions.

Depression and Chronic Pain

It is very common for persons who suffer from chronic pain and disability to feel depressed. In most cases, problems with depression develop as a result of the chronic pain condition. However, studies have shown that some chronic pain sufferers had problems with depression prior to the onset of their pain condition. Irrespective of which came first, the fact remains that the combination of depression and chronic pain, makes the problem all that much worse. This occurs because, when you are depressed, pain and other physical problems become magnified and your ability to cope with pain becomes greatly impaired. While your pain may create physical disability, depression creates mental disability.

Identifying Depression

In order to do something about depression, you first have to recognize its existence. Although depression can take different forms, it often affects you physically, mentally, emotionally, and behaviorally. Following are some signs and symptoms of depression.

Physical

- decreased energy, feeling tired and listless
- sleep problems (insomnia or excessive sleeping)
- decreased appetite or excessive eating
- decreased interest in sex
- increased awareness of pain

Mental

- pessimism regarding the future
- thoughts and memories focus on failures and disappointments

- doubt, excessive self-blame
- decreased satisfaction and enjoyment of activities you used to do
- decreased interest in being around other people
- thoughts of hopelessness and helplessness
- thoughts of suicide
- difficulties concentrating and remembering
- difficulties making decisions

Emotional

- feelings of sadness and discouragement
- tearfulness
- guilt feelings
- increased irritability and low tolerance for frustration
- feeling anxious and restless

Behavioral

- decreased activity level and motivation to do things
- withdrawal from family and friends
- procrastination and neglect of normal responsibilities

It is not necessary to have all these symptoms to be depressed. The specific signs and symptoms of depression can vary from one person to the next. You should keep in mind, however, that it is common and even normal to experience mild and temporary fluctuations in your mood. Many persons feel sad or blue at times but then snap out of it. Depression, on the other hand, becomes a problem when it lasts for an excessive amount of time or becomes so severe that it takes over your life and keeps you from functioning like a normal person.

Sources of Depression

No one chooses to become depressed. Rather, it just seems to happen. Sometimes feelings of depression are triggered by something specific like a particular loss or disappointment, or even an unhappy memory. At other times, it may seem to come out of nowhere. You may even wake up feeling sad or blue.

For those with chronic pain, depression can arise from several sources. Following are some sources of depression.

Losses: It is natural to feel sad when you lose something or someone of value to you. We refer to this type of sadness as mourning or grief. Losses and disappointments are a part of nearly everyone's life. Certainly it is true that some people seem to have a lot more misfortune than others. People with chronic pain and disability can experience a number of significant losses and disappointments. While grief in response to loss is normal, depression can result when one fails to cope with the losses. It is important to keep in mind that depression is not a necessary direct consequence of misfortune. Rather, one of the key factors is how one perceives (thinks about) misfortunes when they do occur.

Learned helplessness: This is the type of depression which develops when pain and disability persist and you feel that there is absolutely nothing you can do about it. No matter how many doctors you see or medical treatments you try, nothing seems to work. After awhile, you feel no sense of control over the pain and feel totally at its mercy. This feeling of helplessness can then generalize to other areas of your life as well.

Chemical imbalances in the brain: Many doctors believe that chemical imbalances in the brain cause depression. It is also possible that depression itself can cause chemical imbalances in the brain. Although in some cases it may be a chicken and egg question as to which comes first, current psychiatric thinking is that some people are biologically prone (genetically predisposed) to develop problems with depression.

Depression as a Self-Perpetuating Process

When depression is left unchecked, it tends to be a self-perpetuating process. Some feel that depression is like a trap because once you are in it, it is difficult to break free. Unfortunately, all the feelings, thoughts, and actions which go along with depression serve to reinforce and magnify each other. For example, the more you withdraw into your depressed shell, the more you tend to dwell on your pain and other negative thoughts. Likewise, the more you avoid taking care of responsibilities as well as activities that you previously found enjoyable, the more depressed you feel. You can also make matters even worse by berating yourself for feeling depressed. It is clear that depression frequently involves interacting vicious cycles.

Breaking Free of Depression

There are two key principles in managing all distressing feelings including depression. These are acceptance and constructive action.

Acceptance: The first step is to recognize and accept the fact that you are depressed. Some people are depressed and either don't know it or will not admit it to themselves or others. It's hard to do anything about a problem if you aren't aware that it exists or deny its presence. Become familiar with the various signs of depression. In particular, become familiar with the many voices of depression. Some common examples are, "what's the use," "why bother," "nothing ever works out right," "things will never get better," "I'm no good," I'm a failure," "nobody cares," and so on.

Acceptance simply means that you recognize your depression and acknowledge the fact that you cannot get rid of it by simply turning off a depression switch. It does no good to block, suppress, or deny depressed feelings. Likewise, it does no good to harshly judge yourself for feeling that way. At the same time, you don't need to hold on to, amplify, or identify with your depression. You are more than your depressed feelings. Feelings, like a wave, come and go, ebb and flow.

Constructive action: Any constructive action that runs counter to the self-perpetuating process of depression is a step in the right direction. Depression tries to convince you that there is absolutely nothing you can do to feel better, so why even bother trying. Another common depressive trap is to wait until you feel better before taking any constructive action. Unfortunately, if you wait until you feel better before you start doing something about it, you may be waiting a long time. Ask yourself, what is this depression trying to get me to do (or not do)? Then do the opposite of what depression is telling you. For example, if depression is telling you to stay in bed rather than get up in the morning, neglect your personal hygiene and attire, not do routine household chores, isolate yourself from other people, and generally avoid doing anything that might bring a sense of accomplishment or satisfaction, then you should do just the opposite.

Following are some additional constructive steps that you might take to break free from the trap of depression:

- The voices of depression always distort your thinking and fool you into thinking that things are much worse than they really are. Learn to identify and forcefully dispute the irrational and distorted ways of thinking that underlie depression.

- Talk to a trusted friend or a professional counselor. Allow them to give you feedback regarding your distorted thinking.

- Do your best to continue meeting your normal daily responsibilities, even if you don't feel like doing them.

- If you feel like having a good cry, go ahead and let the tears flow. After you are done crying, get up and do something constructive.

- Do some form of physical exercise. It is hard to be depressed and physically active at the same time.

- When you are really stuck, remember the phrase: "Move your muscles, change your thoughts." Do something to distract yourself from depressive thoughts. If it means just going through the motions, do it anyway.

- Write down your depressed thoughts and feelings on a piece of paper. Later, you may want to crumble the paper and throw it in the garbage, because that is probably where it belongs.

- Stay away from alcohol and other non-prescribed drugs (including stimulants such as cocaine). Although you may feel better in the short run, they will only make you feel worse in the long run.

- Remind yourself that feelings of depression won't last. Although you may not be able to simply snap your fingers and make the depression go away, you can do everything in your power to keep it from getting worse or persisting longer than necessary.

- Make a list of all the things in your life that you have to feel grateful for.

- Learn and recite to yourself the "Serenity Prayer."

- See your doctor about getting on antidepressant medication. A number of effective antidepressant medications are now available.

- Develop a depression self-management action plan. You can develop a list of specific things to do or think about when you are experiencing depression. This list should be kept handy so you can readily pull it out and review it whenever you are feeling depressed. It could be titled, "My personal depression action plan: Things to do or think about when I am experiencing depression."

Chapter 5

Pain Research

Chapter Contents

Section 5.1

Treatment Blocks Pain without Disrupting Other Functions

"Researchers Develop Targeted Approach to Pain Management," written by Alyssa Kneller. Harvard Medical School Office of Public Affairs, © 2007. Reprinted with permission.

Findings: Scientists have combined a normally inactive lidocaine derivative with capsaicin, the heat-generating ingredient in chili peppers, to produce pain-specific local anesthesia. When injected into rats, this combination completely blocked pain without interfering with either motor function or sensitivity to non-painful stimuli.

Relevance: This technique could revolutionize pain management, as it specifically targets pain-sensing neurons. Current local anesthetics block all neurons, not just pain-sensing ones, and produce dramatic side effects such as temporary paralysis and complete numbness.

Targeted Approach to Pain Management Developed

Imagine an epidural or a shot of Novocain that doesn't paralyze your legs or make you numb, yet totally blocks your pain. This type of pain management is now within reach. As a result, childbirth, surgery, and trips to the dentist might be less traumatic in the future, thanks to researchers at Massachusetts General Hospital (MGH) and Harvard Medical School, who have succeeded in selectively blocking pain-sensing neurons in rats without interfering with other types of neurons.

The pint-sized subjects received injections near their sciatic nerves, which run down their hind limbs, and subsequently lost the ability to feel pain in their paws. But they continued to move normally and react to touch. The injections contained QX-314, a normally inactive derivative of the local anesthetic lidocaine, and capsaicin, the active ingredient in hot peppers. In combination, these chemicals targeted only pain-sensing neurons, preventing them from sending signals to the brain.

"We've introduced a local anesthetic selectively into specific populations of neurons," explains Harvard Medical School Professor Bruce Bean, an author on the paper, which appeared in *Nature* on Oct. 4, 2007. "Now we can block the activity of pain-sensing neurons without disrupting other kinds of neurons that control movements or non-painful sensations."

"We're optimistic that this method will eventually be applied to humans and change our experience during procedures ranging from knee surgery to tooth extractions," adds Professor Clifford Woolf of Massachusetts General Hospital, who is senior author on the study.

Despite enormous investments by industry, surgical pain management has changed little since the first successful demonstration of ether general anesthesia at MGH in 1846. General and local anesthetics work by interfering with the excitability of all neurons, not just pain-sensing ones. Thus, these drugs produce dramatic side effects, such as loss of consciousness in the case of general anesthetics or temporary paralysis for local anesthetics.

"We're offering a targeted approach to pain management that avoids these problems," says Woolf. The new work builds on research done since the 1970s showing how electrical signaling in the nervous system depends on the properties of ion channels, that is, proteins that make pores in the membranes of neurons.

"This project is a perfect illustration of how research trying to understand very basic biological principles can have practical applications," says Bean. The new method exploits a membrane-spanning protein called TRPV1, which is unique to pain-sensing neurons. TRPV1 forms a large channel, where molecules can enter and exit the cell. But a "gate" typically blocks this opening. The gate opens when cells are exposed to heat or the chili-pepper ingredient capsaicin. Thus, bathing pain-sensing neurons in capsaicin leaves these channels open, but non-pain sensing neurons are unaffected because they do not possess TRPV1.

The new method then takes advantage of a special property of the lidocaine derivative QX-314. Unlike most local anesthetics, QX-314 can't penetrate cell membranes to block the excitability of the cell, so it typically lingers outside neurons where it can't affect them. For this reason, it is not used clinically.

When pain-sensing neurons are exposed to capsaicin, however, and the gates guarding the TRPV1 channels disappear, QX-314 can enter the cells and shut them down. But the drug remains outside other types of neurons that do not contain these channels. As a result, these cells fully retain their ability to send and receive signals.

The team first tested their method in the Petri dish. Alexander Binshtok, a postdoctoral researcher in Woolf's lab, applied capsaicin and QX-314 (separately and in combination) to isolated pain-sensing and other neurons and measured their responses. Indeed, the combination of capsaicin and QX-314 selectively blocked the excitability of pain-sensing neurons, leaving the others unaffected.

Next, Binshtok injected these chemicals into the paws of rats and measured their ability to sense pain by placing them on an uncomfortable heat source. The critters tolerated much more heat than usual. He then injected the chemicals near the sciatic nerve of the animals and pricked their paws with stiff nylon probes. The animals ignored the provocation. Although the rats seemed immune to pain, they continued to move normally and respond to other stimuli, indicating that QX-314 failed to penetrate their motor neurons.

The team must overcome several hurdles before this method can be applied to humans. They must figure out how to open the TRPV1 channels without producing even a transient burning pain before QX-314 enters and blocks the neurons, and they must tinker with the formulation to prolong the effects of the drugs. Both Bean and Woolf are confident they'll succeed.

"Eventually this method could completely transform surgical and post-surgical analgesia, allowing patients to remain fully alert without experiencing pain or paralysis," says Woolf. "In fact, the possibilities seem endless. I could even imagine using this method to treat itch, as itch-sensitive neurons fall into the same group as pain-sensing ones."

Reference

Alexander M. Binshtok,[1] Bruce P. Bean,[2] and Clifford J. Woolf.[1] "Inhibition of nociceptors by TRPV1-mediated entry of impermeant sodium channel blockers," *Nature*, Oct. 4, 2007.

[1] Department of Anesthesia and Critical Care, Massachusetts General Hospital and Harvard Medical School, Charlestown, MA.

[2] Department of Neurobiology, Harvard Medical School, Boston, MA.

Section 5.2

Gene Variation Affects Pain Sensitivity and Risk of Chronic Pain

Excerpted from "Gene Variation Affects Pain Sensitivity and Risk of Chronic Pain," National Institutes of Health (NIH), October 2006.

A National Institutes of Health (NIH)-funded study shows that a specific gene variant in humans affects both sensitivity to short-term (acute) pain in healthy volunteers and the risk of developing chronic pain after one kind of back surgery. Blocking increased activity of this gene after nerve injury or inflammation in animals prevented development of chronic pain.

The gene in this study, GCH1, codes for an enzyme called GTP cyclohydrolase. The study suggests that inhibiting GTP cyclohydrolase activity might help to prevent or treat chronic pain which affects as many as 50 million people in the United States. Doctors also may be able to screen people for the gene variant to predict their risk of chronic post-surgical pain before they undergo surgery. The results appeared in the October 22, 2006, advance online publication of *Nature Medicine*.

"This is a completely new pathway that contributes to the development of pain," says Clifford J. Woolf, M.D., of Massachusetts General Hospital and Harvard Medical School in Boston, who led the research. "The study shows that we inherit the extent to which we feel pain, both under normal conditions and after damage to the nervous system."

Dr. Woolf carried out the study in collaboration with Mitchell B. Max, M.D., of the National Institute of Dental and Craniofacial Research (NIDCR) in Bethesda, Maryland, and colleagues at the National Institute on Alcoholism Abuse and Alcoholism (NIAAA) and elsewhere. The researchers originally identified GCH1 by preclinical screening for genes that undergo significant changes in expression after sciatic nerve injury. GCH1 is one of several genes that code for enzymes needed to produce a chemical called tetrahydrobiopterin (BH4). Previous studies have shown that BH4 is an essential ingredient in the process that produces dopamine and several other nerve-signaling chemicals (neurotransmitters). It also plays other important roles in the body. However, this study is the first to show that GCH1 and BH4 play a role in pain.

The investigators tested the effects of GTP cyclohydrolase and BH4 in several animal models of pain. They found that rats with neuropathic pain (pain caused by nerve damage) had greatly increased levels of GCH1 gene activity and BH4, and that injecting a GTP cyclohydrolase inhibitor called 2,4-diamino-6-hydroxypyrimidine (DAHP) alleviated hypersensitivity to pain in animal models of both neuropathic pain and inflammatory pain. In contrast, injecting BH4 greatly increased pain sensitivity.

Next, the researchers looked for GCH1 gene variations in people. They found that a specific variant of the gene, identified by combinations of one-base-pair changes in the deoxyribonucleic acid (DNA) called single nucleotide polymorphisms (SNP), protected against development of chronic post-surgical pain in people who had participated in a study of surgical diskectomy for back pain. About 28 percent of people in the surgical study had at least one copy of the pain-protective variant of the gene (people have two copies of every gene). The researchers found that people with two copies of the protective version of GCH1 had the lowest risk of developing chronic pain, while those with just one copy had an intermediate risk, and those with no copies of the variant had the highest risk.

The researchers then found that the gene variant also appeared to reduce sensations of acute pain in normal volunteers. Normal volunteers with two copies of the protective gene variant were less sensitive to temporary pain induced by pressure and other stimuli than those with one or no copies.

Analysis of blood cells from the people who had undergone back surgery showed that, under normal conditions, the amounts of GTP cyclohydrolase and BH4 were not significantly different in people with and without the gene variant. When the cells were subjected to a chemical that increases GCH1 gene activity, however, the amount of gene activity increased much less in people with the pain-protective variant of the gene than it did in other people.

The variation that affects pain sensitivity is in a region of the gene that may control when the gene is switched on. This, coupled with the results of the blood study, makes the researchers suspect that the protective version of the gene is less likely to be switched on during stressful conditions such as nerve damage and inflammation. "We often hear about gene mutations that are harmful, but here is a mutation that's actually protective," says Dr. Woolf.

The GTP cyclohydrolase inhibitor used in this study, DAHP, is not very strong and is unlikely to be useful as a human drug, Dr. Woolf says. Researchers are now looking for other substances that might work as GTP cyclohydrolase inhibitor drugs in humans.

Screening people for the pain-protective gene variant could allow doctors to identify people at high risk of developing chronic pain before they undergo surgery, Dr. Woolf says. Doctors might then be able to reduce the risk of chronic pain by providing more aggressive pain relief or choosing less invasive surgical procedures for people at high risk of chronic pain. Several studies have suggested that specific pain drugs or combinations of drugs can reduce the risk of chronic pain after surgery.

Dr. Woolf and his colleagues are now planning studies to define exactly how GCH1 is switched on by nerve injury and inflammation and how it regulates pain. They also hope to identify other gene variants that affect pain sensitivity and the risk of chronic pain. "We think this gene accounts for some of the inherited differences in pain, but other genes may also play a role," Dr. Woolf says.

Part Two

Types of Pain and Disorders Characterized by Pain

Chapter 6

Arthritis

Many people start to feel pain and stiffness in their bodies over time. Sometimes their hands or knees or shoulders get sore and are hard to move and may become swollen. These people may have arthritis. Arthritis may be caused by inflammation of the tissue lining the joints. Some signs of inflammation include redness, heat, pain, and swelling. These problems are telling you that something is wrong.

Joints are places where two bones meet, such as your elbow or knee. Over time, in some types of arthritis but not in all, the joints involved can become severely damaged.

There are different types of arthritis. In some diseases in which arthritis occurs, other organs, such as your eyes, chest, or skin, can also be affected. Some people may worry that arthritis means they won't be able to work or take care of their children and their family. Others think that you just have to accept things like arthritis. It's true that arthritis can be painful. But there are things you can do to feel better.

Types of Arthritis

There are several types of arthritis. The two most common ones are osteoarthritis and rheumatoid arthritis.

"Living with Arthritis," National Institute of Arthritis and Musculoskeletal and Skin Diseases (NIAMS), NIH Publication No. 07–7050, January 2007.

Osteoarthritis is the most common form of arthritis. This condition usually comes with age and most often affects the fingers, knees, and hips. Sometimes osteoarthritis follows an injury to a joint. For example, a young person might hurt his knee badly playing soccer. Or someone might fall or be injured in a car accident. Then, years after the individual's knee has apparently healed, he might get arthritis in his knee joint.

Rheumatoid arthritis happens when the body's own defense system doesn't work properly. It affects joints and bones (often of the hands and feet), and may also affect internal organs and systems. You may feel sick or tired, and you may have a fever.

Gout is another common type of arthritis that is caused by crystals that build up in the joints. It usually affects the big toe, but many other joints may be affected.

Other conditions where arthritis is seen include lupus in which the body's defense system can harm the joints, the heart, the skin, the kidneys, and other organs; or an infection that gets into a joint and destroys the cushion between the bones.

Symptoms

Pain is the way your body tells you that something is wrong. Most types of arthritis cause pain in your joints. You might have trouble moving around. Some kinds of arthritis can affect different parts of your body. So, along with pain in your joints, you may:

- have a fever,
- lose weight,
- have trouble breathing, or
- get a rash or itch.

These symptoms may also be signs of other illnesses.

Treatment

Go see a doctor. Many people use herbs or medicines that you can buy without a prescription for pain. You should tell your doctor if you do. Only a doctor can tell if you have arthritis or a related condition, and what to do about it. It is important not to wait.

You will need to tell the doctor how you feel and where you hurt. The doctor will examine you and may take x-rays of your bones or joints. The x-rays do not hurt and are not dangerous. You may also have to give a little blood for tests that will help the doctor decide what kind of arthritis you may have.

After the doctor knows what kind of arthritis you have, he or she will talk with you about the best way to treat it. The doctor may give you a prescription for medicine that will help with the pain, stiffness, and inflammation. Health insurance or public assistance may help you pay for the medicine, doctor visits, tests, and x-rays.

Using Medicine

Before you leave the doctor's office, make sure you ask about the best way to take the medicine the doctor prescribes. For example, you may need to take some medicines with milk, or you may need to eat something just before or after taking them, to make sure they don't upset your stomach. You should also ask how often to take the medicine or to put cream on the spots that bother you. Creams might make your skin and joints feel better. Sometimes, though, they can make your skin burn or break out in a rash. If this happens, call the doctor.

If It Still Hurts

Sometimes you might still have pain after using your medicine. Here are some things to try:

- Take a warm shower.
- Do some gentle stretching exercises.
- Use an ice pack on the sore area.
- Rest the sore joint.

If you still hurt after using your medicine correctly and doing one or more of these things, call your doctor. Another kind of medicine might work better for you. Some people can also benefit from surgery, such as joint replacement.

You Can Feel Better

Arthritis can damage your joints, internal organs, and skin. There are things you can do to keep the damage from getting worse. They might also make you feel better:

47

- Try to keep your weight down. Too much weight can make your knees and hips hurt.

- Exercise. Moving all of your joints will help you. The doctor or nurse can show you how to move more easily. Going for a walk every day will help, too.

- Take your medicines when and how you are supposed to. They can help reduce pain and stiffness.

- Try taking a warm shower in the morning.

- See your doctor regularly.

- Seek information that can help you.

Chapter 7

Back Pain

Back pain is an all-too-familiar problem that can range from a dull, constant ache to a sudden, sharp pain that leaves you incapacitated. It can come on suddenly—from an accident, a fall, or lifting something too heavy—or it can develop slowly, perhaps as the result of age-related changes to the spine. Regardless of how it happens or how it feels, you know it when you have it. And chances are, if you don't have it now, you will eventually. At some point, back pain affects an estimated eight out of ten people. It is one of our society's most common medical problems.

Causes of Back Pain

It is important to understand that back pain is a symptom of a medical condition, not a diagnosis itself. Medical problems that can cause back pain include the following:

Mechanical problems: A mechanical problem is a problem with the way your spine moves or the way you feel when you move your spine in certain ways. Perhaps the most common mechanical cause of back pain is a condition called intervertebral disc degeneration, which simply means that the discs located between the vertebrae of the spine are breaking down with age. Other mechanical causes of

Excerpted from "Handout on Health: Back Pain," National Institute of Arthritis and Musculoskeletal and Skin Diseases (NIAMS), NIH Publication No. 05–5282, September 2005.

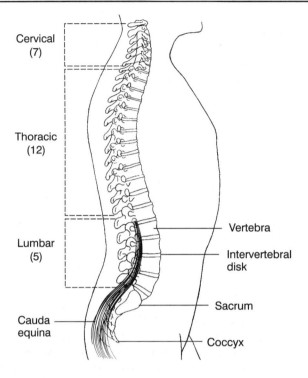

Figure 7.1. *Side View of Spine*

back pain include spasms, muscle tension, and ruptured discs, which are also called herniated discs.

Injuries: Spine injuries such as sprains and fractures can cause either short-lived or chronic pain. Sprains are tears in the ligaments that support the spine, and they can occur from twisting or lifting improperly. Fractured vertebrae are often the result of osteoporosis, a condition that causes weak, porous bones. Less commonly, back pain may be caused by more severe injuries that result from accidents and falls.

Acquired conditions and diseases: Many medical problems can cause or contribute to back pain. They include scoliosis, which causes curvature of the spine and does not usually cause pain until mid-life; spondylolisthesis; various forms of arthritis, including osteoarthritis, rheumatoid arthritis, and ankylosing spondylitis; and spinal stenosis, a narrowing of the spinal column that puts pressure on the spinal cord and nerves. While osteoporosis itself is not painful, it can lead

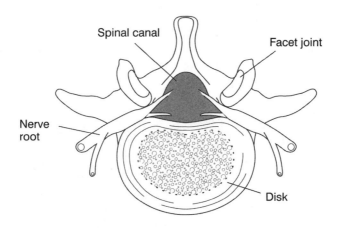

Figure 7.2. *Cross Section of Normal Vertebra*

to painful fractures of the vertebrae. Other causes of back pain include pregnancy, kidney stones or infections, endometriosis (the buildup of uterine tissue in places outside the uterus), and fibromyalgia which causes fatigue and widespread muscle pain.

Infections and tumors: Although they are not common causes of back pain, infections can cause pain when they involve the vertebrae (osteomyelitis), or when they involve the discs that cushion the vertebrae (discitis). Tumors are also relatively rare causes of back pain. Occasionally, tumors begin in the back, but more often they appear in the back as a result of cancer that has spread from elsewhere in the body.

Emotional stress: Although the causes of back pain are usually physical, it is important to know that emotional stress can play a role in how severe pain is and how long it lasts. Stress can affect the body in many ways, including causing back muscles to become tense and painful.

Seeing a Doctor for Pain

In most cases, it is not necessary to see a doctor for back pain because pain usually goes away with or without treatment. However, a trip to the doctor is probably a good idea if you have numbness or tingling, if your pain is severe and doesn't improve with medications and rest, or if you have pain after a fall or an injury. It is also important

51

to see your doctor if you have pain along with any of the following problems: trouble urinating; weakness, pain, or numbness in your legs; fever; or unintentional weight loss. Such symptoms could signal a serious problem that requires treatment soon.

Diagnosing Back Pain

Diagnosing the cause of back pain requires a medical history and a physical exam. If necessary, your doctor may also order medical tests, which may include x-rays. During the medical history, your doctor will ask questions about the nature of your pain and about any health problems you and close family members have or have had.

Often a doctor can find the cause of your pain with a physical and medical history alone. However, depending on what the history and exam show, your doctor may order medical tests to help find the cause.

It is important to understand that medical tests alone may not diagnose the cause of back pain. In fact, experts say that up to 90 percent of all magnetic resonance imaging (MRI) scans of the spine show some type of abnormality, and sometimes the x-rays and computed tomography (CT) scans of people without pain show problems. Similarly, even some healthy, pain-free people can have elevated blood sedimentation rates.

Only with a medical history and exam—and sometimes medical tests—can a doctor diagnose the cause of back pain. Many times, the precise cause of back pain is never known. In these cases, it may be comforting to know that most back pain gets better whether or not you find out what is causing it.

Nonoperative Back Pain Treatments

Hot or cold: Hot or cold packs—or sometimes a combination of the two—can be soothing to chronically sore, stiff backs. Heat dilates the blood vessels, improving the supply of oxygen that the blood takes to the back and reducing muscle spasms. Heat also alters the sensation of pain. Cold may reduce inflammation by decreasing the size of blood vessels and the flow of blood to the area. Although cold may feel painful against the skin, it numbs deep pain. Applying heat or cold may relieve pain, but it does not cure the cause of chronic back pain.

Exercise: Although exercise is usually not advisable for acute back pain, proper exercise can help ease chronic pain and perhaps reduce its risk of returning. Exercise is important to general physical fitness and may be helpful for certain specific causes of back pain. Ask your doctor or physical therapist for guidance about appropriate exercises for your situation.

Medications: A wide range of medications are used to treat chronic back pain. Some you can try on your own. Others are available only with a doctor's prescription. The main types of medications used for back pain include analgesics, nonsteroidal anti-inflammatory drugs (NSAID), muscle relaxants, and certain antidepressants.

Traction: Traction involves using pulleys and weights to stretch the back. The rationale behind traction is to pull the vertebrae apart to allow a bulging disc to slip back into place. Some people experience pain relief while in traction, but that relief is usually temporary. Once traction is released, the stretch is not sustained and back pain is likely to return. There is no scientific evidence that traction provides any long-term benefits for people with back pain.

Corsets and braces: Corsets and braces include a number of devices, such as elastic bands and stiff supports with metal stays, that are designed to limit the motion of the lumbar spine, provide abdominal support, and correct posture. While these may be appropriate after certain kinds of surgery, there is little, if any, evidence that they help treat chronic low back pain. In fact, by keeping you from using your back muscles, they may actually cause more problems than they solve by causing lower back muscles to weaken from lack of use.

Behavioral modification: Developing a healthy attitude and learning to move your body properly while you do daily activities—particularly those involving heavy lifting, pushing, or pulling—are sometimes part of the treatment plan for people with back pain. Other behavior changes that might help pain include adopting healthy habits, such as exercise, relaxation, and regular sleep, and dropping bad habits, such as smoking and eating poorly.

Injections: When medications and other nonsurgical treatments fail to relieve chronic back pain, doctors may recommend injections for pain relief. Some of the most commonly used injections include nerve root blocks, facet joint injections, trigger point injections, and prolotherapy.

Complementary and alternative treatments: When back pain becomes chronic or when medications and other conventional therapies do not relieve it, many people try complementary and alternative treatments. While such therapies won't cure diseases or repair the injuries that cause pain, some people find them useful for managing or relieving pain. Some of the most commonly used complementary therapies include manipulation, transcutaneous electrical nerve stimulation (TENS), acupuncture, acupressure, or Rolfing—a type of massage that involves using strong pressure on deep tissues in the back.

Operative Back Pain Treatments

Depending on the diagnosis, surgery may either be the first treatment of choice—although this is rare—or it is reserved for chronic back pain for which other treatments have failed. You may be a candidate for surgery if you are in constant pain or if pain reoccurs frequently and interferes with your ability to sleep, to function at your job, or to perform daily activities.

In general, there are two groups of people who may require surgery to treat their spinal problems. People in the first group have chronic low back pain and sciatica, and they are often diagnosed with a herniated disc, spinal stenosis, spondylolisthesis, or vertebral fractures with nerve involvement. People in the second group are those with only predominant low back pain (without leg pain). These are people with discogenic low back pain (degenerative disc disease) in which discs wear with age. Usually, the outcome of spine surgery is much more predictable in people with sciatica than in those with predominant low back pain.

Some of the diagnoses that may need surgery include herniated discs, spinal stenosis, spondylolisthesis, vertebral fractures, and discogenic low back pain (degenerative disc disease).

Surgery for Herniated Discs

Laminectomy/discectomy: In this operation, part of the lamina, a portion of the bone on the back of the vertebrae, is removed as well as a portion of a ligament. The herniated disc is then removed through the incision which may extend two or more inches.

Microdiscectomy: As with traditional discectomy, this procedure involves removing a herniated disc or damaged portion of a disc through an incision in the back. The difference is that the incision is much smaller and the doctor uses a magnifying microscope or lenses to locate the disc through the incision. The smaller incision may reduce pain and the disruption of tissues, and it reduces the size of the surgical scar. It appears to take about the same time to recuperate from a microdiscectomy as from a traditional discectomy.

Laser surgery: Technological advances in recent decades have led to the use of lasers for operating on patients with herniated discs accompanied by lower back and leg pain. During this procedure, the surgeon inserts a needle in the disc that delivers a few bursts of laser energy to vaporize the tissue in the disc. This reduces its size and relieves pressure on the nerves. Although many patients return to daily activities within 3–5 days after laser surgery, pain relief may not be apparent until several weeks or even months after the surgery. The usefulness of laser discectomy is still being debated.

Surgery for Spinal Stenosis

Laminectomy: When narrowing of the spine compresses the nerve roots causing pain and/or affecting sensation, doctors sometimes open up the spinal column with a procedure called a laminectomy. In a laminectomy, the doctor makes a large incision down the affected area of the spine and removes the lamina and any bone spurs—overgrowths of bone that may have formed in the spinal canal as the result of osteoarthritis. The procedure is major surgery that requires a short hospital stay and physical therapy afterwards to help regain strength and mobility.

Surgery for Spondylolisthesis

Spinal fusion: When a slipped vertebra leads to the enlargement of adjacent facet joints, surgical treatment generally involves both laminectomy and spinal fusion. In spinal fusion, two or more vertebrae are joined together using bone grafts, screws, and rods to stop slippage of the affected vertebrae. Bone used for grafting comes from another area of the body, usually the hip or pelvis. In some cases, donor bone is used. Although the surgery is generally successful, either type of graft has its drawbacks. Using your own bone means surgery at a second site on your body. With donor bone, there is a slight risk of disease transmission or rejection. In recent years, a new development has eliminated those risks for some people undergoing spinal fusion—proteins called bone morphogenic proteins are being used to stimulate bone generation, eliminating the need for grafts. The proteins are placed in the affected area of the spine, often in collagen putty or sponges. Regardless of how spinal fusion is performed, the fused area of the spine becomes immobilized.

Surgery for Vertebral Osteoporotic Fractures

This surgery is used only if standard care, rest, corsets, braces, or analgesics fail.

Vertebroplasty: When back pain is caused by a compression fracture of a vertebra due to osteoporosis or trauma, doctors may make a small incision in the skin over the affected area and inject a cement-like mixture called polymethyacrylate into the fractured vertebra to relieve pain and stabilize the spine. The procedure is generally performed on an outpatient basis under a mild anesthetic.

Kyphoplasty: Much like vertebroplasty, kyphoplasty is used to relieve pain and stabilize the spine following fractures due to osteoporosis. Kyphoplasty is a two-step process. In the first step, the doctor inserts a balloon device to help restore the height and shape of the spine. In the second step, he or she injects polymethyacrylate to repair the fractured vertebra. The procedure is done under anesthesia, and in some cases it is performed on an outpatient basis.

Surgery for Discogenic Low Back Pain (Degenerative Disc Disease)

Intradiscal electrothermal therapy (IDT): One of the newest and least invasive therapies for low back pain involves inserting a heating wire through a small incision in the back and into a disc. An electrical current is then passed through the wire to strengthen the collagen fibers that hold the disc together. The procedure is done on an outpatient basis, often under local anesthesia. The usefulness of IDT is debatable.

Spinal fusion: When the degenerated disc is painful, the surgeon may recommend removing it and fusing the disc to help with the pain. This fusion can be done through the abdomen, a procedure known as anterior lumbar interbody fusion, or through the back, called posterior fusion. Theoretically, fusion surgery should eliminate the source of pain. The procedure is successful in about 60 to 70 percent of cases. Fusion for low back pain or any spinal surgeries should only be done as a last resort, and the patient should be fully informed of risks.

Disc replacement: When a disc is herniated, one alternative to a discectomy—in which the disc is simply removed—is removing it and replacing it with a synthetic disc. Replacing the damaged one with an artificial one restores disc height and movement between the vertebrae. Artificial discs come in several designs.

Chapter 8

Burns

Burn pain can be profound and poses an extreme challenge to the medical community. First-degree burns are the least severe; with third-degree burns, the skin is lost. Depending on the injury, pain accompanying burns can be excruciating, and even after the wound has healed patients may have chronic pain at the burn site.

Background Information

- Each year in the United States, 1.1 million burn injuries require medical attention (American Burn Association, 2002).

  - Approximately 50,000 burn injuries require hospitalization

  - Approximately 20,000 are major burns involving at least 25 percent of the total body surface

  - Approximately 4,500 of these people die

- Up to 10,000 people in the United States die every year of burn-related infections.

This chapter includes an excerpt from "Pain: Hope through Research," National Institute of Neurological Disorders and Stroke (NINDS), NIH Publication No. 01–2406, updated January 10, 2008; and text from "Mass Casualties: Burns," Centers for Disease Control and Prevention (CDC), July 18, 2006.

First Aid for Burns

What you do to treat a burn in the first few minutes after it occurs can make a huge difference in the severity of the injury.

Immediate Treatment for Burn Victims

1. Stop, drop, and roll to smother flames.

2. Remove all burned clothing. If clothing adheres to the skin, cut or tear around burned area.

3. Remove any jewelry, belts, or tight clothing from the burned areas or from around the victim's neck. This is very important because burned areas swell immediately.

First-Degree Burns

First-degree burns involve the top layer of skin. Sunburn is a first-degree burn. Signs include the following:

- Red
- Painful to touch
- Skin will show mild swelling

Treatment for First Degree Burns

- Apply cool, wet compresses, or immerse in cool, fresh water. Continue until pain subsides.
- Cover the burn with a sterile, nonadhesive bandage or clean cloth.
- Do not apply ointments or butter to burn; these may cause infection.
- Over-the-counter pain medications may be used to help relieve pain and reduce inflammation.
- First degree burns usually heal without further treatment. However, if a first-degree burn covers a large area of the body, or the victim is an infant or elderly, seek emergency medical attention.

Second-Degree Burns

Second-degree burns involve the first two layers of skin. Signs include the following:

- Deep reddening of the skin
- Pain
- Blisters
- Glossy appearance from leaking fluid
- Possible loss of some skin

Treatment for Second Degree Burns

- Immerse in fresh, cool water, or apply cool compresses. Continue for 10 to 15 minutes.
- Dry with clean cloth and cover with sterile gauze.
- Do not break blisters.
- Do not apply ointments or butter to burns; these may cause infection.
- Elevate burned arms or legs.
- Take steps to prevent shock. Lay the victim flat, elevate the feet about 12 inches, and cover the victim with a coat or blanket. Do not place the victim in the shock position if a head, neck, back, or leg injury is suspected, or if it makes the victim uncomfortable.
- Further medical treatment is required. Do not attempt to treat serious burns unless you are a trained health professional.

Third-Degree Burns

A third-degree burn penetrates the entire thickness of the skin and permanently destroys tissue. Signs include the following:

- Loss of skin layers
- Often painless—pain may be caused by patches of first- and second-degree burns which often surround third-degree burns
- Skin is dry and leathery
- Skin may appear charred or have patches which appear white, brown, or black

Treatment for Third Degree Burns

- Cover burn lightly with sterile gauze or clean cloth. (Do not use material that can leave lint on the burn).

- Do not apply ointments or butter to burns; these may cause infection.

- Take steps to prevent shock. Lay the victim flat and elevate the feet about 12 inches.

- Have person sit up if face is burned. Watch closely for possible breathing problems.

- Elevate burned area higher than the victim's head when possible. Keep person warm and comfortable, and watch for signs of shock.

- Do not place a pillow under the victim's head if the person is lying down and there is an airway burn. This can close the airway.

- Immediate medical attention is required. Do not attempt to treat serious burns unless you are a trained health professional.

Escape Information

Safeguard Your Home

- Install smoke alarms on each floor of your home. One alarm must be outside a bedroom where you sleep.

- Change batteries in smoke alarms at least once a year. (Never borrow smoke alarm batteries for other purposes).

- Keep emergency phone numbers and other pertinent information posted close to your telephone.

- Draw a floor plan and find two exits from each room. Windows can serve as emergency exits.

- Practice getting out of the house through the various exits.

- Designate a meeting place at a safe distance outside the home.

- Respond to every alarm as if it were a real fire.

- Call the fire department after escaping. Tell them your address and do not hang up until you are told to do so. Let them know if anyone is trapped inside.

- Never go back into a burning building to look for missing people, pets, or property. Wait for firefighters.

If You Are Trapped in a Burning Building

- Smoke rises, so crawl low to the ground where the air will be cleanest.

- Get out quickly if it is safe to leave. Cover your nose and mouth with a cloth (moist if possible).

- Test doorknobs and spaces around doors with the back of your hand. If the door is warm, try another escape route. If it is cool, open it slowly. Check to make sure your escape path is clear of fire and smoke.

- Use the stairs. Never use an elevator during a fire.

- Call the fire department for assistance if you are trapped. If you cannot get to a phone, yell for help out the window. Wave or hang a sheet or other large object to attract attention.

- Close as many doors as possible between yourself and the fire. Seal all doors and vents between you and the fire with rags, towels, or sheets. Open windows slightly at the top and bottom, but close them if smoke comes in.

For More Information

American Burn Association
625 N. Michigan Ave., Suite 2550
Chicago, IL 60611
Toll-Free: 800-548-2876
Phone: 312-642-9260
Fax: 312-642-9130
Website: http://www.ameriburn.org
E-mail: info@ameriburn.org

Phoenix Society for Burn Survivors, Inc.
1835 R W Berends Dr. S.W.
Grand Rapids, MI 49519-4955
Toll-Free: 800-888-2876
Phone: 616-458-2773
Fax: 616-458-2831
Website: http://www.phoenix-society.org
E-mail: info@phoenix-society.org

Chapter 9

Bursitis and Tendonitis

Bursitis and tendonitis are both common conditions that involve inflammation of the soft tissue around muscles and bones, most often in the shoulder, elbow, wrist, hip, knee, or ankle.

A bursa is a small, fluid-filled sac that acts as a cushion between a bone and other moving parts: muscles, tendons, or skin. Bursae are found throughout the body. Bursitis occurs when a bursa becomes inflamed (redness and increased fluid in the bursa).

A tendon is a flexible band of fibrous tissue that connects muscles to bones. Tendonitis is inflammation of a tendon. Tendons transmit the pull of the muscle to the bone to cause movement. They are found throughout the body, including the hands, wrists, elbows, shoulders, hips, knees, ankles, and feet. Tendons can be small, like those found in the hand, or large, like the Achilles tendon in the heel.

Bursitis is commonly caused by overuse or direct trauma to a joint. Bursitis may occur at the knee or elbow, for example, from kneeling or leaning on the elbows longer than usual on a hard surface. Tendonitis is most often the result of a repetitive injury in the affected area. These conditions occur more often with age. Tendons become less flexible with age, and therefore, more prone to injury.

People such as carpenters, gardeners, musicians, and athletes who perform activities that require repetitive motions or place stress on

Excerpted from "Questions and Answers about Bursitis and Tendonitis," National Institute of Arthritis and Musculoskeletal and Skin Diseases (NIAMS), NIH Publication No. 07–6240, April 2007.

joints are at higher risk for tendonitis and bursitis. An infection, arthritis, gout, thyroid disease, and diabetes can also bring about inflammation of a bursa or tendon.

Tendonitis causes pain and tenderness just outside a joint. Some common names for tendonitis identify with the sport or movement that typically increases risk for tendon inflammation. They include tennis elbow, golfer's elbow, pitcher's shoulder, swimmer's shoulder, and jumper's knee.

Tennis Elbow and Golfer's Elbow

Tennis elbow refers to an injury to the outer elbow tendon. Golfer's elbow is an injury to the inner tendon of the elbow. These conditions can also occur with any activity that involves repetitive wrist turning or hand gripping, such as tool use, hand shaking, or twisting movements. Carpenters, gardeners, painters, musicians, manicurists, and dentists are at higher risk for these forms of tendonitis. Pain occurs near the elbow, sometimes radiating into the upper arm or down to the forearm. Another name for tennis elbow is lateral epicondylitis. Golfer's elbow is also called medial epicondylitis.

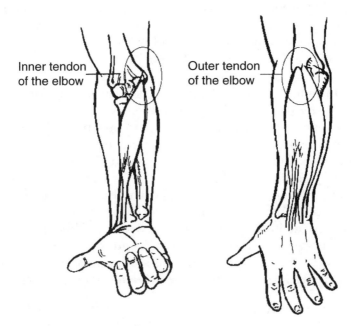

Figure 9.1. *Structure of the Elbow*

Shoulder Tendonitis, Bursitis, and Impingement Syndrome

Two types of tendonitis can affect the shoulder. Biceps tendonitis causes pain in the front or side of the shoulder and may travel down to the elbow and forearm. Pain may also occur when the arm is raised overhead. The biceps muscle, in the front of the upper arm, helps stabilize the upper arm bone (humerus) in the shoulder socket. It also helps accelerate and decelerate the arm during overhead movement in activities like tennis or pitching.

Rotator cuff tendonitis causes shoulder pain at the tip of the shoulder and the upper, outer arm. The pain can be aggravated by reaching, pushing, pulling, lifting, raising the arm above shoulder level, or lying on the affected side. The rotator cuff is primarily a group of four muscles that attach the arm to the shoulder girdle/shoulder blade. The rotator cuff attaches the arm to the shoulder joint and allows the arm to rotate and elevate. If the rotator cuff and bursa are irritated, inflamed, and swollen, they may become compressed between the head of the humerus and the acromion, the outer edge of the shoulder blade. Repeated motion involving the arms, or the aging process involving

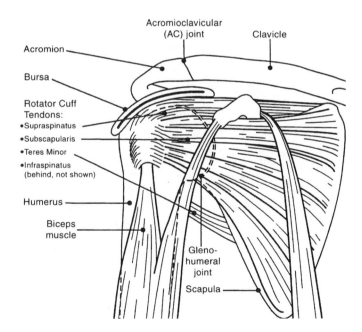

Figure 9.2. *Structure of the Shoulder*

65

shoulder motion over many years, may also irritate and wear down the tendons, muscles, and surrounding structures. Squeezing of the rotator cuff is called shoulder impingement syndrome.

Inflammation caused by rheumatoid arthritis may cause rotator cuff tendonitis and bursitis. Sports involving overuse of the shoulder and occupations requiring frequent overhead reaching are other potential causes of irritation to the rotator cuff or bursa, and may lead to inflammation and impingement.

Knee Tendonitis or Jumper's Knee

If a person overuses a tendon during activities such as dancing, cycling, or running, it may elongate or undergo microscopic tears and become inflamed. Trying to break a fall may also cause the quadriceps muscles to contract and tear the quadriceps tendon above the knee cap (patella) or the patellar tendon below it. This type of injury is most likely to happen in older people whose tendons tend to be

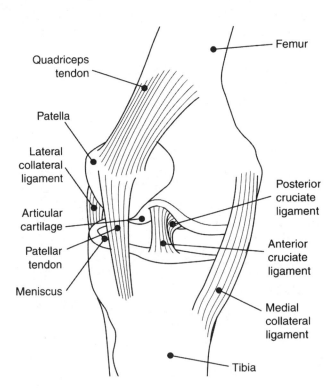

Figure 9.3. *Lateral View of the Knee*

weaker and less flexible. Tendonitis of the patellar tendon is sometimes called jumper's knee because in sports that require jumping,
such as basketball, the muscle contraction and force of hitting the
ground after a jump strain the tendon. After repeated stress, the tendon may become inflamed or tear.

People with tendonitis of the knee may feel pain during running,
hurried walking, or jumping. Knee tendonitis can increase risk for rup-
tures or large tears to the tendon. A complete rupture of the quadriceps or patellar tendon is not only painful, but also makes it difficult
for a person to bend, extend, lift, or bear weight with the involved leg.

Achilles Tendonitis

Achilles tendon injuries involve an irritation, stretch, or tear to the
tendon connecting the calf muscle to the back of the heel. Achilles tendonitis is a common overuse injury, but can also be caused by tight or
weak calf muscles or any condition that causes the tendon to become

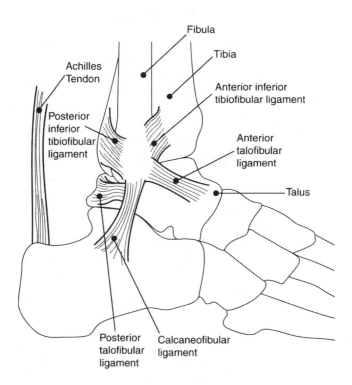

Figure 9.4. Lateral View of the Ankle

less flexible and more rigid, such as reactive arthritis or normal aging.

Achilles tendon injuries can happen to anyone who regularly participates in an activity that causes the calf muscle to contract, like climbing stairs or using a stair-stepper, but are most common in middle-aged weekend warriors who may not exercise regularly or take time to warm up and stretch properly before an activity. Among professional athletes, most Achilles injuries seem to occur in quick-acceleration or jumping sports like football, tennis, and basketball, and almost always end the season's competition for the athlete.

Achilles tendonitis can be a chronic condition. It can also cause what appears to be a sudden injury. Tendonitis is the most common factor contributing to Achilles tendon tears. When a tendon is weakened by age or overuse, trauma can cause it to rupture. These injuries can be so sudden and agonizing that they have been known to bring down charging professional football players in shocking fashion.

Diagnosis of Tendonitis and Bursitis

Diagnosis of tendonitis and bursitis begins with a medical history and physical examination. The patient will describe the pain and circumstances in which pain occurs. The location and onset of pain, whether it varies in severity throughout the day, and the factors that relieve or aggravate the pain are all important diagnostic clues. Therapists and physicians will use manual tests called selective tissue tension tests to determine which tendon is involved, and then will palpate (a form of touching the tendon) specific areas of the tendon to pinpoint the area of inflammation. X-rays do not show tendons or bursae, but may be helpful in ruling out problems in the bone or arthritis. In the case of a torn tendon, x-rays may help show which tendon is affected. In a knee injury, for example, an x-ray will show that the patella is lower than normal in a quadriceps tendon tear and higher than normal in a patellar tendon tear. The doctor may also use magnetic resonance imaging (MRI) to confirm a partial or total tear. MRI detects both bone and soft tissues like muscles, tendons and their coverings (sheaths), and bursae.

An anesthetic-injection test is another way to confirm a diagnosis of tendonitis. A small amount of anesthetic (lidocaine hydrochloride) is injected into the affected area. If the pain is temporarily relieved, the diagnosis is confirmed. To rule out infection, the doctor may remove and test fluid from the inflamed area.

Treatment

A primary care physician or a physical therapist can treat the common causes of tendonitis and bursitis. Complicated cases or those resistant to conservative therapies may require referral to a specialist, such as an orthopaedist or rheumatologist.

Treatment focuses on healing the injured bursa or tendon. The first step in treating both of these conditions is to reduce pain and inflammation with rest, compression, elevation, and anti-inflammatory medicines such as aspirin, naproxen (for example, Naprosyn, Aleve), or ibuprofen (for example, Advil, Motrin, or Nuprin). Ice may also be used in acute injuries, but most cases of bursitis or tendonitis are considered chronic, and ice is not helpful. When ice is needed, an ice pack can be applied to the affected area for 15–20 minutes every 4–6 hours for 3–5 days. Longer use of ice and a stretching program may be recommended by a health care provider. Activity involving the affected joint is also restricted to encourage healing and prevent further injury.

In some cases (for example, in tennis elbow), elbow bands may be used to compress the forearm muscle to provide some pain relief, limiting the pull of the tendon on the bone. Other protective devices, such as foot orthoses for the ankle and foot or splints for the knee or hand, may temporarily reduce stress to the affected tendon or bursa and facilitate quicker healing times, while allowing general activity levels to continue as usual.

The doctor or therapist may use ultrasound to warm deep tissues and improve blood flow. Iontophoresis may also be used. This involves using an electrical current to push a corticosteroid medication through the skin directly over the inflamed bursa or tendon. Gentle stretching and strengthening exercises are added gradually. Massage of the soft tissue may be helpful. These may be preceded or followed by use of an ice pack. The type of exercises recommended may vary depending on the location of the affected bursa or tendon.

If there is no improvement, the doctor may inject a corticosteroid medicine into the area surrounding the inflamed bursa or tendon. While corticosteroid injections are a common treatment, they must be used with caution because they may lead to weakening or rupture of the tendon (especially weight-bearing tendons such as the Achilles [ankle], posterior tibial [arch of the foot], and patellar [knee] tendons). If there is still no improvement after 6–12 months, the doctor may perform either arthroscopic or open surgery to repair damage and relieve pressure on the tendons and bursae.

If the bursitis is caused by an infection, the doctor will prescribe antibiotics. If a tendon is completely torn, surgery may be needed to repair the damage. After surgery on a quadriceps or patellar tendon, for example, the patient will wear a cast for 3–6 weeks and use crutches. For a partial tear, the doctor might apply a cast without performing surgery.

Rehabilitating a partial or complete tear of a tendon requires an exercise program to restore the ability to bend and straighten the knee and to strengthen the leg to prevent repeat injury. A rehabilitation program may last six months, although the patient can return to many activities before then.

Prevention

To help prevent inflammation or reduce the severity of its recurrence:[1]

- Warm up or stretch before physical activity.

- Strengthen muscles around the joint.

- Take frequent breaks from repetitive tasks.

- Cushion the affected joint. Use foam for kneeling or elbow pads. Increase the gripping surface of tools with gloves or padding. Apply grip tape or an oversized grip to golf clubs.

- Use two hands to hold heavy tools; use a two-handed backhand in tennis.

- Do not sit still for long periods.

- Practice good posture and position the body properly when going about daily activities.

- Begin new activities or exercise regimens slowly. Gradually increase physical demands following several well-tolerated exercise sessions.

- If a history of tendonitis is present, consider seeking guidance from your doctor or therapist before engaging in new exercises and activities.[1]

[1] Adapted from MayoClinic.com

Chapter 10

Cancer Pain Management

Cancer pain can be managed effectively in most patients with cancer or with a history of cancer. Although cancer pain cannot always be relieved completely, therapy can lessen pain in most patients. Pain management improves the patient's quality of life throughout all stages of the disease.

Flexibility is important in managing cancer pain. As patients vary in diagnosis, stage of disease, responses to pain and treatments, and personal likes and dislikes, management of cancer pain must be individualized. Patients, their families, and their health care providers must work together closely to manage a patient's pain effectively.

Assessment

To treat pain, it must be measured. The patient and the doctor should measure pain levels at regular intervals after starting cancer treatment, at each new report of pain, and after starting any type of treatment for pain. The cause of the pain must be identified and treated promptly.

Text in this chapter is from PDQ® Cancer Information Summary. National Cancer Institute, Bethesda, MD. "Pain (PDQ®) Supportive Care–Patient." Updated February 2008. Available at http://cancergov. Accessed March 5, 2008. Text under the heading "Relaxation Exercises for Pain Relief," was published in *Pain: Clinical Manual for Nursing Practice, First Edition*, 1989, pages 177, 201, and 206. © 1989 Elsevier. These exercises are still deemed pertinent. Reprinted with permission.

Patient Self-Report

To help the health care provider determine the type and extent of the pain, cancer patients can describe the location and intensity of their pain, any aggravating or relieving factors, and their goals for pain control. The family or caregiver may be asked to report for a patient who has a communication problem involving speech, language, or a thinking impairment. The health care provider should help the patient describe the following:

- **Pain:** The patient describes the pain, when it started, how long it lasts, and whether it is worse during certain times of the day or night.

- **Location:** The patient shows exactly where the pain is on his or her body or on a drawing of a body and where the pain goes if it travels.

- **Intensity or severity:** The patient keeps a diary of the degree or severity of pain.

- **Aggravating and relieving factors:** The patient identifies factors that increase or decrease the pain.

- **Personal response to pain:** Feelings of fear, confusion, or hopelessness about cancer, its prognosis, and the causes of pain can affect how a patient responds to and describes the pain. For example, a patient who thinks pain is caused by cancer spreading may report more severe pain or more disability from the pain.

- **Behavioral response to pain:** The health care provider and/ or caregivers note behaviors that may suggest pain in patients who have communication problems.

- **Goals for pain control:** With the health care provider, the patient decides how much pain he or she can tolerate and how much improvement he or she may achieve. The patient uses a daily pain diary to increase awareness of pain, gain a sense of control of the pain, and receive guidance from health care providers on ways to manage the pain.

Assessment of the Outcomes of Pain Management

The results of pain management should be measured by monitoring for a decrease in the severity of pain and improvement in thinking ability, emotional well-being, and social functioning. The results of taking pain medication should also be monitored. Drug addiction is rare in cancer patients. Developing a higher tolerance for a drug and becoming physically dependent on the drug for pain relief does not mean that the patient is addicted. Patients should take pain medication as prescribed by the doctor. Patients who have a history of drug abuse may tolerate higher doses of medication to control pain.

Management with Drugs

Basic Principles of Cancer Pain Management

The World Health Organization developed a three-step approach for pain management based on the severity of the pain:

- For mild to moderate pain, the doctor may prescribe a Step 1 pain medication such as aspirin, acetaminophen, or a nonsteroidal anti-inflammatory drug (NSAID). Patients should be monitored for side effects, especially those caused by NSAIDs, such as kidney, heart and blood vessel, or stomach and intestinal problems.

- When pain lasts or increases, the doctor may change the prescription to a Step 2 or Step 3 pain medication. Most patients with cancer-related pain will need a Step 2 or Step 3 medication. The doctor may skip Step 1 medications if the patient initially has moderate to severe pain.

- At each step, the doctor may prescribe additional drugs or treatments (for example, radiation therapy).

- The patient should take doses regularly, "by mouth, by the clock" (at scheduled times), to maintain a constant level of the drug in the body; this will help prevent recurrence of pain. If the patient is unable to swallow, the drugs are given by other routes (for example, by infusion or injection).

- The doctor may prescribe additional doses of drug that can be taken as needed for pain that occurs between scheduled doses of drug.

- The doctor will adjust the pain medication regimen for each patient's individual circumstances and physical condition.

Note: Part III of *Pain Sourcebook, Third Edition* has separate chapters which address the use of specific medications and delivery methods for the relief of pain.

Drugs Used with Pain Medications

Other drugs may be given at the same time as the pain medication. This is done to increase the effectiveness of the pain medication, treat symptoms, and relieve specific types of pain. These drugs include antidepressants, anticonvulsants, local anesthetics, corticosteroids, bisphosphonates, and stimulants. There are great differences in how patients respond to these drugs. Side effects are common and should be reported to the doctor. Certain bisphosphonates given for bone pain are linked to a risk of bone loss after dental work. Patients taking bisphosphonates should check with their doctor before having dental work done.

Physical and Psychosocial Interventions

Noninvasive physical and psychological methods can be used along with drugs and other treatments to manage pain during all phases of cancer treatment. The effectiveness of the pain interventions depends on the patient's participation in treatment and his or her ability to tell the health care provider which methods work best to relieve pain.

Physical Interventions

Weakness, muscle wasting, and muscle and bone pain may be treated with heat (a hot pack or heating pad); cold (flexible ice packs); massage, pressure, and vibration (to improve relaxation); exercise (to strengthen weak muscles, loosen stiff joints, help restore coordination and balance, and strengthen the heart); changing the position of the patient; restricting the movement of painful areas or broken bones; stimulation; controlled low-voltage electrical stimulation; or acupuncture.

Thinking and Behavioral Interventions

Thinking and behavior interventions are also important in treating pain. These interventions help give patients a sense of control and help them develop coping skills to deal with the disease and its symptoms. Beginning these interventions early in the course of the disease is useful so that patients can learn and practice the skills while they have enough strength and energy. Several methods should be tried, and one or more should be used regularly.

- **Relaxation and imagery:** Simple relaxation techniques may be used for episodes of brief pain (for example, during cancer treatment procedures).

- **Hypnosis:** Hypnotic techniques may be used to encourage relaxation and may be combined with other thinking/behavior methods.

- **Redirecting thinking:** Focusing attention on triggers other than pain or negative emotions that come with pain may involve distractions that are internal (for example, counting, praying, or saying things like "I can cope") or external (for example, music, television, talking, listening to someone read, or looking at something specific).

- **Patient education:** Health care providers can give patients and their families information and instructions about pain and pain management and assure them that most pain can be controlled effectively. Health care providers should also discuss the major barriers that interfere with effective pain management.

- **Psychological support:** Short-term psychological therapy helps some patients. Patients who develop clinical depression or adjustment disorder may see a psychiatrist for diagnosis.

- **Support groups and religious counseling:** Support groups help many patients. Religious counseling may also help by providing spiritual care and social support.

Relaxation Exercises for Pain Relief

Exercise 1: Slow, Rhythmic Breathing for Relaxation

1. Breathe in slowly and deeply, keeping your stomach and shoulders relaxed.

2. As you breathe out slowly, feel yourself beginning to relax; feel the tension leaving your body.

3. Breathe in and out slowly and regularly at a comfortable rate. Let the breath come all the way down to your stomach, as it completely relaxes.

4. To help you focus on your breathing and to breathe slowly and rhythmically: Breathe in as you say silently to yourself, "in, two, three;" or, each time you breathe out, say silently to yourself a word such as "peace" or "relax."

5. Do steps 1–4 only once or repeat steps 3–4 for up to 20 minutes.

6. End with a slow deep breath. As you breathe out say to yourself, "I feel alert and relaxed."

Exercise 2: Simple Touch, Massage, or Warmth for Relaxation

Touch and massage are traditional methods of helping others relax. Some examples are:

• Brief touch or massage, such as hand holding or briefly touching or rubbing a person's shoulders.

• Soaking feet in a basin of warm water or wrapping the feet in a warm, wet towel.

• Massage (3–10 minutes) of the whole body or just the back, feet, or hands. If the patient is modest or cannot move or turn easily in bed, consider massage of the hands and feet.

• Use a warm lubricant. A small bowl of hand lotion may be warmed in the microwave oven or a bottle of lotion may be warmed in a sink of hot water for about ten minutes.

• Massage for relaxation is usually done with smooth, long, slow strokes. Try several degrees of pressure along with different types of massage, such as kneading and stroking, to determine which is preferred.

Especially for the elderly person, a back rub that effectively produces relaxation may consist of no more than three minutes of slow, rhythmic stroking (about 60 strokes per minute) on both sides of the spine, from the crown of the head to the lower back. Continuous hand contact is maintained by starting one hand down the back as the other hand stops at the lower back and is raised. Set aside a regular time for the massage. This gives the patient something pleasant to anticipate.

Exercise 3: Peaceful Past Experiences

Something may have happened to you a while ago that brought you peace or comfort. You may be able to draw on that experience to bring you peace or comfort now. Think about these questions:

• Can you remember any situation, even when you were a child, when you felt calm, peaceful, secure, hopeful, or comfortable?

- Have you ever daydreamed about something peaceful? What were you thinking?

- Do you get a dreamy feeling when you listen to music? Do you have any favorite music?

- Do you have any favorite poetry that you find uplifting or reassuring?

- Have you ever been active religiously? Do you have favorite readings, hymns, or prayers? Even if you haven't heard or thought of them for many years, childhood religious experiences may still be very soothing.

Additional points: Some of the things that may comfort you, such as your favorite music or a prayer, can probably be recorded for you. Then you can listen to the tape whenever you wish. Or, if your memory is strong, you may simply close your eyes and recall the events or words.

Exercise 4: Active Listening to Music

1. Obtain a cassette player, tape recorder, compact disk (CD) or MP3 player with earphones or a headset and music you like. Other options for listening include comedy routines, sporting events, old radio shows, or audio-books.

2. Mark time to the music; for example, tap out the rhythm with your finger or nod your head. This helps you concentrate on the music rather than on your discomfort.

3. Keep your eyes open and focus on a fixed spot or object. If you wish to close your eyes, picture something about the music.

4. Listen to the music at a comfortable volume. If the discomfort increases, try increasing the volume; decrease the volume when the discomfort decreases.

5. If this is not effective enough, try adding or changing one or more of the following: massage your body in rhythm to the music; try other music; or mark time to the music in more than one manner, such as tapping your foot and finger at the same time.

Additional points: Many patients have found this technique to be helpful. It tends to be very popular, probably because the equipment is usually readily available and is a part of daily life. Other advantages are that it is easy to learn and not physically or mentally demanding.

If you are very tired, you may simply listen to the music and omit marking time or focusing on a spot.

Anticancer Interventions

Radiation therapy, radiofrequency ablation, and surgery may be used for pain relief rather than as treatment for primary cancer. Certain chemotherapy drugs may also be used to manage cancer-related pain.

Local or whole-body radiation therapy may increase the effectiveness of pain medication and other noninvasive therapies by directly affecting the cause of the pain (for example, by reducing tumor size). A single injection of a radioactive agent may relieve pain when cancer spreads extensively to the bones. Radiation therapy also helps reduce pain-related interference with walking and other functions in patients who have cancer that has spread to the bones.

Radiofrequency ablation uses a needle electrode to heat tumors and destroy them. This minimally invasive procedure may provide significant pain relief in patients who have cancer that has spread to the bones.

Surgery may be used to remove part or all of a tumor to reduce pain directly, relieve symptoms of obstruction or compression, and improve outcome, even increasing long-term survival.

Invasive Interventions

Less invasive methods should be used for relieving pain before trying invasive treatment. Some patients, however, may need invasive therapy.

A nerve block is the injection of either a local anesthetic or a drug that inactivates nerves to control otherwise uncontrollable pain. Nerve blocks can be used to determine the source of pain, to treat painful conditions that respond to nerve blocks, to predict how the pain will respond to long-term treatments, and to prevent pain following procedures.

Neurologic interventions include surgery to implant devices that deliver drugs or electrically stimulate the nerves. In rare cases, surgery may be done to destroy a nerve or nerves that are part of the pain pathway.

Chapter 11

Carpal Tunnel Syndrome

You're working at your desk, trying to ignore the tingling or numbness you've had for months in your hand and wrist. Suddenly, a sharp, piercing pain shoots through the wrist and up your arm. Just a passing cramp? More likely you have carpal tunnel syndrome, a painful progressive condition caused by compression of a key nerve in the wrist.

What is carpal tunnel syndrome?

Carpal tunnel syndrome occurs when the median nerve, which runs from the forearm into the hand, becomes pressed or squeezed at the wrist. The median nerve controls sensations to the palm side of the thumb and fingers (although not the little finger), as well as impulses to some small muscles in the hand that allow the fingers and thumb to move. The carpal tunnel—a narrow, rigid passageway of ligament and bones at the base of the hand—houses the median nerve and tendons. Sometimes, thickening from irritated tendons or other swelling narrows the tunnel and causes the median nerve to be compressed. The result may be pain, weakness, or numbness in the hand and wrist, radiating up the arm. Although painful sensations may indicate other conditions, carpal tunnel syndrome is the most common and widely known of the entrapment neuropathies in which the body's peripheral nerves are compressed or traumatized.

Excerpted from "Carpal Tunnel Syndrome Fact Sheet," National Institute of Neurological Disorders and Stroke (NINDS), NIH Publication No. 03–4898, updated December 11, 2007.

What are the symptoms of carpal tunnel syndrome?

Symptoms usually start gradually, with frequent burning, tingling, or itching numbness in the palm of the hand and the fingers, especially the thumb and the index and middle fingers. Some carpal tunnel sufferers say their fingers feel useless and swollen, even though little or no swelling is apparent. The symptoms often first appear in one or both hands during the night, since many people sleep with flexed wrists. A person with carpal tunnel syndrome may wake up feeling the need to shake out the hand or wrist. As symptoms worsen, people might feel tingling during the day. Decreased grip strength may make it difficult to form a fist, grasp small objects, or perform other manual tasks. In chronic or untreated cases, the muscles at the base of the thumb may waste away. Some people are unable to tell between hot and cold by touch.

What are the causes of carpal tunnel syndrome?

Carpal tunnel syndrome is often the result of a combination of factors that increase pressure on the median nerve and tendons in the carpal tunnel, rather than a problem with the nerve itself. Most likely the disorder is due to a congenital predisposition—the carpal tunnel is simply smaller in some people than in others. Other contributing factors include trauma or injury to the wrist that cause swelling, such as sprain or fracture; overactivity of the pituitary gland; hypothyroidism; rheumatoid arthritis; mechanical problems in the wrist joint; work stress; repeated use of vibrating hand tools; fluid retention during pregnancy or menopause; or the development of a cyst or tumor in the canal. In some cases no cause can be identified.

There is little clinical data to prove whether repetitive and forceful movements of the hand and wrist during work or leisure activities can cause carpal tunnel syndrome. Repeated motions performed in the course of normal work or other daily activities can result in repetitive motion disorders such as bursitis and tendonitis. Writer's cramp—a condition in which a lack of fine motor skill coordination and ache and pressure in the fingers, wrist, or forearm is brought on by repetitive activity—is not a symptom of carpal tunnel syndrome.

How is carpal tunnel syndrome diagnosed?

Early diagnosis and treatment are important to avoid permanent damage to the median nerve. A physical examination of the hands, arms, shoulders, and neck can help determine if the patient's complaints are related to daily activities or to an underlying disorder, and can rule out other painful conditions that mimic carpal tunnel syndrome. The wrist is examined for tenderness, swelling, warmth, and discoloration. Each finger should be tested for sensation, and the muscles at the base of the hand should be examined for strength and signs of atrophy. Routine laboratory tests and x-rays can reveal diabetes, arthritis, and fractures.

Physicians can use specific tests to try to produce the symptoms of carpal tunnel syndrome. In the Tinel test, the doctor taps on or presses on the median nerve in the patient's wrist. The test is positive when tingling in the fingers or a resultant shock-like sensation occurs. The Phalen, or wrist-flexion, test involves having the patient hold his or her forearms upright by pointing the fingers down and pressing the backs of the hands together. The presence of carpal tunnel syndrome is suggested if one or more symptoms, such as tingling or increasing numbness, is felt in the fingers within one minute. Doctors may also ask patients to try to make a movement that brings on symptoms.

Often it is necessary to confirm the diagnosis by use of electrodiagnostic tests. In a nerve conduction study, electrodes are placed on the hand and wrist. Small electric shocks are applied and the speed with which nerves transmit impulses is measured. In electromyography, a fine needle is inserted into a muscle; electrical activity viewed on a screen can determine the severity of damage to the median nerve. Ultrasound imaging can show impaired movement of the median nerve. Magnetic resonance imaging (MRI) can show the anatomy of the wrist but to date has not been especially useful in diagnosing carpal tunnel syndrome.

Treatment for Carpal Tunnel Syndrome

Treatments for carpal tunnel syndrome should begin as early as possible, under a doctor's direction. Underlying causes such as diabetes or arthritis should be treated first. Initial treatment generally involves resting the affected hand and wrist for at least two weeks, avoiding activities that may worsen symptoms, and immobilizing the wrist in a splint to avoid further damage from twisting or bending. If there is inflammation, applying cool packs can help reduce swelling.

Non-Surgical Treatments

Drugs: In special circumstances, various drugs can ease the pain and swelling associated with carpal tunnel syndrome. Nonsteroidal anti-inflammatory drugs, such as aspirin, ibuprofen, and other non-prescription pain relievers, may ease symptoms that have been present for a short time or have been caused by strenuous activity. Orally administered diuretics (water pills) can decrease swelling. Corticosteroids (such as prednisone) or the drug lidocaine can be injected directly into the wrist or taken by mouth (in the case of prednisone) to relieve pressure on the median nerve and provide immediate, temporary relief to persons with mild or intermittent symptoms. Additionally, some studies show that vitamin B$_6$ (pyridoxine) supplements may ease the symptoms of carpal tunnel syndrome.

Exercise: Stretching and strengthening exercises can be helpful in people whose symptoms have abated. These exercises may be supervised by a physical therapist trained to use exercises to treat physical impairments, or an occupational therapist trained in evaluating people with physical impairments and helping them build skills to improve their health and well-being.

Alternative therapies: Acupuncture and chiropractic care have benefited some patients but their effectiveness remains unproved. An exception is yoga, which has been shown to reduce pain and improve grip strength among patients with carpal tunnel syndrome.

Surgery

Carpal tunnel release is one of the most common surgical procedures in the United States. Generally recommended if symptoms last for six months, surgery involves severing the band of tissue around the wrist to reduce pressure on the median nerve. Surgery is done under local anesthesia and does not require an overnight hospital stay. Many patients require surgery on both hands. The following are types of carpal tunnel release surgery:

Open release surgery, the traditional procedure used to correct carpal tunnel syndrome, consists of making an incision up to two inches in the wrist and then cutting the carpal ligament to enlarge the carpal tunnel. The procedure is generally done under local anesthesia on an outpatient basis, unless there are unusual medical considerations.

Endoscopic surgery may allow faster functional recovery and less postoperative discomfort than traditional open release surgery.

The surgeon makes two incisions (about one-half inch each) in the wrist and palm, inserts a camera attached to a tube, observes the tissue on a screen, and cuts the carpal ligament (the tissue that holds joints together). This two-portal endoscopic surgery, generally performed under local anesthesia, is effective and minimizes scarring and scar tenderness, if any. One-portal endoscopic surgery for carpal tunnel syndrome is also available.

Recovery from Carpal Tunnel Surgery

Although symptoms may be relieved immediately after surgery, full recovery from carpal tunnel surgery can take months. Some patients may have infection, nerve damage, stiffness, and pain at the scar. Occasionally the wrist loses strength because the carpal ligament is cut. Patients should undergo physical therapy after surgery to restore wrist strength. Some patients may need to adjust job duties or even change jobs after recovery from surgery. Recurrence of carpal tunnel syndrome following treatment is rare. The majority of patients recover completely.

Prevention of Carpal Tunnel Syndrome

At the workplace, workers can do on-the-job conditioning, perform stretching exercises, take frequent rest breaks, wear splints to keep wrists straight, and use correct posture and wrist position. Wearing fingerless gloves can help keep hands warm and flexible. Workstations, tools and tool handles, and tasks can be redesigned to enable the worker's wrist to maintain a natural position during work. Jobs can be rotated among workers. Employers can develop programs in ergonomics, the process of adapting workplace conditions and job demands to the capabilities of workers. However, research has not conclusively shown that these workplace changes prevent the occurrence of carpal tunnel syndrome.

Chapter 12

Chest Pain

Definition

Chest pain is discomfort or pain that you feel anywhere along the front of your body between your neck and upper abdomen.

Considerations

Many people with chest pain fear a heart attack. However, there are many possible causes of chest pain. Some causes are mildly inconvenient, while other causes are serious, even life-threatening. Any organ or tissue in your chest can be the source of pain, including your heart, lungs, esophagus, muscles, ribs, tendons, or nerves.

Angina is a type of heart-related chest pain. This pain occurs because your heart is not getting enough blood and oxygen. Angina pain can be similar to the pain of a heart attack.

Angina is called stable angina when your chest pain begins at a predictable level of activity (for example, when you walk up a steep hill). However, if your chest pain happens unexpectedly after light activity or occurs at rest, this is called unstable angina. This is a more dangerous form of angina and you need to be seen in an emergency room right away.

Causes

Other causes of chest pain include:

- Asthma, which is generally accompanied by shortness of breath, wheezing, or cough.

- Pneumonia, a blood clot to the lung (pulmonary embolism), the collapse of a small area of a lung (pneumothorax), or inflammation of the lining around the lung (pleurisy). In these cases, the chest pain often worsens when you take a deep breath or cough and usually feels sharp.

- Strain or inflammation of the muscles and tendons between the ribs.

- Anxiety and rapid breathing.

Chest pain can also be related to problems with your digestive system. These include stomach ulcer, gallbladder disease, gallstones, indigestion, heartburn, or gastroesophageal reflux (when acid from your stomach backs up into your esophagus).

Ulcer pain burns if your stomach is empty and feels better with food. Gallbladder pain often gets worse after a meal, especially a fatty meal.

In children, most chest pain is not caused by the heart.

Home Care

If injury, over-exertion, or coughing have caused muscle strain, your chest wall is often tender or painful when you press a finger at the location of the pain. This can often be treated at home. Try acetaminophen or ibuprofen, ice, heat, and rest.

If you know you have asthma or angina, follow the instructions of your doctor and take your medications regularly to avoid flare-ups.

When to Contact a Medical Professional

Call 911 if:

- You have sudden crushing, squeezing, tightening, or pressure in your chest.

- Pain radiates to your jaw, left arm, or between your shoulder blades.

- You have nausea, dizziness, sweating, a racing heart, or shortness of breath.

- You know you have angina and your chest discomfort is suddenly more intense, brought on by lighter activity, or lasts longer than usual.

- Your angina symptoms occur at rest.

- You have sudden sharp chest pain with shortness of breath, especially after a long trip, a stretch of bedrest (for example, following an operation), or other lack of movement that can lead to a blood clot in your leg.

Know that your risk of heart attack is greater if you have a family history of heart disease, you smoke, use cocaine, are overweight, or you have high cholesterol, high blood pressure, or diabetes.

Call your doctor if:

- You have a fever or a cough that produces yellow-green phlegm.

- Chest wall pain persists for longer than three to five days.

What to Expect at Your Office Visit

Emergency measures will be taken, if necessary. Hospitalization will be required in difficult or serious cases or when the cause of the pain is unclear.

The doctor will perform a physical examination and monitor your vital signs (temperature, pulse, rate of breathing, blood pressure). The physical examination will focus on the chest wall, lungs, and heart. Your doctor may ask questions like the following:

- Is the pain between the shoulder blades? Is it under the breastbone? Does the pain change location? Is it on one side only?

- How would you describe the pain? (Severe, tearing or ripping, sharp, stabbing, burning, squeezing, constricting, tight, pressure-like, crushing, aching, dull, heavy)

- Does it come on suddenly? Does the pain occur at the same time each day?

- Is the pain getting worse? How long does the pain last?

- Does the pain go from your chest into your shoulder, arm, neck, jaw, or back?

- Is the pain worse when you are breathing deeply, coughing, eating, bending?

- When you are exercising? Is the pain better after you rest? Is it completely relieved or just less pain?

- Is the pain better after you take nitroglycerin medication? After you drink milk or take antacids? After belching?

- What other symptoms are also present?

  Diagnostic tests that may be performed include:

- Blood tests (such as lactate dehydrogenase (LDH), LDH isoenzymes, creatine phosphokinase (CPK), CPK isoenzymes, troponin, complete blood count (CBC), and blood differential)

- Cardiac catheterization

- Electrocardiogram (ECG)

- Exercise ECG

- Lung scan

- X-rays of the chest

More complex tests may be required depending on the difficulty of diagnosis or the suspected cause of the chest pain.

Prevention

Make healthy lifestyle choices to prevent chest pain from heart disease:

- Achieve and maintain normal weight.

- Control high blood pressure, high cholesterol, and diabetes.

- Avoid cigarette smoking and second-hand smoke.

- Eat a diet low in saturated and hydrogenated fats and cholesterol, and high in starches, fiber, fruits, and vegetables.

- Get at least 30 minutes of moderate intensity exercise on most days of the week.

- Reduce stress.

References

Altman EM, Smith SC Jr., Alpert JS, et al. ACC/AHA Guidelines for the Management of Patients with ST-Elevation Myocardial Infarction Executive Summary: A Report of the American College of Cardiology/ American Heart Association Task Force on Practice Guidelines (Writing Committee to Revise the 1999 Guidelines for the Management of

Patients with Acute Myocardial Infarction). *Circulation*. 2004;110: 588–636.

Braunwald E, Artman EM, Beasley JW, et al. ACC/AHA Guidelines for the Management of Patients with Unstable Angina and Non-ST-Segment Elevation Myocardial Infarction: A Report of the American College of Cardiology/American Heart Association Task Force on Practice Guidelines (Committee on the Management of Patients with Unstable Angina). *Journal of the American College of Cardiology*. 2000; 36(3):970–1062.

Smith SD Jr., Blair SN, Bonow RD, et al. AHA/ACC Guidelines for Preventing Heart Attack and Death in Patients with Atherosclerotic Cardiovascular Disease: 2001 Update: A Statement for Healthcare Professionals From the American Heart Association and the American College of Cardiology. *Circulation*. 2001;104:1577–1759.

Chapter 13

Childbirth: Pain during Labor and Delivery

If you're like most women, the pain of labor and delivery is one of the things that worry you about having a baby. This is certainly understandable, because labor is painful for most women.

It's possible to have labor with relatively little pain, but it's wise to prepare yourself by planning some strategies for coping with pain. Alleviating your anxiety about pain is one of the best ways to ensure that you'll be able to deal with it when the time comes.

Pain during Labor and Delivery

Pain during labor is caused primarily by uterine muscle contractions and somewhat by pressure on the cervix. This pain manifests itself as cramping in the abdomen, groin, and back, as well as a tired, achy feeling all over. Some women experience pain in their sides or thighs as well.

Other causes of pain during labor include pressure on the bladder and bowels by the baby's head and the stretching of the birth canal and vagina.

Although labor is often thought of as one of the more painful events in human experience, it ranges widely from woman to woman and

"Dealing with Pain during Childbirth," February 2008, reprinted with permission from www.kidshealth.org. Copyright © 2008 The Nemours Foundation. This information was provided by KidsHealth, one of the largest resources online for medically reviewed health information written for parents, kids, and teens. For more articles like this one, visit www.KidsHealth.org, or www.TeensHealth.org.

even from pregnancy to pregnancy. Women experience labor pain differently—for some, it resembles menstrual cramps; for others, severe pressure; and for others, extremely strong waves that feel like diarrheal cramps. In addition, first-time mothers are more likely to give their pain a higher rating than women who've had babies before.

The intensity of labor pain isn't always the determining factor that drives women to seek pain management—often it's the repetitive nature and length of time the pain persists with each contraction.

Preparing for Pain

To reduce pain during labor, here are some things you can start doing before or during your pregnancy:

Regular and reasonable exercise (unless your health care provider recommends against it) can help strengthen your muscles and prepare your body for the stress of labor. Exercise can also increase your endurance, which will come in handy if you have a long labor. The important thing to remember with any exercise is not to overdo it— and this is especially true if you're pregnant. Talk to your health care provider about what he or she considers to be a safe regimen, given your prepregnancy fitness level and the history of your pregnancy.

If you and your partner attend childbirth classes, you'll learn different techniques for handling pain, from visualization to stretches designed to strengthen the muscles that support your uterus. The two most common childbirth philosophies in the United States are the Lamaze technique and the Bradley method.

The Lamaze technique is the most widely used method in the United States. The Lamaze philosophy teaches that birth is a normal, natural, and healthy process and that women should be empowered to approach it with confidence. Lamaze classes educate women about the ways they can decrease their perception of pain, such as through relaxation techniques, breathing exercises, distraction, or massage by a supportive coach. Lamaze approach takes a neutral position toward pain medication, encouraging women to make an informed decision about whether it's right for them.

The Bradley method (also called Husband-Coached Birth) emphasizes a natural approach to birth and the active participation of the baby's father as birth coach. A major goal of this method is the avoidance of medications unless absolutely necessary. The Bradley method also focuses on good nutrition and exercise during pregnancy and relaxation and deep-breathing techniques as a method of coping with labor. Although the Bradley method advocates a medication-free birth experience, the classes do prepare parents for unexpected complications or situations, like emergency cesarean sections.

Other ways to handle pain during labor include:

- hypnosis;
- yoga;
- meditation;
- walking;
- massage or counterpressure;
- changing position;
- taking a bath or shower;
- distracting yourself by counting or performing an activity that keeps your mind otherwise occupied.

Pain Medications

A variety of pain medications could potentially be used during labor and delivery, depending on the situation. Talk to your health care provider about the risks and benefits of each.

Analgesics: Pain medications, including the drugs like morphine and meperidine, can be given intravenously or through a shot that's re-administered as needed. Either way, these medications act systemically—meaning they affect the whole body. These medicines don't usually slow down labor or interfere with contractions, but can cause side effects in the mother, including drowsiness and nausea. Analgesics may be administered well into labor but several hours before the expected birth.

If pain medications are given systemically, the baby's also going to get those medications. The effect on the baby depends on how much and how close to delivery the drug is given to the mother—some babies show signs of sleepiness immediately after birth. And some women find that the drowsiness and nausea they experience with systemic analgesics makes them less helpful than regional anesthesia. Talk to your health care provider about the risks and benefits of taking analgesics systemically.

Tranquilizers: These drugs don't relieve pain, but they may help to calm and relax seriously anxious women. Sometimes they are used in conjunction with analgesics. These drugs can have significant effects on both the mother and baby, and should be used cautiously. Women's reactions to these drugs vary—some feel a loss of control that is unnerving, whereas others do not. These drugs can sometimes make it difficult for women to remember the details of the birth. You should discuss the risks of taking tranquilizers first with your health care provider.

Regional anesthesia: This is what most women think of when they consider pain medication during labor. Nerve blocks deaden the sensation in specific regions of the body and can be used in both vaginal and cesarean section deliveries.

Epidurals, a form of local anesthesia, provide continuous pain relief to the entire body below the belly button, including the vaginal walls, during the entire process of labor. An epidural involves medication given by an anesthesiologist through a thin, tube-like catheter that's inserted in the woman's lower back (in the same location where a spinal tap would be performed). The amount of medication can be regulated according to a woman's needs. Some medication does reach the baby, but it's much less than what the baby would get intravenously or under general anesthesia (which sedates the baby as well as the mother and is almost exclusively reserved for emergency surgical births). Epidurals are usually given once a woman is in active labor.

Epidurals do have some drawbacks—they may make it more difficult for the woman to push the baby out, and they can cause her blood pressure to drop. They can also cause itching, nausea, and headaches in the mother. The risks to the baby are minimal, but include possible distress caused by the mother's lowered blood pressure.

Natural Childbirth

Some women choose to give birth using no medication at all, relying instead on relaxation techniques and controlled breathing for pain. If you'd like to experience childbirth without pain medication, make your wishes known to your health care provider.

Things to Consider

Here are some things to think about when considering pain control during labor:

* Medications can relieve much of your pain, but probably won't relieve all of it.

- Labor often hurts more than you anticipated. Some women who have previously said they want no pain medicine whatsoever end up changing their minds once they're actually in labor.

- Pain medications can affect your labor—your blood pressure may drop, your labor may slow down or speed up, you may become nauseous, and you may feel a sense of lack of control.

- Pain medications can affect your baby, the baby may be drowsy or have changes in the heart rate.

- If you end up needing a cesarean section, you'll be given regional or general anesthesia for the birth. General anesthesia is given in emergencies when a life-threatening condition has developed in the pregnant woman or baby.

Talking to Your Health Care Provider

You'll want to review your pain control options with the person who'll be delivering your baby. Find out what pain control methods are available, how effective they're likely to be, and when it's best not to use certain medications.

If you want to use pain-control methods other than medication, make sure your health care provider and the hospital staff know. You might want to also consider writing a birth plan that makes your preferences clear.

Remember, too, that many women make decisions about pain relief during labor that they abandon—often for very good reason—at the last minute. Try not to confuse your ability to endure the pain of childbirth with your worth as a mother. Your best bet is to educate yourself about all of your options for pain relief to make a choice about what's best for you and then to be flexible about that decision.

Chapter 14

Chronic Fatigue Syndrome

Chronic fatigue syndrome (CFS) is a debilitating and complex disorder characterized by profound fatigue that is not improved by bed rest and that may be worsened by physical or mental activity. Persons with CFS most often function at a substantially lower level of activity than they were capable of before the onset of illness. In addition to these key defining characteristics, patients report various nonspecific symptoms, including weakness, muscle pain, impaired memory and/or mental concentration, insomnia, and post-exertional fatigue lasting more than 24 hours. In some cases, CFS can persist for years. The cause or causes of CFS have not been identified and no specific diagnostic tests are available. Moreover, since many illnesses have incapacitating fatigue as a symptom, care must be taken to exclude other known and often treatable conditions before a diagnosis of CFS is made.

Definition of CFS

A great deal of debate has surrounded the issue of how best to define CFS. In an effort to resolve these issues, an international panel of CFS research experts convened in 1994 to draft a definition of CFS that would be useful both to researchers studying the illness and to clinicians diagnosing it. In essence, in order to receive a diagnosis of chronic fatigue syndrome, a patient must satisfy two criteria:

Excerpted from "CFS Basic Facts," Centers for Disease Control and Prevention (CDC), May 9, 2006.

1. Have severe chronic fatigue of six months or longer duration with other known medical conditions excluded by clinical diagnosis.

2. Concurrently have four or more of the following symptoms: substantial impairment in short-term memory or concentration; sore throat; tender lymph nodes; muscle pain; multi-joint pain without swelling or redness; headaches of a new type, pattern, or severity; sleep that does not refresh; and post-exertional malaise lasting more than 24 hours.

The symptoms must have persisted or recurred during six or more consecutive months of illness and must not have predated the fatigue.

Similar Medical Conditions

A number of illnesses have been described that have a similar spectrum of symptoms to CFS. These include fibromyalgia syndrome, myalgic encephalomyelitis, neurasthenia, multiple chemical sensitivities, and chronic mononucleosis. Although these illnesses may present with a primary symptom other than fatigue, chronic fatigue is commonly associated with all of them.

Other Conditions That May Cause Similar Symptoms

In addition, there are a large number of clinically defined, frequently treatable illnesses that can result in fatigue. Diagnosis of any of these conditions would exclude a definition of CFS unless the condition has been treated sufficiently and no longer explains the fatigue and other symptoms. These include hypothyroidism, sleep apnea and narcolepsy, major depressive disorders, chronic mononucleosis, bipolar affective disorders, schizophrenia, eating disorders, cancer, autoimmune disease, hormonal disorders, subacute infections, obesity, alcohol or substance abuse, and reactions to prescribed medications.

Other Commonly Observed Symptoms in CFS

In addition to the eight primary defining symptoms of CFS, a number of other symptoms have been reported by some CFS patients. The frequencies of occurrence of these symptoms vary from 20% to 50% among CFS patients. They include abdominal pain, alcohol intolerance, bloating, chest pain, chronic cough, diarrhea, dizziness, dry eyes or mouth, earaches, irregular heartbeat, jaw pain, morning stiffness, nausea, night sweats, psychological problems (depression, irritability, anxiety, panic attacks), shortness of breath, skin sensations, tingling sensations, and weight loss.

Prevalence of CFS

Chronic fatigue syndrome affects more than one million people in the United States. There are tens of millions of people with similar fatiguing illnesses who do not fully meet the strict research definition of CFS.

Risk Factors for CFS

- People of every age, gender, ethnicity, and socioeconomic group can have CFS.

- CFS affects women at four times the rate of men.

- Research indicates that CFS is most common in people in their 40s and 50s.

- Although CFS is much less common in children than in adults, children can develop the illness, particularly during the teen years.

Diagnosis of CFS

- There are no physical signs that identify CFS.

- There are no diagnostic laboratory tests for CFS.

- People who suffer the symptoms of CFS must be carefully evaluated by a physician because many treatable medical and psychiatric conditions are hard to distinguish from CFS. Common conditions that should be ruled out through a careful medical history and appropriate testing include mononucleosis, Lyme disease, thyroid conditions, diabetes, multiple sclerosis, various cancers, depression and bipolar disorder.

- Research conducted by the Centers for Disease Control and Prevention (CDC) indicates that less than 20% of CFS patients in the U.S. have been diagnosed.

Treatment of CFS

- Since there is no known cure for CFS, treatment is aimed at symptom relief and improved function. A combination of drug and nondrug therapies is usually recommended.

- No single therapy exists that helps all CFS patients.

- Lifestyle changes, including prevention of overexertion, reduced stress, dietary restrictions, gentle stretching, and nutritional supplementation, are frequently recommended in addition to drug therapies used to treat sleep, pain, and other specific symptoms.

- Carefully supervised physical therapy may also be part of treatment for CFS. However, symptoms can be exacerbated by overly ambitious physical activity. A very moderate approach to exercise and activity management is recommended to avoid overactivity and to prevent deconditioning.

- Although health care professionals may hesitate to give patients a diagnosis of CFS for various reasons, it's important to receive an appropriate and accurate diagnosis to guide treatment and further evaluation.

- Delays in diagnosis and treatment are thought to be associated with poorer long-term outcomes. For example, CDC research has shown that those who have CFS for two years or less were more likely to improve. It's not known if early intervention is responsible for this more favorable outcome; however, the longer a person is ill before diagnosis, the more complicated the course of the illness appears to be.

Recovery from CFS

CFS affects each individual differently. Some people with CFS remain homebound and others improve to the point that they can resume work and other activities, even though they continue to experience symptoms. Recovery rates for CFS are unclear. Improvement rates varied from 8% to 63% in a 2005 review of published studies, with a median of 40% of patients improving during follow-up. However, full recovery from CFS may be rare, with an average of only 5% to 10% sustaining total remission.

Chapter 15

Complex Regional Pain Syndrome (Reflex Sympathetic Dystrophy Syndrome)

Complex regional pain syndrome (CRPS) is a chronic pain condition that is believed to be the result of dysfunction in the central or peripheral nervous systems. Typical features include dramatic changes in the color and temperature of the skin over the affected limb or body part, accompanied by intense burning pain, skin sensitivity, sweating, and swelling. CRPS I is frequently triggered by tissue injury; the term describes all patients with the above symptoms but with no underlying nerve injury. Patients with CRPS II experience the same symptoms, but their cases are clearly associated with a nerve injury.

Older terms used to describe CRPS are "reflex sympathetic dystrophy syndrome" and "causalgia," a term first used during the Civil War to describe the intense, hot pain felt by some veterans long after their wounds had healed.

CRPS can strike at any age and affects both men and women, although most experts agree that it is more common in young women.

Symptoms of CRPS

The key symptom of CRPS is continuous, intense pain out of proportion to the severity of the injury (if an injury has occurred), which

---

Text in this chapter is from "Complex Regional Pain Syndrome Fact Sheet," National Institute of Neurological Disorders and Stroke (NINDS), NIH Publication No. 04–4173, updated January 10, 2008.

gets worse rather than better over time. CRPS most often affects one of the extremities (arms, legs, hands, or feet) and is also often accompanied by:

- burning pain,
- increased skin sensitivity,
- changes in skin temperature (warmer or cooler compared to the opposite extremity),
- changes in skin color (often blotchy, purple, pale, or red),
- changes in skin texture (shiny and thin, and sometimes excessively sweaty),
- changes in nail and hair growth patterns,
- swelling and stiffness in affected joints, or
- motor disability with decreased ability to move the affected body part.

Often the pain spreads to include the entire arm or leg, even though the initiating injury might have been only to a finger or toe. Pain can sometimes even travel to the opposite extremity. It may be heightened by emotional stress.

The symptoms of CRPS vary in severity and length. Some experts believe there are three stages associated with CRPS, marked by progressive changes in the skin, muscles, joints, ligaments, and bones of the affected area, although this progression has not yet been validated by clinical research studies.

Stage one is thought to last from 1–3 months and is characterized by severe, burning pain, along with muscle spasm, joint stiffness, rapid hair growth, and alterations in the blood vessels that cause the skin to change color and temperature.

Stage two lasts from 3–6 months and is characterized by intensifying pain, swelling, decreased hair growth, cracked, brittle, grooved, or spotty nails, softened bones, stiff joints, and weak muscle tone.

In stage three the syndrome progresses to the point where changes in the skin and bone are no longer reversible. Pain becomes unyielding and may involve the entire limb or affected area. There may be marked muscle loss (atrophy), severely limited mobility, and involuntary contractions of the muscles and tendons that flex the joints. Limbs may become contorted.

Causes of CRPS

Doctors are not sure what causes CRPS. In some cases the sympathetic nervous system plays an important role in sustaining the pain. The most recent theories suggest that pain receptors in the affected part of the body become responsive to a family of nervous system messengers known as catecholamines. Animal studies indicate that norepinephrine, a catecholamine released from sympathetic nerves, acquires the capacity to activate pain pathways after tissue or nerve injury. The incidence of sympathetically maintained pain in CRPS is not known. Some experts believe that the importance of the sympathetic nervous system depends on the stage of the disease.

Another theory is that post-injury CRPS (CRPS II) is caused by a triggering of the immune response, which leads to the characteristic inflammatory symptoms of redness, warmth, and swelling in the affected area. CRPS may therefore represent a disruption of the healing process. In all likelihood, CRPS does not have a single cause, but is rather the result of multiple causes that produce similar symptoms.

Diagnosis of CRPS

CRPS is diagnosed primarily through observation of the signs and symptoms. Because many other conditions have similar symptoms, it can be difficult for doctors to make a firm diagnosis of CRPS early in the course of the disorder when symptoms are few or mild. Or, for example, a simple nerve entrapment can sometimes cause pain severe enough to resemble CRPS. Diagnosis is further complicated by the fact that some people will improve gradually over time without treatment.

Since there is no specific diagnostic test for CRPS, the most important role for testing is to help rule out other conditions. Some clinicians apply a stimulus (such as touch, pinprick, heat, or cold) to the area to see if it causes pain. Doctors may also use triple-phase bone scans to identify changes in the bone and in blood circulation.

Prognosis

The prognosis for CRPS varies from person to person. Spontaneous remission from symptoms occurs in certain people. Others can have unremitting pain and crippling, and irreversible changes in spite of treatment. Some doctors believe that early treatment is helpful in limiting the disorder, but this belief has not yet been supported by evidence from clinical studies. More research is needed to understand the causes of CRPS, how it progresses, and the role of early treatment.

Treatment for CRPS

Since there is no cure for CRPS, treatment is aimed at relieving painful symptoms so that people can resume their normal lives. The following therapies are often used:

- **Physical therapy:** A gradually increasing exercise program to keep the painful limb or body part moving may help restore some range of motion and function.

- **Psychotherapy:** CRPS often has profound psychological effects on people and their families. Those with CRPS may suffer from depression, anxiety, or post-traumatic stress disorder, all of which heighten the perception of pain and make rehabilitation efforts more difficult.

- **Sympathetic nerve block:** Some patients will get significant pain relief from sympathetic nerve blocks. Sympathetic blocks can be done in a variety of ways. One technique involves intravenous administration of phentolamine, a drug that blocks sympathetic receptors. Another technique involves placement of an anesthetic next to the spine to directly block the sympathetic nerves.

- **Medications:** Many different classes of medication are used to treat CRPS including: topical analgesic drugs that act locally on painful nerves, skin, and muscles; antiseizure drugs; and anti-depressants, corticosteroids, and opioids. However, no single drug or combination of drugs has produced consistent long-lasting improvement in symptoms.

- **Surgical sympathectomy:** The use of surgical sympathectomy, a technique that destroys the nerves involved in CRPS, is contro-versial. Some experts think it is unwarranted and makes CRPS worse; others report a favorable outcome. Sympathectomy should be used only in patients whose pain is dramatically relieved (al-though temporarily) by selective sympathetic blocks.

- **Spinal cord stimulation:** The placement of stimulating elec-trodes next to the spinal cord provides a pleasant tingling sensa-tion in the painful area. This technique appears to help many patients with their pain.

- **Intrathecal drug pumps:** These devices administer drugs direct-ly to the spinal fluid, so that opioids and local anesthetic agents can be delivered to pain-signaling targets in the spinal cord at doses far lower than those required for oral administration. This technique decreases side effects and increases drug effectiveness.

Chapter 16

Earaches: A Painful Problem for Many Children

How does the ear work?

The ear works by receiving sound waves and sending messages to the brain. The outer ear includes the part of the ear you can see and the ear canal. The sound waves go through the ear canal and hit the eardrum and cause it to vibrate.

The vibration of the eardrum causes the tiny bones in the ear to move. This movement sends the sound waves to the inner ear.

What causes earaches?

A tube called the eustachian (say: "you-stay-shun") tube connects the middle ear with the back of the nose. Normally this tube lets fluid drain out of the middle ear. If bacteria or viruses infect the lining of your child's eustachian tube, the tube gets swollen and fills with thick mucus. This keeps fluid in the ear from draining normally. Bacteria can grow in the fluid, increasing pressure behind the eardrum and causing pain.

The eustachian tubes can become blocked because of allergies, or a cold or other infection. In other cases, the adenoids (glands near the ear) become enlarged and block the eustachian tubes.

Acute ear infections usually clear up within one or two weeks. Sometimes, ear infections last longer and become chronic. After an infection, fluid may stay in the middle ear. This may lead to more infections and hearing loss.

What are the symptoms of ear infections?

The most common symptoms of an acute ear infection are ear pain and fever. If your child is too young to tell you what hurts, he or she may cry or pull at his or her ear. Your child may also be irritable or listless, have trouble hearing, or not feel like eating or sleeping.

What is the treatment for ear infections?

The treatment for ear infections may include any of the following:

- If your doctor thinks the infection is caused by bacteria, he or she may prescribe an antibiotic. (Antibiotics don't work for infections caused by viruses.) It's very important to follow the directions for giving your child the medicine.

- Pain relievers like acetaminophen (brand names: Children's or Infants' Tylenol) and ibuprofen (brand names: Children's Advil or Children's Motrin) can help make your child feel better and reduce fever. Never give your child aspirin, as it has been linked to Reye syndrome.

- A warm, not hot, heating pad held over the ear can also help relieve the earache.

- Ear drops to relieve pain are sometimes prescribed.

Why are earaches so common in children?

This may be because children's eustachian tubes are shorter and more narrow than those of adults. Most children will have at least one ear infection by their third birthday.

Children may be at higher risk for ear infections if they:

- Are around people who smoke.

- Have had previous ear infections.

- Have a family history of ear infections.

- Attend day care (because they are exposed to more germs and viruses).

- Were born prematurely or with a low birth weight.

- Have frequent colds or other infections.

- Take a bottle to bed.

- Use a pacifier.

- Are male (boys tend to get more ear infections than girls).

- Have nasal speech (caused by large adenoids that block the eustachian tube).

- Have allergies with nasal congestion.

What can be done to prevent ear infections from returning?

Some children seem to get many ear infections. If your child has had three ear infections in six months or four in one year, your doctor may suggest that your child take a low dose of antibiotic every day, usually during the winter when these infections are most common.

Your doctor may want to see your child a few times when he or she is taking the antibiotic to make sure another ear infection does not happen.

Will earaches hurt my child's hearing?

Middle ear infections and fluid in the ear are the most common causes of temporary hearing loss in children. Children who have ongoing problems with hearing may have trouble developing their speech and language skills. For this reason, it is important to talk with your doctor if your child has repeated ear infections.

What about fluid that stays in the middle ear?

Your child's hearing may be affected if fluid stays in the middle ear after an infection. This is called otitis media with effusion. (Effusion is another word for fluid buildup.) Usually the fluid goes away in two to three months, and hearing returns to normal. Your doctor may want to check your child again at this time to see if fluid is still present.

If the fluid stays for more than a few months, your doctor may want to check your child's hearing. Your doctor may recommend ear tubes (also called tympanostomy tubes) to drain the fluid if your child's hearing is decreased a lot. Ear tubes may also decrease the number of ear infections your child gets.

What are ear tubes?

Ear tubes are tiny plastic tubes that help balance the pressure in your child's ears. They allow air into the middle ear so that fluid can drain out down the eustachian tube. They're put into the eardrum (which is also called the tympanic membrane) during surgery and stay in place for an average of six to nine months.

The tubes are usually left in place until they fall out on their own or your doctor decides your child no longer needs them. Sometimes, another set of tubes may be needed.

Placing tubes in the ears is an operation and has some risks. Your child will need general anesthesia when the tube is inserted. Your doctor will talk with you about the risks if he or she thinks your child needs tubes.

Chapter 17

Fibromyalgia

Fibromyalgia syndrome is a common and chronic disorder characterized by widespread muscle pain, fatigue, and multiple tender points. Tender points are specific places on the body—on the neck, shoulders, back, hips, and upper and lower extremities—where people with fibromyalgia feel pain in response to slight pressure.

Although fibromyalgia is often considered an arthritis-related condition, it is not truly a form of arthritis (a disease of the joints) because it does not cause inflammation or damage to the joints, muscles, or other tissues. Like arthritis, however, fibromyalgia can cause significant pain and fatigue, and it can interfere with a person's ability to carry on daily activities. Also like arthritis, fibromyalgia is considered a rheumatic condition. In medicine, the term rheumatic means a medical condition that impairs the joints and/or soft tissues and causes chronic pain.

In addition to pain and fatigue, people who have fibromyalgia may experience:

- sleep disturbances,

- morning stiffness,

This chapter includes text from "Questions and Answers about Fibromyalgia," National Institute of Arthritis and Musculoskeletal and Skin Diseases (NIAMS), NIH Publication No. 04–5326, revised June 2004; and an excerpt titled "First Drug Approved for Fibromyalgia Treatment," from "Living with Fibromyalgia, First Drug Approved," *Consumer Update*, U.S. Food and Drug Administration (FDA), June 21, 2007.

- headaches,

- irritable bowel syndrome,

- painful menstrual periods,

- numbness or tingling of the extremities,

- restless legs syndrome,

- temperature sensitivity,

- cognitive and memory problems, or

- a variety of other symptoms.

Fibromyalgia is a syndrome rather than a disease. Unlike a disease, which is a medical condition with a specific cause or causes and recognizable signs and symptoms, a syndrome is a collection of signs, symptoms, and medical problems that tend to occur together but are not related to a specific, identifiable cause.

According to a paper published by the American College of Rheumatology (ACR), fibromyalgia affects 3–6 million—or as many as one in 50—Americans. For unknown reasons, between 80 and 90 percent of those diagnosed with fibromyalgia are women; however, men and children also can be affected. Most people are diagnosed during middle age, although the symptoms often become present earlier in life. The causes of fibromyalgia are unknown, but there are probably a number of factors involved.

How is fibromyalgia diagnosed?

Research shows that people with fibromyalgia typically see many doctors before receiving the diagnosis. One reason for this may be that pain and fatigue, the main symptoms of fibromyalgia, overlap with many other conditions. Therefore, doctors often have to rule out other potential causes of these symptoms before making a diagnosis of fibromyalgia. Another reason is that there are currently no diagnostic laboratory tests for fibromyalgia; standard laboratory tests fail to reveal a physiologic reason for pain. Because there is no generally accepted, objective test for fibromyalgia, some doctors unfortunately may conclude a patient's pain is not real, or they may tell the patient there is little they can do.

A doctor familiar with fibromyalgia, however, can make a diagnosis based on two criteria established by the ACR: a history of widespread pain lasting more than three months and the presence of tender points.

Pain is considered to be widespread when it affects all four quadrants of the body; that is, you must have pain in both your right and left sides as well as above and below the waist to be diagnosed with fibromyalgia. The ACR also has designated 18 sites on the body as possible tender points. For a fibromyalgia diagnosis, a person must have 11 or more tender points. One of these predesignated sites is considered a true tender point only if the person feels pain upon the application of four kilograms of pressure to the site. People who have fibromyalgia certainly may feel pain at other sites, too, but those 18 standard possible sites on the body are the criteria used for classification.

How is fibromyalgia treated?

Fibromyalgia can be difficult to treat. Not all doctors are familiar with fibromyalgia and its treatment, so it is important to find a doctor who treats fibromyalgia. Fibromyalgia treatment often requires a team approach, with your doctor, a physical therapist, possibly other health professionals, and most importantly, yourself, all playing an active role. It can be hard to assemble this team, and you may struggle to find the right professionals to treat you. However, when you do, the combined expertise of these various professionals can help you improve your quality of life. A place to begin is through pain clinics that specialize in pain and rheumatology clinics that specialize in arthritis and other rheumatic diseases, including fibromyalgia.

In June 2007, the U.S. Food and Drug Administration approved Lyrica (pregabalin) as the first drug to treat fibromyalgia. Doctors also treat fibromyalgia with a variety of medications developed and approved for other purposes. Following are some of the most commonly used categories of drugs for fibromyalgia:

Analgesics: Analgesics are painkillers. They range from over-the-counter acetaminophen (Tylenol) to prescription medicines, such as tramadol (Ultram), and even stronger narcotic preparations. For a subset of people with fibromyalgia, narcotic medications are prescribed for severe muscle pain. However, there is no solid evidence showing that narcotics actually work to treat the chronic pain of fibromyalgia, and most doctors hesitate to prescribe them for long-term use because of the potential that the person taking them will become physically or psychologically dependent on them.

Nonsteroidal anti-inflammatory drugs (NSAIDs): As their name implies, nonsteroidal anti-inflammatory drugs, including aspirin, ibuprofen (Advil, Motrin), and naproxen sodium (Anaprox, Aleve), are used to treat inflammation. Although inflammation is not a symptom of fibromyalgia, NSAIDs also relieve pain. The drugs work by inhibiting substances in the body called prostaglandins which play a role in pain and inflammation. These medications, some of which are available without a prescription, may help ease the muscle aches of fibromyalgia. They may also relieve menstrual cramps and the headaches often associated with fibromyalgia.

Antidepressants: Perhaps the most useful medications for fibromyalgia are several in the antidepressant class. Antidepressants elevate the levels of certain chemicals in the brain, including serotonin and norepinephrine (which was formerly called adrenaline). Low levels of these chemicals are associated not only with depression, but also with pain and fatigue. Increasing the levels of these chemicals can reduce pain in people who have fibromyalgia. Doctors prescribe several types of antidepressants for people with fibromyalgia including:

- **Tricyclic antidepressants:** When taken at bedtime in dosages lower than those used to treat depression, tricyclic antidepressants can help promote restorative sleep in people with fibromyalgia. They also can relax painful muscles and heighten the effects of the body's natural pain-killing substances called endorphins. Tricyclic medications used to treat fibromyalgia include amitriptyline and cyclobenzaprine which have been proven useful for the treatment of fibromyalgia.

- **Selective serotonin reuptake inhibitors:** If a tricyclic antidepressant fails to bring relief, doctors sometimes prescribe a newer type of antidepressant called a selective serotonin reuptake inhibitor (SSRI). As with tricyclics, doctors usually prescribe these for people with fibromyalgia in lower dosages than are used to treat depression. By promoting the release of serotonin, these drugs may reduce fatigue and some other symptoms associated with fibromyalgia. SSRIs may be prescribed along with a tricyclic antidepressant. Doctors rarely prescribe SSRIs alone. Because they make people feel more energetic, they also interfere with sleep, which often is already a problem for people with fibromyalgia. Studies have shown that a combination therapy of the tricyclic amitriptyline and the SSRI fluoxetine resulted in greater improvements in the study participants' fibromyalgia symptoms than either drug alone.

- **Mixed reuptake inhibitors:** Some newer antidepressants raise levels of both serotonin and norepinephrine, and are therefore called mixed reuptake inhibitors. Researchers are actively studying the efficacy of these newer medications in treating fibromyalgia.

Benzodiazepines: Benzodiazepines help some people with fibromyalgia by relaxing tense, painful muscles and stabilizing the erratic brain waves that can interfere with deep sleep. Benzodiazepines also can relieve the symptoms of restless legs syndrome, which is common among people with fibromyalgia. Restless legs syndrome is characterized by unpleasant sensations in the legs as well as twitching, particularly at night. Because of the potential for addiction, doctors usually prescribe benzodiazepines only for people who have not responded to other therapies.

Other medications: In addition to the previously described general categories of drugs, doctors may prescribe others, depending on a person's specific symptoms or fibromyalgia-related conditions.

Other treatments: People with fibromyalgia also may benefit from a combination of physical and occupational therapy, from learning pain-management and coping techniques, and from properly balancing rest and activity.

- **Complementary and alternative therapies:** Many people with fibromyalgia also report varying degrees of success with complementary and alternative therapies, including massage, movement therapies (such as Pilates and the Feldenkrais method), chiropractic treatments, acupuncture, and various herbs and dietary supplements for different fibromyalgia symptoms. Though some of these supplements are being studied for fibromyalgia, there is little, if any, scientific proof yet that they help.

Will fibromyalgia get better with time?

Fibromyalgia is a chronic condition, meaning it lasts a long time—possibly a lifetime. However, it may comfort you to know that fibromyalgia is not a progressive disease. It is never fatal, and it won't cause damage to your joints, muscles, or internal organs. In many people, the condition does improve over time.

What can I do to try to feel better?

Besides taking medicine prescribed by your doctor, there are many things you can do to minimize the impact of fibromyalgia on your life. These include:

- **Getting enough sleep:** Getting enough sleep and the right kind of sleep can help ease the pain and fatigue of fibromyalgia. Even so, many people with fibromyalgia have problems such as pain, restless legs syndrome, or brain-wave irregularities that interfere with restful sleep.

- **Exercising:** Though pain and fatigue may make exercise and daily activities difficult, it's crucial to be as physically active as possible. Research has repeatedly shown that regular exercise is one of the most effective treatments for fibromyalgia. People who have too much pain or fatigue to do vigorous exercise should begin with walking or other gentle exercise and build their endurance and intensity slowly.

- **Making changes at work:** Most people with fibromyalgia continue to work, but they may have to make big changes to do so; for example, some people cut down the number of hours they work, switch to a less demanding job, or adapt a current job. If you face obstacles at work, such as an uncomfortable desk chair that leaves your back aching or difficulty lifting heavy boxes or files, your employer may make adaptations that will enable you to keep your job. An occupational therapist can help you design a more comfortable workstation or find more efficient and less painful ways to lift. If you are unable to work at all due to a medical condition, you may qualify for disability benefits through your employer, Social Security Disability Insurance (SSDI), or Supplemental Security Insurance (SSI).

- **Eating well:** Although some people with fibromyalgia report feeling better when they eat or avoid certain foods, no specific diet has been proven to influence fibromyalgia. Of course, it is important to have a healthy, balanced diet. Not only will proper nutrition give you more energy and make you generally feel better, it will also help you avoid other health problems.

First Drug Approved for Fibromyalgia Treatment

People with fibromyalgia have typically turned to pain medicines, antidepressants, muscle relaxants, and sleep medicines. On June 21,

2007, Lyrica (pregabalin) became the first U.S. Food and Drug Administration (FDA)-approved drug for specifically treating fibromyalgia. Marketed by Pfizer Inc., Lyrica reduces pain and improves function in patients with fibromyalgia. While patients with fibromyalgia have been shown to experience pain differently from other people, the mechanism by which Lyrica produces its effects is unknown. The drug was already approved to treat seizures, as well as pain from damaged nerves that can happen in people with diabetes and in those who develop pain following the rash of shingles.

"People who take Lyrica should be aware of important side effects, including sleepiness and dizziness," says Jeffrey Siegel, M.D., clinical team leader in FDA's Division of Anesthesia, Analgesia, and Rheumatology Products. Other side effects seen in patients taking Lyrica include swelling of the hands and feet, and allergic reactions.

"Studies showed that a substantial number of patients with fibromyalgia received good pain relief with Lyrica, but there are other patients who didn't benefit," Siegel says. "This new approval marks an important advance, and we think it's reason for optimism. But we still have much more progress to make."

Chapter 18

Gout

Gout is a painful condition that occurs when the bodily waste product uric acid is deposited as needle-like crystals in the joints or soft tissues. In the joints, these uric acid crystals cause inflammatory arthritis, which in turn leads to intermittent swelling, redness, heat, pain, and stiffness in the joints.

In many people gout initially affects the joints of the big toe (a condition called podagra). But many other joints and areas around the joints can be affected in addition to or instead of the big toe. These include the insteps, ankles, heels, knees, wrists, fingers, and elbows. Chalky deposits of uric acid, also known as tophi, can appear as lumps under the skin that surrounds the joints and covers the rim of the ear. Uric acid crystals can also collect in the kidneys and cause kidney stones.

Uric acid is a substance that results from the breakdown of purines. A normal part of all human tissue, purines are found in many foods. Normally, uric acid is dissolved in the blood and passed through the kidneys into the urine, where it is eliminated.

If there is an increase in the production of uric acid or if the kidneys do not eliminate enough uric acid from the body, levels of it build up in the blood (a condition called hyperuricemia). Hyperuricemia also may result when a person eats too many high-purine foods, such as

Excerpted from "Questions and Answers about Gout," National Institute of Arthritis and Musculoskeletal and Skin Diseases (NIAMS), NIH Publication No. 07–5027, December 2006.

liver, dried beans and peas, anchovies, and gravies. Hyperuricemia is not a disease, and by itself it is not dangerous. However, if excess uric acid crystals form as a result of hyperuricemia, gout can develop. The crystals form and accumulate in the joint, causing inflammation.

Four Stages of Gout

Literally translated, arthritis means joint inflammation. It refers to more than 100 different diseases that affect the joints. Gout accounts for approximately five percent of all cases of arthritis. The disease can progress through four stages:

1. **Asymptomatic (without symptoms) hyperuricemia:** In this stage, a person has elevated levels of uric acid in the blood (hyperuricemia), but no other symptoms. Treatment is usually not required.

2. **Acute gout, or acute gouty arthritis:** In this stage, hyperuricemia has caused the deposit of uric acid crystals in joint spaces. This leads to a sudden onset of intense pain and swelling in the joints, which also may be warm and very tender. An acute attack commonly occurs at night and can be triggered by stressful events, alcohol or drugs, or the presence of another illness. Attacks usually subside within 3–10 days, even without treatment, and the next attack may not occur for months or even years. Over time, however, attacks can last longer and occur more frequently.

3. **Interval or intercritical gout:** This is the period between acute attacks. In this stage, a person does not have any symptoms.

4. **Chronic tophaceous gout:** This is the most disabling stage of gout. It usually develops over a long period, such as ten years. In this stage, the disease may have caused permanent damage to the affected joints and sometimes to the kidneys. With proper treatment, most people with gout do not progress to this advanced stage.

When It's Not Gout, It May Be Pseudogout

Gout is sometimes confused with other forms of arthritis because the symptoms—acute and episodic attacks of joint warmth, pain, swelling, and stiffness—can be similar. One form of arthritis often confused with gout is called pseudogout. The pain, swelling, and redness of pseudogout can also come on suddenly and may be severe, closely resembling the symptoms of gout. However, the crystals that irritate the joint are calcium phosphate crystals, not uric acid. Therefore, pseudogout is treated somewhat differently and is not reviewed in this chapter.

Causes of Gout

A number of risk factors are associated with hyperuricemia and gout.

- **Genetics:** Twenty percent of people with gout have a family history of the disease.

- **Gender and age:** It is more common in men than in women and more common in adults than in children.

- **Weight:** Being overweight increases the risk of developing hyperuricemia and gout because there is more tissue available for turnover or breakdown, which leads to excess uric acid production.

- **Alcohol consumption:** Drinking too much alcohol can lead to hyperuricemia, because alcohol interferes with the removal of uric acid from the body.

- **Diet:** Eating too many foods that are rich in purines can cause or aggravate gout in some people.

- **Lead exposure:** In some cases, exposure to lead in the environment can cause gout.

- **Other health problems:** Renal insufficiency, or the inability of the kidneys to eliminate waste products, is a common cause of gout in older people. Other medical problems that contribute too high blood levels of uric acid include the following:

  - high blood pressure

  - hypothyroidism (underactive thyroid gland)

  - conditions that cause an excessively rapid turnover of cells, such as psoriasis, hemolytic anemia, or some cancers

  - Kelley-Seegmiller syndrome or Lesch-Nyhan syndrome—two rare conditions in which the enzyme that helps control uric acid levels either is not present or is found in insufficient quantities

- **Medications:** A number of medications may put people at risk for developing hyperuricemia and gout. They include the following:

  - diuretics, such as furosemide (Lasix), hydrochlorothiazide (Esidrix, Hydro-chlor), and metolazone (Diulo, Zaroxolyn)

  - salicylate-containing drugs, such as aspirin

  - niacin, a vitamin also known as nicotinic acid

  - cyclosporine (Sandimmune, Neoral), a medication that suppresses the body's immune system

  - levodopa (Larodopa), a medicine used to support communication along nerve pathways in the treatment of Parkinson disease

Gout Statistics

Gout occurs in 8.4 of every 1,000 people. It is rare in children and young adults. Men, particularly those between the ages of 40 and 50, are more likely to develop gout than women, who rarely develop the disorder before menopause. People who have had an organ transplant are more susceptible to gout.

Diagnosing Gout

Gout may be difficult for doctors to diagnose because the symptoms can be vague, and gout often mimics other conditions. Although most people with gout have hyperuricemia at some time during the course of their disease, it may not be present during an acute attack. In addition, having hyperuricemia alone does not mean that a person will get gout. In fact, most people with hyperuricemia do not develop the disease.

To confirm a diagnosis of gout, a doctor may insert a needle into an inflamed joint and draw a sample of synovial fluid, the substance that lubricates a joint. The joint fluid is placed on a slide and examined under a microscope for uric acid crystals. Their absence, however, does not completely rule out the diagnosis.

The doctor also may find it helpful to look for uric acid crystals around joints to diagnose gout. Gout attacks may mimic joint infections, and a doctor who suspects a joint infection (rather than gout) may also culture the joint fluid to see whether bacteria are present.

Treatments for Gout

With proper treatment, most people who have gout are able to control their symptoms and live productive lives. Gout can be treated with one or a combination of therapies. The goals of treatment are to ease the pain associated with acute attacks, to prevent future attacks, and to avoid the formation of tophi and kidney stones. Successful treatment can reduce discomfort caused by the symptoms of gout, as well as long-term damage to the affected joints. Treatment will help to prevent disability due to gout.

The most common treatments for an acute attack of gout are nonsteroidal anti-inflammatory drugs (NSAIDs) taken orally (by mouth), or corticosteroids which are taken orally or injected into the affected joint. NSAIDs reduce the inflammation caused by deposits of uric acid crystals, but have no effect on the amount of uric acid in the body. The NSAIDs most commonly prescribed for gout are indomethacin (Indocin) and naproxen (Anaprox, Naprosyn), which are taken orally every day. Corticosteroids are strong anti-inflammatory hormones. The most commonly prescribed corticosteroid is prednisone. Patients often begin to improve within a few hours of treatment with a corticosteroid, and the attack usually goes away completely within a week or so.

When NSAIDs or corticosteroids do not control symptoms, the doctor may consider using colchicine. This drug is most effective when taken within the first 12 hours of an acute attack. Doctors may ask patients to take oral colchicine as often as every hour until joint symptoms begin to improve or side effects such as nausea, vomiting, abdominal cramps, or diarrhea make it uncomfortable to continue the drug.

For some patients, the doctor may prescribe either NSAIDs or oral colchicine in small daily doses to prevent future attacks. The doctor also may consider prescribing medicine such as allopurinol (Zyloprim) or probenecid (Benemid) to treat hyperuricemia and reduce the frequency of sudden attacks and the development of tophi.

People who have other medical problems, such as high blood pressure or high blood triglycerides (fats), may find that the drugs they take for those conditions can also be useful for gout. Both losartan (Cozaar), a blood pressure medication, and fenofibrate (TriCor), a triglyceride-lowering drug, also help reduce blood levels of uric acid.

The doctor may also recommend losing weight, for those who are overweight; limiting alcohol consumption; and avoiding or limiting high-purine foods, which can increase uric acid levels.

Controlling Gout

Fortunately, gout can be controlled. People with gout can decrease the severity of attacks and reduce their risk of future attacks by taking their medications as prescribed. Acute gout is best controlled if medications are taken at the first sign of pain or inflammation. Other steps you can take to stay healthy and minimize gout's effect on your life include the following:

- Tell your doctor about all the medicines and vitamins you take. He or she can tell you if any of them increase your risk of hyperuricemia.

- Plan follow-up visits with your doctor to evaluate your progress.

- Drink plenty of nonalcoholic fluids, especially water. Nonalcoholic fluids help remove uric acid from the body. Alcohol, on the other hand, can raise the levels of uric acid in your blood.

- Exercise regularly and maintain a healthy body weight. Lose weight if you are overweight, but avoid low-carbohydrate diets that are designed for quick weight loss. When carbohydrate intake is insufficient, your body cannot completely burn its own fat. As a consequence, substances called ketones form and are released into the bloodstream, resulting in a condition called ketosis. After a short time, ketosis can increase the level of uric acid in your blood.

- Avoid foods that are high in purines including, anchovies, asparagus, beef kidneys, brains, dried beans and peas, game meats, gravy, herring, liver, mackerel, mushrooms, sardines, scallops, and sweetbreads.

Chapter 19

Gynecological Pain

Chapter Contents

Section 19.1

Menstrual Pain

Painful menstrual periods are marked by crampy lower abdominal pain. A woman may feel sharp pain that comes and goes, or have dull, aching pain. Painful menstrual periods may also cause back pain.

Considerations

Painful menstruation affects many women. For a small number of women, such discomfort makes it next to impossible to perform normal household, job, or school-related activities for a few days during each menstrual cycle. Painful menstruation is the leading cause of lost time from school and work among women in their teens and 20s.

The pain may begin several days before or just at the start of your period. It generally subsides as menstrual bleeding tapers off.

Although some pain during menstruation is normal, excessive pain is not. The medical term for excessively painful periods is dysmenorrhea.

There are two general types of dysmenorrhea:

- Primary dysmenorrhea refers to menstrual pain that occurs in otherwise healthy women. This type of pain is not related to any specific problems with the uterus or other pelvic organs.

- Secondary dysmenorrhea is menstrual pain that is attributed to some underlying disease or structural abnormality either within or outside the uterus.

Activity of the hormone prostaglandin, produced in the uterus, is thought to be a factor in primary dysmenorrhea. This hormone causes contraction of the uterus and levels tend to be much higher in women with severe menstrual pain than in women who experience mild or no menstrual pain.

Causes

- Premenstrual syndrome (PMS)
- Stress and anxiety
- Endometriosis
- Pelvic inflammatory disease
- Sexually transmitted diseases
- Fibroids
- Ovarian cysts
- Intrauterine Device (IUD)

Home Care

The following steps may allow you to avoid prescription medications:

- Apply a heating pad to your lower abdomen (below your belly-button). Be careful not to fall asleep with it on.
- Take warm showers or baths.
- Drink warm beverages.
- Do light circular massage with your fingertips around your lower abdomen.
- Walk or exercise regularly, including pelvic rocking exercises.
- Follow a diet rich in complex carbohydrates such as whole grains, fruits, and vegetables, but low in salt, sugar, alcohol, and caffeine.
- Eat light but frequent meals.
- Try over-the-counter anti-inflammatory medicine, such as ibuprofen.
- Practice relaxation techniques like meditation or yoga.
- Try vitamin B_6, calcium, and magnesium supplements, especially if your pain is from premenstrual syndrome (PMS).
- Keep your legs elevated while lying down. Or lie on your side with knees bent.

If these self-care measures do not work, your doctor may prescribe medications such as:

- Stronger anti-inflammatories like diclofenac (Cataflam)
- Antidepressants
- Birth control pills
- Antibiotics
- Stronger pain relievers (even narcotics such as codeine, for brief periods)

When to Contact a Medical Professional

Call your doctor right away if:

- You have a fever.
- Vaginal discharge is increased in amount or foul-smelling.
- Your pain is significant, your period is over one week late, and you have been sexually active.

Also call your doctor if:

- Your pain is severe or sudden.
- Self-care measures don't relieve your pain after three months.
- You pass blood clots or have other symptoms with the pain.
- Your pain occurs at times other than menstruation, begins more than five days prior to your period, or continues after your period is over.
- You have an intrauterine device (IUD) that was placed more than three months ago.

What to Expect at Your Office Visit

Your doctor will examine you, paying close attention to your pelvis and abdomen, and ask questions about your medical history and current symptoms, such as:

- How old were you when your periods started?
- Have they always been painful? If not, when did the pain begin?
- When in your menstrual cycle do you experience the pain?
- Is the pain sharp, dull, intermittent, constant, aching, or cramping?

- Are you sexually active?

- Do you use birth control? What type?

- When was your last menstrual period?

- Was the flow of your last menstrual period a normal amount for you?

- Do your periods tend to be heavy or prolonged (lasting longer than 5 days)?

- Have you passed blood clots?

- Are your periods generally regular and predictable?

- Do you use tampons with menstruation?

- What have you done to try to relieve the discomfort? How effective was it?

- Does anything make the pain worse?

- Do you have any other symptoms?

Diagnostic tests that may be performed include:

- Blood tests including complete blood count (CBC)

- Ultrasound

- Laparoscopy

- Cultures (may be taken to rule out sexually transmitted diseases such as gonorrhea, primary syphilis, or chlamydia infections)

Birth control pills may be prescribed to alleviate menstrual pain. If not needed for birth control, they may be discontinued after 6–12 months. Many women note continued freedom from symptoms despite stopping the medication.

Surgery may be necessary for women who are unable to obtain adequate pain relief or pain control. Procedures may range from removal of cysts, polyps, adhesions, or fibroids to complete hysterectomy in cases of extreme endometriosis.

Prescription medications may be used for endometriosis. For pain caused by an IUD, removal of the IUD and alternative birth control methods may be needed.

Antibiotics are necessary for pelvic inflammatory disease.

References

Mahutte NG. Medical management of endometriosis-associated pain. *Obstet Gynecol Clin North Am.* 2003; 30(1): 133–150.

French L. Dysmenorrhea. *Am Fam Physician.* 2005; 71(2): 285–291.

Rakel D. *Integrative Medicine. 1st edition.* Philadelphia, Pa: WB Saunders; 2003:385.

Section 19.2

Pelvic Pain from Uterine Fibroids, Endometriosis, or Vulvodynia

This chapter includes text from "Pelvic Pain," National Institute of Child Health and Human Development (NICHD), May 2007; and "The Vexing Pain of Vulvodynia," *NIH News in Health*, National Institutes of Health (NIH), November 2007.

Pelvic Pain

Pelvic pain is a general term that health care providers use to describe pain that occurs mostly or only in the lower abdomen area. It may be steady pain, or pain that comes and goes. In some cases the pain may be severe and might get in the way of daily activities. In other cases, the pain might be dull and occur only during the menstrual cycle. Pelvic pain also describes pain that occurs during sexual intercourse.

What conditions cause pelvic pain?

In general, pelvic pain signals that there might be a problem with one of the organs in your pelvic area: uterus, ovaries, fallopian tubes, cervix, vagina, urinary tract, lower intestines, or rectum. Or the pain might be a symptom of infection. Sometimes pelvic pain can be caused by muscular and skeletal problems.

There are some common health conditions that are often associated with pelvic pain.

- **Vulvodynia** is chronic pain or discomfort of the vulva (the external female genitalia). Vulvodynia can cause burning, stinging, irritation, or rawness of the vulva. The type of pain can be different for each woman. Pain may move around or always be in the same place. It can be constant, or come and go.

- **Endometriosis** occurs when tissues that usually line a woman's uterus instead grow outside the uterus. These tissues often grow on the surfaces of organs in the pelvis or abdomen, where they are not supposed to grow. The two most common symptoms of endometriosis are pain and infertility.

- **Uterine fibroids** are the most common, non-cancerous tumors in women of childbearing age. The fibroids are made of muscle cells and other tissues that grow within and around the wall of the uterus. Symptoms can include heavy or painful periods, pain during sex, and lower back pain, among others.

What is the treatment for pelvic pain?

It may be difficult to find the cause of your pelvic pain. Your health care provider will likely run a number of tests to find the cause of your pain. Treatment will depend on what is causing your pelvic pain, how intense the pain is, and how often the pain occurs.

Your health care provider may prescribe pain medication or antibiotics to treat the pain. For other conditions, treatment may be more involved, such as surgery for endometriosis.

Uterine Fibroids

Uterine fibroids are the most common, non-cancerous tumors in women of childbearing age. The fibroids are made of muscle cells and other tissues that grow within and around the wall of the uterus.

There are several risk factors for uterine fibroids:

- African American woman are at three- to five-times greater risk than white women for fibroids.

- Women who are overweight or obese for their height are at greater risk.

- Women who have given birth are a lower risk.

What are the symptoms of uterine fibroids?

Many women with uterine fibroids have no symptoms. Symptoms of uterine fibroids can include the following:

- Heavy or painful periods, or bleeding between periods
- Feeling full in the lower abdomen
- Urinating often
- Pain during sex
- Lower back pain
- Reproductive problems, such as infertility, multiple miscarriages, or early labor

Most women with fibroids do not have problems with fertility and can get pregnant. Some women with fibroids may not be able to get pregnant naturally. But advances in treatments for infertility may help some of these women get pregnant.

What are the treatments for fibroids?

If you have uterine fibroids, but show no symptoms, you many not need any treatment. Women who have pain and other symptoms might benefit from these treatments:

- Medications can offer relief from the symptoms of fibroids and even slow or stop their growth. But, once you stop taking the medicine, the fibroids often grow back.
- There are several types of fibroid surgery:
  - Myomectomy: Removes only the fibroids and leaves the healthy areas of the uterus in place.
  - Uterine artery embolization (UAE): Cuts off the blood supply to the uterus and fibroids, making them shrink.
  - Hysterectomy: A major procedure that removes the uterus; this type of surgery is the only sure way to cure fibroids.

Endometriosis

Endometriosis occurs when tissues that usually grow inside uterus instead grow on the outside. These tissues often grow on the surfaces of organs in the pelvis or abdomen, where they are not supposed to grow. Endometriosis is one of the most common gynecological diseases, affecting more than 5.5 million women in North America. An estimated 2%–10% of women of reproductive age have endometriosis, and about 30%–40% of women with endometriosis are infertile. It is one of the top three causes for female infertility.

What are the symptoms of endometriosis?

The two most common symptoms of endometriosis are pain and infertility. Symptoms can include the following:

- Pain before or after menstrual periods, as well as during or after sex
- Lower back, intestinal, or pelvic pain
- Heavy menstrual periods, or spotting and bleeding between periods
- Painful bowel movements or painful urination during menstrual periods
- Infertility

In most cases, the symptoms of endometriosis become milder after menopause because the growths begin to get smaller.

What are the treatments for endometriosis?

There is currently no cure for endometriosis. But a variety of treatment options exist, and there are ways to minimize the symptoms caused by the condition. There are several ways to treat the pain of endometriosis.

- Pain medication may be used to relieve symptoms.
- Hormone therapy may be used to control the growth of endometriosis.
- Surgery may be used to remove growths or control the size of very large endometriosis and to relieve pain.

Hormone treatments and surgery may help women who are unable to become pregnant. There are also other treatments for infertility associated with endometriosis.

The Vexing Pain of Vulvodynia: Giving Attention to a Private Problem

If you've never heard of the term vulvodynia, you're not alone. You're more likely to hear women refer to it as "the pain down there" or "feminine pain." Although an estimated 14 million American women may have it at one point in their lives, few people are aware that the condition has a name. Even health care providers may not be familiar with it. This can lead to multiple doctor visits and delayed diagnosis and treatment for some women.

Women with vulvodynia have lasting and unexplained pain in their genitals—specifically in the vulva, the outer area around the opening of the vagina. Vulvodynia can greatly interfere with a woman's life. It may feel uncomfortable to exercise, have sex, or take part in social activities. The most common symptom is a burning feeling. Women also report stabbing pain, stinging, or irritation. Symptoms are most common in women 18–25 years old. They're less likely to appear after age 35, although older women have also reported symptoms.

No one knows for sure what causes vulvodynia, in part because it hasn't been studied much in the past. Some researchers think it stems from irritation of the nerves around the vulva or an abnormal response to infection or injury. Medical researchers continue to investigate possible causes and treatments.

If you experience pain in the genital area, it's important to see your doctor and discuss your symptoms. Your health care provider should ask for your thorough medical history and give you a pelvic exam. The doctor may also conduct laboratory tests to rule out bacterial and fungal infections, which can have similar painful symptoms.

Although there is no cure for vulvodynia, some of its symptoms can be treated. Experts often recommend a combination of treatments. You and your health care provider should work together to develop a treatment strategy that reduces your pain and discomfort.

Treating Vulvodynia

Health care professionals may recommend several approaches for treating vulvodynia:

Lifestyle Changes

- Avoid using perfumed tampons and pads, bubble baths, soaps, sprays and douches that may irritate genital tissue.

132

- Use laundry detergent designed for sensitive skin.

- Rinse the vulva with cool to lukewarm water after urination and in the shower.

- Try wearing white, 100% cotton underwear and loose-fitting pants or skirts.

- For some women, it helps to eliminate highly acidic and sugary foods from the diet. Talk with your doctor before making dietary changes.

Medical Approaches

- Pain-relief cream, like lidocaine ointment, can be applied to the vulva.

- Oral medicines, especially different types of antidepressants, sometimes help with pain relief. Other medicines, like antiseizure drugs, are sometimes used for their pain-blocking properties, although they are not U.S. Food and Drug Administration (FDA)-approved for treating vulvodynia. Ask your doctor about various medications and their side effects.

- Physical therapy, including pelvic muscle exercises, may help prevent muscle spasms and pain.

- Complementary and alternative medical approaches—including acupuncture, hypnosis, massage therapy, relaxation techniques, and biofeedback—may help with long-lasting pain. Discuss these options with your health care provider.

Section 19.3

Dyspareunia: Painful Sexual Intercourse

What is dyspareunia?

Dyspareunia (say: "dis-par-oon-ya") is painful sexual intercourse for women. The pain can be in the genital area or deep inside the pelvis. The pain is often described as sharp, burning, or similar to menstrual cramps. It can have many causes. It is important to talk to your doctor if you have this problem because there are effective treatments for many of the causes.

What are some of the causes of dyspareunia?

Any part of the genitals can cause pain during sex. Some conditions affect the skin around the vagina. The pain from these conditions is usually felt when a tampon or penis is inserted into the vagina, but pain can also occur even when sitting or wearing pants. Inflammation or infection may be the cause (such as a yeast infection, urinary tract infection, or inflammation of the vagina). Injury to the vagina and the surrounding area can also cause pain. If a diaphragm or cervical cap (which are types of birth control) does not fit correctly, sex may also be painful. Vaginismus (say: "vag-in-is-mus") is a spasm of the muscles around the vagina. In some women, the pain of the spasms is so severe that penile penetration is impossible. Vaginal dryness can also cause painful sex. This dryness may be caused by menopause and changes in estrogen levels, or from a lack of foreplay before intercourse.

Pain during intercourse may feel like it is coming from deep in the pelvis. Women often report the feeling that "something is being bumped into." The uterus may hurt if there are fibroid growths, the uterus is tilted, or if the uterus prolapses (falls) into the vagina. Certain conditions or infections of the ovaries may also cause pain, especially in certain sexual positions. Past surgeries may leave scar tissue that can cause pain. Because the bladder and intestines are close to the vagina, they may also cause pain during sex. Endometriosis and pelvic inflammatory disease may also cause pain.

We know that the mind and the body work together. This is also seen with sexual problems. Often the problem that first caused the pain may go away, but you have learned to expect the pain. This can lead to further problems because you may be tense during sex or you may be unable to become aroused. The problem can then become a cycle and you are caught in the middle.

Negative attitudes about sex, misinformation about sex, and misinformation about the functions of the woman's body are often associated with some types of pain. Is painful sex all in your head? No. But it is important to discuss feelings and difficulties with your partner and your doctor.

How can my doctor tell what is causing my pain?

Your doctor may ask you to describe your pain, where it is located, and when it began. He or she may also ask you to describe what you have tried in the past. For example, have you tried a sexual lubricant or more foreplay? Is it painful every time you try to have sex? Are there other problems associated with sex? These are some of the questions that your doctor will need to discuss with you. Your doctor may want to examine your genital area or give you a pelvic exam.

What will the exam be like?

During the exam, your doctor may apply a cotton-tipped swab to the area to see if the area around the vagina is painful. A gentle exam of the vagina and cervix is done with a speculum, similar to the way you get a Pap smear. For some women, this part of the exam may be painful. Your doctor may use a smaller speculum to decrease the discomfort. Or, your doctor may delay the exam until the pain has decreased.

It is important to let your doctor know if the exam becomes too painful. Discuss this with your doctor ahead of time. Many women find it useful to hold a mirror during the exam to see the appearance of their genital structures.

During the final part of the exam, your doctor will feel your uterus and ovaries with one hand on the abdomen and one finger in your vagina. This is similar to exams performed during a pelvic exam.

Will I need any tests?

If your symptoms and exam suggest an infection, tests may be needed done to check for yeast or bacteria. If there is no infection, your doctor may do some other tests, such as urine or allergy tests.

Where can I turn for help?

Discuss your symptoms with your doctor. Depending on the situation, you may need to see a doctor who specializes in women's problems. Various support groups are also available.

Chapter 20

Headache

What hurts when you have a headache? The bones of the skull and tissues of the brain itself never hurt, because they lack pain-sensitive nerve fibers. Several areas of the head can hurt, including a network of nerves which extends over the scalp and certain nerves in the face, mouth, and throat. Also sensitive to pain, because they contain delicate nerve fibers, are the muscles of the head and blood vessels found along the surface and at the base of the brain.

The ends of these pain-sensitive nerves, called nociceptors, can be stimulated by stress, muscular tension, dilated blood vessels, and other triggers of headache. Once stimulated, a nociceptor sends a message up the length of the nerve fiber to the nerve cells in the brain, signaling that a part of the body hurts. The message is determined by the location of the nociceptor. A person who suddenly realizes "My toe hurts," is responding to nociceptors in the foot that have been stimulated by the stubbing of a toe.

A number of chemicals help transmit pain-related information to the brain. Some of these chemicals are natural painkilling proteins called endorphins, Greek for "the morphine within." One theory suggests that people who suffer from severe headache and other types of chronic pain have lower levels of endorphins than people who are generally pain free.

Excerpted from "Headache: Hope Through Research," National Institute of Neurological Disorders and Stroke (NINDS), NIH Publication No. 02–158, updated January 10, 2008. The full text of this document is available at http://www.ninds.nih.gov/disorders/headache/detail_headache.htm.

When should you see a physician?

Not all headaches require medical attention. Some result from missed meals or occasional muscle tension and are easily remedied. But some types of headache are signals of more serious disorders, and call for prompt medical care. These include the following:

- Sudden, severe headache

- Sudden, severe headache associated with a stiff neck

- Headache associated with fever

- Headache associated with convulsions

- Headache accompanied by confusion or loss of consciousness

- Headache following a blow on the head

- Headache associated with pain in the eye or ear

- Persistent headache in a person who was previously headache free

- Recurring headache in children

- Headache which interferes with normal life

A headache sufferer usually seeks help from a family practitioner. If the problem is not relieved by standard treatments, the patient may then be referred to a specialist—perhaps an internist or neurologist. Additional referrals may be made to psychologists.

What tests are used to diagnose headache?

Diagnosing a headache is like playing *Twenty Questions*. Experts agree that a detailed question-and-answer session with a patient can often produce enough information for a diagnosis. Many types of headaches have clear-cut symptoms which fall into an easily recognizable pattern.

Patients may be asked: How often do you have headaches? Where is the pain? How long do the headaches last? When did you first develop headaches? The patient's sleep habits and family and work situations may also be probed.

Most physicians will also obtain a full medical history from the patient, inquiring about past head trauma or surgery, eye strain, sinus problems, dental problems, difficulties with opening and closing of the jaw, and the use of medications. This may be enough to suggest strongly that the patient has migraine or cluster headaches. A complete and careful physical and neurological examination will exclude many possibilities and the suspicion of aneurysm, meningitis, or certain brain tumors. A blood test may be ordered to screen for thyroid disease, anemia, or infections which might cause a headache.

A test called an electroencephalogram (EEG) may be given to measure brain activity. EEG's can indicate a malfunction in the brain, but they cannot usually pinpoint a problem that might be causing a headache. A physician may suggest that a patient with unusual headaches undergo a computed tomographic (CT) scan and/or a magnetic resonance imaging (MRI) scan. The scans enable the physician to distinguish, for example, between a bleeding blood vessel in the brain and a brain tumor, and are important diagnostic tools in cases of headache associated with brain lesions or other serious disease. CT scans produce x-ray images of the brain that show structures or variations in the density of different types of tissue. MRI scans use magnetic fields and radio waves to produce an image that provides information about the structure and biochemistry of the brain.

If an aneurysm—an abnormal ballooning of a blood vessel—is suspected, a physician may order a CT scan to examine for blood and then an angiogram. In this test, a special fluid which can be seen on an x-ray is injected into the patient and carried in the bloodstream to the brain to reveal any abnormalities in the blood vessels there.

A physician analyzes the results of all these diagnostic tests along with a patient's medical history and examination in order to arrive at a diagnosis.

Headaches are diagnosed as

- vascular,
- muscle contraction (tension),
- traction, or
- inflammatory.

Vascular headaches—a group that includes the well-known migraine—are so named because they are thought to involve abnormal function of the brain's blood vessels or vascular system. Muscle contraction headaches appear to involve the tightening or tensing of facial and neck muscles. Traction and inflammatory headaches are symptoms of other disorders, ranging from stroke to sinus infection. Some people have more than one type of headache.

Migraine Headaches

The most common type of vascular headache is migraine. Migraine headaches are usually characterized by severe pain on one or both sides of the head, an upset stomach, and at times disturbed vision.

Symptoms of Migraine

Sensitivity to light is a standard symptom of the two most prevalent types of migraine-caused headache—classic and common. The major difference between the two types is the appearance of neurological symptoms 10–30 minutes before a classic migraine attack. These symptoms are called an aura. The person may see flashing lights or zigzag lines, or may temporarily lose vision. Other classic symptoms include speech difficulty, weakness of an arm or leg, tingling of the face or hands, and confusion.

The pain of a classic migraine headache may be described as intense, throbbing, or pounding and is felt in the forehead, temple, ear, jaw, or around the eye. Classic migraine starts on one side of the head but may eventually spread to the other side. An attack lasts 1–2 pain-wracked days.

Common migraine—a term that reflects the disorder's greater occurrence in the general population—is not preceded by an aura. But some people experience a variety of vague symptoms beforehand, including mental fuzziness, mood changes, fatigue, and unusual retention of fluids. During the headache phase of a common migraine, a person may have diarrhea and increased urination, as well as nausea and vomiting. Common migraine pain can last three or four days.

Both classic and common migraine can strike as often as several times a week, or as rarely as once every few years. Both types can occur at any time. Some people, however, experience migraines at predictable times—for example, near the days of menstruation or every Saturday morning after a stressful week of work.

The Migraine Process

Research scientists are unclear about the precise cause of migraine headaches. There seems to be general agreement, however, that a key element is blood flow changes in the brain. People who get migraine headaches appear to have blood vessels that overreact to various triggers.

Women and Migraine

Although both males and females seem to be equally affected by migraine, the condition is more common in adult women. Both sexes may develop migraine in infancy, but most often the disorder begins between the ages of five and thirty-five.

The relationship between female hormones and migraine is still unclear. Women may have "menstrual migraine"—headaches around the time of their menstrual period—which may disappear during pregnancy. Other women develop migraine for the first time when they are pregnant. Some are first affected after menopause.

The effect of oral contraceptives on headaches is perplexing. Scientists report that some women with migraine who take birth control pills experience more frequent and severe attacks. However, a small percentage of women have fewer and less severe migraine headaches when they take birth control pills. And normal women who do not suffer from headaches may develop migraines as a side effect when they use oral contraceptives. Investigators around the world are studying hormonal changes in women with migraine in the hope of identifying the specific ways these naturally occurring chemicals cause headaches.

Triggers of Headache

Although many sufferers have a family history of migraine, the exact hereditary nature of this condition is still unknown. People who get migraines are thought to have an inherited abnormality in the regulation of blood vessels.

"It's like a cocked gun with a hair trigger," explains one specialist. "A person is born with a potential for migraine and the headache is triggered by things that are really not so terrible."

These triggers include stress and other normal emotions, as well as biological and environmental conditions. Fatigue, glaring or flickering lights, changes in the weather, and certain foods can set off migraine. It may seem hard to believe that eating such seemingly harmless foods as yogurt, nuts, and lima beans can result in a painful migraine headache. However, some scientists believe that these foods and several others contain chemical substances, such as tyramine, which constrict arteries—the first step of the migraine process. Other scientists believe that foods cause headaches by setting off an allergic reaction in susceptible people.

While a food-triggered migraine usually occurs soon after eating, other triggers may not cause immediate pain. Scientists report that people can develop migraine not only during a period of stress but also afterwards when their vascular systems are still reacting. For example, migraines that wake people up in the middle of the night are believed to result from a delayed reaction to stress.

Other Forms of Migraine

In addition to classic and common, migraine headache can take several other forms.

Hemiplegic migraine: Patients with hemiplegic migraine have temporary paralysis on one side of the body, a condition known as hemiplegia. Some people may experience vision problems and vertigo—a feeling that the world is spinning. These symptoms begin ten to ninety minutes before the onset of headache pain.

Ophthalmoplegic migraine: In ophthalmoplegic migraine, the pain is around the eye and is associated with a droopy eyelid, double vision, and other problems with vision.

Basilar artery migraine: Involves a disturbance of a major brain artery at the base of the brain. Pre-headache symptoms include vertigo, double vision, and poor muscular coordination. This type of migraine occurs primarily in adolescent and young adult women and is often associated with the menstrual cycle.

Benign exertional headache: Brought on by running, lifting, coughing, sneezing, or bending. The headache begins at the onset of activity, and pain rarely lasts more than several minutes.

Status migrainous: A rare and severe type of migraine that can last 72 hours or longer. The pain and nausea are so intense that people who have this type of headache must be hospitalized. The use of certain drugs can trigger status migrainous. Neurologists report that many of their status migrainous patients were depressed and anxious before they experienced headache attacks.

Headache-free migraine: Characterized by such migraine symptoms as visual problems, nausea, vomiting, constipation, or diarrhea. Patients, however, do not experience head pain. Headache specialists have suggested that unexplained pain in a particular part of the body, fever, and dizziness could also be possible types of headache-free migraine.

Treatment for Migraine Headache

Drug therapy, biofeedback training, stress reduction, and elimination of certain foods from the diet are the most common methods of preventing and controlling migraine and other vascular headaches. Regular exercise, such as swimming or vigorous walking, can also reduce the frequency and severity of migraine headaches. During a migraine headache, temporary relief can sometimes be obtained by applying cold packs to the head or by pressing on the bulging artery found in front of the ear on the painful side of the head.

Drug Therapy

There are two ways to approach the treatment of migraine headache with drugs: prevent the attacks, or relieve symptoms after the headache occurs.

For infrequent migraine, drugs can be taken at the first sign of a headache in order to stop it or to at least ease the pain. People who get occasional mild migraine may benefit by taking aspirin or acetaminophen at the start of an attack. Aspirin raises a person's tolerance to pain and also discourages clumping of blood platelets. Small amounts of caffeine may be useful if taken in the early stages of migraine. But for most migraine sufferers who get moderate to severe headaches, and for all cluster headache patients, stronger drugs may be necessary to control the pain.

Several drugs for the prevention of migraine have been developed in recent years, including serotonin agonists which mimic the action of this key brain chemical. One of the most commonly used drugs for the relief of classic and common migraine symptoms is sumatriptan, which binds to serotonin receptors. For optimal benefit, the drug is taken during the early stages of an attack. If a migraine has been in progress for about an hour after the drug is taken, a repeat dose can be given.

Physicians caution that sumatriptan should not be taken by people who have angina pectoris, basilar migraine, severe hypertension, or vascular, or liver disease.

Another migraine drug is ergotamine tartrate, a vasoconstrictor which helps counteract the painful dilation stage of the headache. Other drugs that constrict dilated blood vessels or help reduce blood vessel inflammation also are available.

For headaches that occur three or more times a month, preventive treatment is usually recommended. Drugs used to prevent classic and common migraine include methysergide maleate, which counteracts blood vessel constriction; propranolol hydrochloride, which stops blood vessel dilation; amitriptyline, an antidepressant; valproic acid, an anticonvulsant; and verapamil, a calcium channel blocker.

Antidepressants called monoamine oxidase (MAO) inhibitors also prevent migraine. These drugs block an enzyme called monoamine oxidase which normally helps nerve cells absorb the artery-constricting brain chemical, serotonin. MAO inhibitors can have potentially serious side effects—particularly if taken while ingesting foods or beverages that contain tyramine, a substance that constricts arteries.

Many antimigraine drugs can have adverse side effects. But like most medicines they are relatively safe when used carefully and under a physician's supervision. To avoid long-term side effects of preventive medications, headache specialists advise patients to reduce the dosage of these drugs and then stop taking them as soon as possible.

Biofeedback and Relaxation Training

Drug therapy for migraine is often combined with biofeedback and relaxation training. Biofeedback refers to a technique that can give people better control over such body function indicators as blood pressure, heart rate, temperature, muscle tension, and brain waves. Thermal biofeedback allows a patient to consciously raise hand temperature. Some patients who are able to increase hand temperature can reduce the number and intensity of migraines. The mechanisms underlying these self-regulation treatments are being studied by research scientists.

In another type of biofeedback called electromyographic or EMG training, the patient learns to control muscle tension in the face, neck, and shoulders. Either kind of biofeedback may be combined with relaxation training, during which patients learn to relax the mind and body.

Biofeedback can be practiced at home with a portable monitor. But the ultimate goal of treatment is to wean the patient from the machine. The patient can then use biofeedback anywhere at the first sign of a headache.

The Antimigraine Diet

Scientists estimate that a small percentage of migraine sufferers will benefit from a treatment program focused solely on eliminating headache-provoking foods and beverages.

Other migraine patients may be helped by a diet to prevent low blood sugar. Low blood sugar, or hypoglycemia, can cause headache.

This condition can occur after a period without food, for example, overnight or when a meal is skipped. People who wake up in the morning with a headache may be reacting to the low blood sugar caused by the lack of food overnight.

Treatment for headaches caused by low blood sugar consists of scheduling smaller, more frequent meals for the patient. A special diet designed to stabilize the body's sugar-regulating system is sometimes recommended. For the same reason, many specialists also recommend that migraine patients avoid oversleeping on weekends. Sleeping late can change the body's normal blood sugar level and lead to a headache.

Other Types of Vascular Headaches besides Migraine

After migraine, the most common type of vascular headache is the toxic headache produced by fever. Pneumonia, measles, mumps, and tonsillitis are among the diseases that can cause severe toxic vascular headaches. Toxic headaches can also result from the presence of foreign chemicals in the body. Other kinds of vascular headaches include "clusters," which cause repeated episodes of intense pain, and headaches resulting from a rise in blood pressure.

Chemical Culprits

Repeated exposure to nitrite compounds can result in a dull, pounding headache that may be accompanied by a flushed face. Nitrite, which dilates blood vessels, is found in such products as heart medicine and dynamite, but is also used as a chemical to preserve meat. Hot dogs and other processed meats containing sodium nitrite can cause headaches.

Eating foods prepared with monosodium glutamate (MSG) can result in headache. Soy sauce, meat tenderizer, and a variety of packaged foods contain this chemical which is touted as a flavor enhancer.

Headache can also result from exposure to poisons, even common household varieties like insecticides, carbon tetrachloride, and lead. Children who ingest flakes of lead paint may develop headaches. So may anyone who has contact with lead batteries or lead-glazed pottery.

Artists and industrial workers may experience headaches after exposure to materials that contain chemical solvents. These solvents, like benzene, are found in turpentine, spray adhesives, rubber cement, and inks.

Drugs such as amphetamines can cause headaches as a side effect. Another type of drug-related headache occurs during withdrawal from long-term therapy with the antimigraine drug ergotamine tartrate.

Jokes are often made about alcohol hangovers but the headache associated with "the morning after" is no laughing matter. Fortunately, there are several suggested treatments for the pain. The hangover headache may also be reduced by taking honey, which speeds alcohol metabolism, or caffeine, a constrictor of dilated arteries. Caffeine, however, can cause headaches as well as cure them. Heavy coffee drinkers often get headaches when they try to break the caffeine habit.

Cluster Headaches

Cluster headaches are a rare form of headache notable for their extreme pain and their pattern of occurring in clusters, usually at the same time(s) of the day for several weeks. A cluster headache usually begins suddenly with excruciating pain on one side of the head, often behind or around one eye. In some individuals, it may be preceded by a migraine-like aura. The pain usually peaks over the next 5–10 minutes, and then continues at that intensity for up to an hour or two before going away.

People with cluster headaches describe the pain as piercing and unbearable. The nose and the eye on the affected side of the face may also get red, swollen, and runny, and some people will experience nausea, restlessness and agitation, or sensitivities to light, sound, or smell. Most affected individuals have one to three cluster headaches a day and two cluster periods a year, separated by periods of freedom from symptoms. Alcohol (especially red wine) provokes attacks in more than half of those with cluster headaches, but has no effect once the cluster period ends. Cluster headaches are also strongly associated with cigarette smoking.

There are medications available to lessen the pain of a cluster headache and suppress future attacks. Oxygen inhalation and triptan drugs (such as those used to treat migraine) administered as a tablet, nasal spray, or injection can provide quick relief from acute cluster headache pain. Lidocaine nasal spray, which numbs the nose and nostrils, may also be effective. Ergotamine and corticosteroids such as prednisone and dexamethasone may be prescribed to break the cluster cycle and then tapered off once headaches end. Verapamil may be used preventively to decrease the frequency and pain level of attacks. Lithium, valproic acid, and topiramate are sometimes also used preventively.

Painful Pressure

Chronic high blood pressure can cause headache, as can rapid rises in blood pressure like those experienced during anger, vigorous exercise, or sexual excitement. The severe orgasmic headache occurs right before orgasm and is believed to be a vascular headache. Since sudden rupture of a cerebral blood vessel can occur, this type of headache should be evaluated by a doctor.

Muscle-Contraction Headaches

Tension headache is named not only for the role of stress in triggering the pain, but also for the contraction of neck, face, and scalp muscles brought on by stressful events. Tension headache is a severe but temporary form of muscle-contraction headache. The pain is mild to moderate and feels like pressure is being applied to the head or neck. The headache usually disappears after the period of stress is over. Ninety percent of all headaches are classified as tension or muscle contraction headaches.

By contrast, chronic muscle-contraction headaches can last for weeks, months, and sometimes years. The pain of these headaches is often described as a tight band around the head or a feeling that the head and neck are in a cast. The pain is steady, and is usually felt on both sides of the head. Chronic muscle-contraction headaches can cause sore scalps—even combing one's hair can be painful.

Occasionally, muscle-contraction headaches will be accompanied by nausea, vomiting, and blurred vision, but there is no pre-headache syndrome as with migraine. Muscle-contraction headaches have not been linked to hormones or foods, nor is there a strong hereditary connection.

Research has shown that for many people, chronic muscle-contraction headaches are caused by depression and anxiety. These people tend to get their headaches in the early morning or evening when conflicts in the office or home are anticipated.

Emotional factors are not the only triggers of muscle-contraction headaches. Certain physical postures that tense head and neck muscles—such as holding one's chin down while reading—can lead to head and neck pain. So can prolonged writing under poor light, or holding a phone between the shoulder and ear, or even gum-chewing.

More serious problems that can cause muscle-contraction headaches include degenerative arthritis of the neck and temporomandibular joint dysfunction (TMD). TMD is a disorder of the joint between the temporal bone (above the ear) and the mandible or lower jaw bone. The disorder results from poor bite and jaw clenching.

Treatment for muscle-contraction headache varies. The first consideration is to treat any specific disorder or disease that may be causing the headache. For example, arthritis of the neck is treated with anti-inflammatory medication and TMD may be helped by corrective devices for the mouth and jaw.

Acute tension headaches not associated with a disease are treated with analgesics like aspirin and acetaminophen. Stronger analgesics, such as propoxyphene and codeine, are sometimes prescribed. As prolonged use of these drugs can lead to dependence, patients taking them should have periodic medical checkups and follow their physicians' instructions carefully.

Nondrug therapy for chronic muscle-contraction headaches includes biofeedback, relaxation training, and counseling. A technique called cognitive restructuring teaches people to change their attitudes and responses to stress. Patients might be encouraged, for example, to imagine that they are coping successfully with a stressful situation. In progressive relaxation therapy, patients are taught to first tense and then relax individual muscle groups. Finally, the patient tries to relax his or her whole body. Many people imagine a peaceful scene—such as lying on the beach or by a beautiful lake. Passive relaxation does not involve tensing of muscles. Instead, patients are encouraged to focus on different muscles, suggesting that they relax.

People with chronic muscle-contraction headaches may also be helped by taking antidepressants or MAO inhibitors. Mixed muscle-contraction and migraine headaches are sometimes treated with barbiturate compounds which slow down nerve function in the brain and spinal cord.

People who suffer infrequent muscle-contraction headaches may benefit from a hot shower or moist heat applied to the back of the neck. Cervical collars are sometimes recommended as an aid to good posture. Physical therapy, massage, and gentle exercise of the neck may also be helpful.

Headache as Warning of a More Serious Condition

Like other types of pain, headaches can serve as warning signals of more serious disorders. This is particularly true for headaches caused by traction or inflammation. Traction headaches can occur if the pain-sensitive parts of the head are pulled, stretched, or displaced, as, for example, when eye muscles are tensed to compensate for eyestrain.

Headaches caused by inflammation include those related to meningitis as well as those resulting from diseases of the sinuses, spine, neck, ears, and teeth. Ear and tooth infections and glaucoma can cause headaches. In oral and dental disorders, headache is experienced as pain in the entire head, including the face. These headaches are treated by curing the underlying problem. This may involve surgery, antibiotics, or other drugs.

Characteristics of the various types of more serious traction and inflammatory headaches vary by disorder:

- **Brain tumor:** As they grow, brain tumors sometimes cause headache by pushing on the outer layer of nerve tissue that covers the brain or by pressing against pain-sensitive blood vessel walls. Headache resulting from a brain tumor may be periodic or continuous. Typically, it feels like a strong pressure is being applied to the head. The pain is relieved when the tumor is treated by surgery, radiation, or chemotherapy.

- **Stroke:** Headache may accompany several conditions that can lead to stroke, including hypertension or high blood pressure, arteriosclerosis, and heart disease. Headaches are also associated with completed stroke, when brain cells die from lack of sufficient oxygen. Many stroke-related headaches can be prevented by careful management of the patient's condition through diet, exercise, and medication. Mild to moderate headaches are associated with transient ischemic attacks (TIA), sometimes called mini-strokes, which result from a temporary lack of blood supply to the brain. The head pain occurs near the clot or lesion that blocks blood flow. The similarity between migraine and symptoms of TIA can cause problems in diagnosis. The rare person under age 40 who suffers a TIA may be misdiagnosed as having migraine; similarly, TIA-prone older patients who suffer migraine may be misdiagnosed as having stroke-related headaches.

- **Spinal tap:** About one-fourth of the people who undergo a lumbar puncture or spinal tap develop a headache. Since headache pain occurs only when the patient stands up, the cure is to remain lying down until the headache runs its course—anywhere from a few hours to several days.

- **Head trauma:** Headaches may develop after a blow to the head, either immediately or months later. There is little relationship between the severity of the trauma and the intensity of headache pain. In most cases, the cause of the headache is not known. Occasionally the cause is ruptured blood vessels which result in an accumulation of blood called a hematoma. This mass of blood can displace brain tissue and cause headaches as well as weakness, confusion, memory loss, and seizures. Hematomas can be drained to produce rapid relief of symptoms.

- **Temporal arteritis:** Arteritis, an inflammation of certain arteries in the head, primarily affects people over age 50. Symptoms include throbbing headache, fever, and loss of appetite. Some patients experience blurring or loss of vision. Prompt treatment with corticosteroid drugs helps to relieve symptoms.

- **Meningitis and encephalitis:** Meningitis and encephalitis headaches are caused by infections of meninges—the brain's outer covering—and in encephalitis, inflammation of the brain itself.

- **Trigeminal neuralgia:** Trigeminal neuralgia, or tic douloureux, results from a disorder of the trigeminal nerve. This nerve supplies the face, teeth, mouth, and nasal cavity with feeling and also enables the mouth muscles to chew. Symptoms are headache and intense facial pain that comes in short, excruciating jabs set off by the slightest touch to or movement of trigger points in the face or mouth. Many trigeminal neuralgia patients are controlled with drugs, including carbamazepine. Patients who do not respond to drugs may be helped by surgery on the trigeminal nerve.

- **Sinus infection:** In a condition called acute sinusitis, a viral or bacterial infection of the upper respiratory tract spreads to the membrane which lines the sinus cavities. When one or more of these cavities are filled with fluid from the inflammation, they become painful. Treatment of acute sinusitis includes antibiotics, analgesics, and decongestants. Chronic sinusitis may be caused by an allergy to such irritants as dust, ragweed, animal hair, and smoke. Research scientists disagree about whether chronic sinusitis triggers headache.

Causes of Headache in Children

Like adults, children experience the infections, trauma, and stresses that can lead to headaches. In fact, research shows that as young people enter adolescence and encounter the stresses of puberty and secondary school, the frequency of headache increases. Migraine headaches often begin in childhood or adolescence. According to recent surveys, as many as half of all schoolchildren experience some type of headache.

150

Children with migraine often have nausea and excessive vomiting. Some children have periodic vomiting, but no headache—the so-called abdominal migraine. Research scientists have found that these children usually develop headaches when they are older.

Physicians have many drugs to treat migraine in children. Different classes that may be tried include analgesics, antiemetics, anticonvulsants, beta-blockers, and sedatives. A diet may also be prescribed to protect the child from foods that trigger headache. Sometimes psychological counseling or even psychiatric treatment for the child and the parents is recommended.

Childhood headache can be a sign of depression. Parents should alert the family pediatrician if a child develops headaches along with other symptoms such as a change in mood or sleep habits. Antidepressant medication and psychotherapy are effective treatments for childhood depression and related headache.

Conclusion

If you suffer from headaches and none of the standard treatments help, do not despair. Some people find that their headaches disappear once they deal with a troubled marriage, pass their certifying board exams, or resolve some other stressful problem. Others find that if they control their psychological reaction to stress, the headaches disappear.

For those who get headaches anyway, today's headache research offers hope. The work of NINDS-supported scientists around the world promises to improve the understanding of this complex disorder and provide better tools to treat it.

Chapter 21

Heartburn, Gastroesophageal Reflux (GER), and Gastroesophageal Reflux Disease (GERD)

Gastroesophageal Reflux Disease (GERD)

Gastroesophageal reflux disease (GERD) is a more serious form of gastroesophageal reflux (GER), which is common. GER occurs when the lower esophageal sphincter (LES) opens spontaneously, for varying periods of time, or does not close properly and stomach contents rise up into the esophagus. GER is also called acid reflux or acid regurgitation, because digestive juices—called acids—rise up with the food. The esophagus is the tube that carries food from the mouth to the stomach. The LES is a ring of muscle at the bottom of the esophagus that acts like a valve between the esophagus and stomach.

When acid reflux occurs, food or fluid can be tasted in the back of the mouth. When refluxed stomach acid touches the lining of the esophagus, it may cause a burning sensation in the chest or throat called heartburn or acid indigestion. Occasional GER is common and does not necessarily mean one has GERD. Persistent reflux that occurs more than twice a week is considered GERD, and it can eventually lead to more serious health problems. People of all ages can have GERD.

Excerpted from "Heartburn, Gastroesophageal Reflux (GER), and Gastroesophageal Reflux Disease (GERD)," National Institute of Diabetes and Digestive and Kidney Diseases (NIDDK), NIH Publication No. 07–0882, May 2007. The full text of this document is available at http://digestive.niddk.nih.gov/ddiseases/pubs/gerd.

Symptoms of GERD

The main symptom of GERD in adults is frequent heartburn, also called acid indigestion—burning-type pain in the lower part of the mid-chest, behind the breast bone, and in the mid-abdomen. Most children under 12 years with GERD, and some adults, have GERD without heartburn. Instead, they may experience a dry cough, asthma symptoms, or trouble swallowing.

Causes of GERD

The reason some people develop GERD is still unclear. However, research shows that in people with GERD, the LES relaxes while the rest of the esophagus is working. Anatomical abnormalities such as a hiatal hernia may also contribute to GERD. A hiatal hernia occurs when the upper part of the stomach and the LES move above the diaphragm, the muscle wall that separates the stomach from the chest. Normally, the diaphragm helps the LES keep acid from rising up into the esophagus. When a hiatal hernia is present, acid reflux can occur more easily. A hiatal hernia can occur in people of any age and is most often a normal finding in otherwise healthy people over age 50. Most of the time, a hiatal hernia produces no symptoms.

Other factors that may contribute to GERD include obesity, pregnancy, and smoking.

Common foods that can worsen reflux symptoms include the following:

- citrus fruits
- chocolate
- drinks with caffeine or alcohol
- fatty and fried foods
- garlic and onions
- mint flavorings
- spicy foods
- tomato-based foods, like spaghetti sauce, salsa, chili, and pizza

GERD in Children

Distinguishing between normal, physiologic reflux and GERD in children is important. Most infants with GER are happy and healthy even if they frequently spit up or vomit, and babies usually outgrow GER by their first birthday. Reflux that continues past one year of age may be GERD. Studies show GERD is common and may be overlooked in infants and children. For example, GERD can present as repeated regurgitation, nausea, heartburn, coughing, laryngitis, or respiratory problems like wheezing, asthma, or pneumonia. Infants and young children may demonstrate irritability or arching of the back, often during or immediately after feedings. Infants with GERD may refuse to feed and experience poor growth.

Talk with your child's health care provider if reflux-related symptoms occur regularly and cause your child discomfort. Your health care provider may recommend simple strategies for avoiding reflux, such as burping the infant several times during feeding or keeping the infant in an upright position for 30 minutes after feeding. If your child is older, your health care provider may recommend that your child eat small, frequent meals and avoid the following foods:

- sodas that contain caffeine
- chocolate
- peppermint
- spicy foods
- acidic foods like oranges, tomatoes, and pizza
- fried and fatty foods

Avoiding food 2–3 hours before bedtime may also help. Your health care provider may recommend raising the head of your child's bed with wood blocks secured under the bedposts. Just using extra pillows will not help. If these changes do not work, your health care provider may prescribe medicine for your child. In rare cases, a child may need surgery.

Treatment for GERD

See your health care provider if you have had symptoms of GERD and have been using antacids or other over-the-counter reflux medications for more than two weeks. Your health care provider may refer you to a gastroenterologist, a doctor who treats diseases of the stomach and intestines. Depending on the severity of your GERD, treatment may involve one or more of the following lifestyle changes, medications, or surgery.

Lifestyle Changes

- If you smoke, stop.

- Avoid foods and beverages that worsen symptoms.

- Lose weight if needed.

- Eat small, frequent meals.

- Wear loose-fitting clothes.

- Avoid lying down for three hours after a meal.

- Raise the head of your bed 6–8 inches by securing wood blocks under the bedposts. Just using extra pillows will not help.

Medications

Your health care provider may recommend over-the-counter antacids or medications that stop acid production or help the muscles that empty your stomach. You can buy many of these medications without a prescription. However, see your health care provider before starting or adding a medication.

- **Antacids,** such as Alka-Seltzer, Maalox, Mylanta, Rolaids, and Riopan, are usually the first drugs recommended to relieve heartburn and other mild GERD symptoms. Antacids, however, can have side effects including diarrhea or constipation.

- **Foaming agents,** such as Gaviscon, work by covering your stomach contents with foam to prevent reflux.

- **H2 blockers,** such as cimetidine (Tagamet HB), famotidine (Pepcid AC), nizatidine (Axid AR), and ranitidine (Zantac 75), decrease acid production. They are available in prescription strength and over-the-counter strength. These drugs provide short-term relief and are effective for about half of those who have GERD symptoms.

- **Proton pump inhibitors** include omeprazole (Prilosec, Zegerid), lansoprazole (Prevacid), pantoprazole (Protonix), rabeprazole (AcipHex), and esomeprazole (Nexium), which are available by prescription. Prilosec is also available in over-the-counter strength. Proton pump inhibitors are more effective than H2 blockers and can relieve symptoms and heal the esophageal lining in almost everyone who has GERD.

- **Prokinetics** help strengthen the LES and make the stomach empty faster. This group includes bethanechol (Urecholine) and metoclopramide (Reglan). Metoclopramide also improves muscle action in the digestive tract. Prokinetics have frequent side effects that limit their usefulness—fatigue, sleepiness, depression, anxiety, and problems with physical movement.

Because drugs work in different ways, combinations of medications may help control symptoms. People who get heartburn after eating may take both antacids and H2 blockers. Your health care provider is the best source of information about how to use medications for GERD.

What if GERD symptoms persist?

If your symptoms do not improve with lifestyle changes or medications, you may need additional tests.

- **Barium swallow radiograph** uses x-rays to help spot abnormalities such as a hiatal hernia and other structural or anatomical problems of the esophagus. With this test, you drink a solution and then x-rays are taken. The test will not detect mild irritation, although strictures—narrowing of the esophagus—and ulcers can be observed.

- **Upper endoscopy** is more accurate than a barium swallow radiograph and may be performed in a hospital or a doctor's office. The doctor may spray your throat to numb it and then, after lightly sedating you, will slide a thin, flexible plastic tube with a light and lens on the end called an endoscope down your throat. Acting as a tiny camera, the endoscope allows the doctor to see the surface of the esophagus and search for abnormalities. If you have had moderate to severe symptoms and this procedure reveals injury to the esophagus, usually no other tests are needed to confirm GERD. The doctor also may perform a biopsy to remove small pieces of tissue from your esophagus. The tissue is then viewed with a microscope to look for damage caused by acid reflux and to rule out other problems if infection or abnormal growths are not found.

- **pH monitoring examination** involves the doctor either inserting a small tube into the esophagus or clipping a tiny device to the esophagus that will stay there for 24 to 48 hours. While you go about your normal activities, the device measures when and how much acid comes up into your esophagus. This test can be useful if combined with a carefully completed diary—recording when, what, and amounts the person eats—which allows the doctor to see correlations between symptoms and reflux episodes. The procedure is sometimes helpful in detecting whether respiratory symptoms, including wheezing and coughing, are triggered by reflux.

A completely accurate diagnostic test for GERD does not exist, and tests have not consistently shown that acid exposure to the lower esophagus directly correlates with damage to the lining.

Surgery

Surgery is an option when medicine and lifestyle changes do not help to manage GERD symptoms. Surgery may also be a reasonable alternative to a lifetime of drugs and discomfort.

Fundoplication is the standard surgical treatment for GERD. Usually a specific type of this procedure, called Nissen fundoplication, is performed. During the Nissen fundoplication, the upper part of the stomach is wrapped around the LES to strengthen the sphincter, prevent acid reflux, and repair a hiatal hernia. The Nissen fundoplication may be performed using a laparoscope. When performed by experienced surgeons, laparoscopic fundoplication is safe and effective in people of all ages, including infants.

Endoscopic techniques used to treat chronic heartburn include the Bard EndoCinch system, NDO Plicator, and the Stretta system. These techniques require the use of an endoscope to perform the anti-reflux operation. The EndoCinch and NDO Plicator systems involve putting stitches in the LES to create pleats that help strengthen the muscle. The Stretta system uses electrodes to create tiny burns on the LES. When the burns heal, the scar tissue helps toughen the muscle. The long-term effects of these three procedures are unknown.

Long-Term Complications of GERD

Chronic GERD that is untreated can cause serious complications. Inflammation of the esophagus from refluxed stomach acid can damage the lining and cause bleeding or ulcers—also called esophagitis. Scars from tissue damage can lead to strictures—narrowing of the esophagus—that make swallowing difficult. Some people develop

Barrett's esophagus, in which cells in the esophageal lining take on an abnormal shape and color. Over time, the cells can lead to esophageal cancer, which is often fatal. Persons with GERD and its complications should be monitored closely by a physician. Studies have shown that GERD may worsen or contribute to asthma, chronic cough, and pulmonary fibrosis.

For More Information

American College of Gastroenterology
P.O. Box 342260
Bethesda, MD 20827–2260
Phone: 301-263-9000
Website: http://www.acg.gi.org

American Gastroenterological Association
National Office
4930 Del Ray Ave.
Bethesda, MD 20814
Phone: 301-654-2055
Fax: 301-654-5920
Website: http://www.gastro.org
E-mail: member@gastro.org

International Foundation for Functional Gastrointestinal Disorders
P.O. Box 170864
Milwaukee, WI 53217–8076
Toll-Free: 888-964-2001
Phone: 414-964-1799
Fax: 414-964-7176
Website: http://www.aboutgerd.org
E-mail: iffgd@iffgd.org

North American Society for Pediatric Gastroenterology, Hepatology, and Nutrition
P.O. Box 6
Flourtown, PA 19031
Phone: 215-233-0808
Fax: 215-233-3918
Website: http://www.naspghan.org
E-mail: naspghan@naspghan.org

Pediatric Adolescent Gastroesophageal Reflux Association, Inc. (PAGER)
P.O. Box 486
Buckeystown, MD 21717–0486
Phone: 301-601-9541
Website: http://www.reflux.org
E-mail: gergroup@aol.com

Chapter 22

Hip Pain

Definition

Hip pain involves any pain in or around the hip joint.

Considerations

Hip-related pain is not always felt directly over the hip. Instead, you may feel it in the middle of your thigh or in your groin. Similarly, pain you feel in the hip may actually reflect a problem in your back, rather than your hip itself.

Causes

Two possible causes of hip pain are fractures and insufficient blood flow to the hip (aseptic necrosis).

A hip fracture can change the quality of your life significantly. Fewer than 50% of those with a hip fracture return to their former level of activity. In addition, while recovering from a hip fracture, several possible complications can be life-threatening. These include pneumonia and a blood clot in the leg, which can dislodge and travel to cause a clot in the lungs. Both are due to immobility following a hip fracture and hip surgery.

Hip fractures become more common as people age because falls are more likely and bones become less dense. People with osteoporosis can get a fracture from simple, everyday activities, not just a dramatic fall or injury.

Aseptic necrosis can happen if you have been on steroids for a long time or you have sickle cell anemia. Injury and regular use of alcohol also increase your risk. Legg-Calve-Perthes disease is a type of aseptic necrosis that happens in children.

Other possible causes of hip pain include:

- Arthritis—often felt in the front part of your thigh or in your groin;

- Trochanteric bursitis—hurts when you get up from a chair, walk, climb stairs, and drive;

- Tendinitis from repetitive or strenuous activity;

- Strain or sprain;

- Low-back pain such as sciatica;

- Infection.

Home Care

- Try to avoid activities that aggravate the pain.

- Take over-the-counter pain medication, like ibuprofen or acetaminophen.

- Sleep on your non-painful side with a pillow between your legs.

A hip fracture is considered a medical emergency. Therefore, if suspected, you should be seen right away.

As the pain improves, gradually begin to exercise. It is best to work with a physical therapist to learn proper exercises and how to advance your activity. Swimming may be a good option because it stretches the muscles and builds good muscle tone without straining your hip joint. However, swimming does not build bone mass. When you are ready (a physical therapist can help determine that), slowly and carefully resume walking or another activity against the resistance of gravity.

When to Contact a Medical Professional

Go to a hospital or call 911 if:

- Your hip pain is caused by a fall or other injury.

- Your hip is misshapen, badly bruised, or bleeding.

- You are unable to move your hip or bear any weight.

Call your doctor if:

- Your hip is still painful after one week of home treatment.

- You also have a fever or rash.

- You have sudden hip pain, plus sickle cell anemia or long-term steroid use.

- You have pain in both hips or other joints.

What to Expect at Your Office Visit

Your health care provider will perform a physical examination, with careful attention to your hips, thighs, back, and gait.

To help diagnose the cause of the problem, your doctor will ask medical history questions, such as:

- Do you have pain in one or both hips?

- Do you have pain elsewhere like your lower back or thigh?

- Do you have pain in other joints?

- Did your pain begin suddenly, or slowly and mildly?

- Did the pain begin after an injury, fall, or accident?

- Does any particular activity make the pain worse?

- Have you done anything to try to relieve the pain? If so, what helps?

- Are you able to walk and bear weight?

- What other medical problems do you have? Osteoporosis or other signs of bone loss? Sickle cell anemia?

- Do you take any medications? If so, which ones? If on steroids, for how long have you been on them?

X-rays of the hip may be necessary.

Your doctor may tell you to take a higher dose of over-the-counter medication, or give you a prescription anti-inflammatory medication.

Surgical repair or hip replacement may be recommended for aseptic necrosis. Hip replacement is necessary for hip fracture and severe arthritis. With current technology, an artificial hip should last at least 10 to 15 years. Expect recovery from surgery to take at least six weeks.

Complications can occur from surgery. A blood clot in the leg is the most common complication, which can lead to a blood clot in the lungs.

Prevention

- Avoid activities that raise one of your hips above the other for extended periods of time, like running on an uneven surface. Running on a treadmill can keep your hips level.

- Warm up before exercising and cool down afterward. Stretch your hips, low back, and thighs.

- Avoid falls.

- Wear hip pads for contact sports like football and hockey. For those at high risk for a hip fracture, pads with a streamline design can be worn in undergarments.

- Learn how to prevent osteoporosis.

References

Wong TK, Lee RY. Effects of low back pain on the relationship between the movements of the lumbar spine and hip. *Hum Mov Sci*. 2004; 23(1): 21–34.

Dohnke B, Knauper B, Muller-Fahrnow W. Perceived self-efficacy gained from, and health effects of, a rehabilitation program after hip joint replacement. *Arthritis Rheum*. 2005; 53(4): 585–592.

Tak E, Staats P, Van Hespen A, Hopman-Rock M. The effects of an exercise program for older adults with osteoarthritis of the hip. *J Rheumatol*. 2005; 32(6): 1106–1113.

Chapter 23

Inflammatory Bowel Disease

Editor's note: This chapter was written for parents of children that have inflammatory bowel disease; however, the information is applicable for all individuals diagnosed with inflammatory bowel disease.

The digestive system is a set of organs (including the stomach, large and small intestines, rectum, and others) that convert the foods we eat into nutrients and absorb these nutrients into the bloodstream to fuel our bodies. We seldom notice its workings unless something goes wrong, as in the case of inflammatory bowel disease (IBD).

It's estimated that up to one million Americans have inflammatory bowel disease. It occurs most frequently in people ages 15 to 30, but it can also affect younger children and older people. And there are significantly more reported cases in western Europe and North America than in other parts of the world.

Text in this chapter is from "Inflammatory Bowel Disease," May 2007, reprinted with permission from www.kidshealth.org. Copyright © 2007 The Nemours Foundation. This information was provided by KidsHealth, one of the largest resources online for medically reviewed health information written for parents, kids, and teens. For more articles like this one, visit www.KidsHealth.org, or www.TeensHealth.org. Figure 23.1 is from "Diagnostic Tests: Lower GI Series," National Institute of Diabetes and Digestive and Kidney Diseases (NIDDK), NIH Publication No. 05–4334, November 2004.

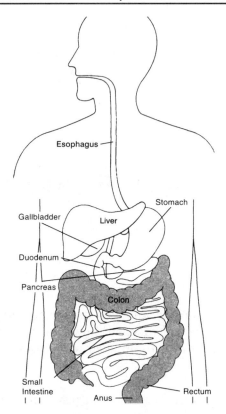

Figure 23.1. *The Digestive System*

What is inflammatory bowel disease?

Inflammatory bowel disease (which is not the same thing as irritable bowel syndrome, or IBS) refers to two chronic diseases that cause inflammation of the intestines: ulcerative colitis and Crohn disease. Although the diseases have some features in common, there are some important differences.

Ulcerative colitis is an inflammatory disease of the large intestine, also called the colon. In ulcerative colitis, the inner lining—or mucosa—of the intestine becomes inflamed (meaning the lining of the intestinal wall reddens and swells) and develops ulcers (an ulcer is a sore, which means it's an open, painful wound). Ulcerative colitis is often the most severe in the rectal area, which can cause frequent diarrhea. Mucus and blood often appear in the stool (feces or poop) if the lining of the colon is damaged.

Crohn disease differs from ulcerative colitis in the areas of the bowel it involves—it most commonly affects the last part of the small intestine (called the terminal ileum) and parts of the large intestine. However, Crohn disease isn't limited to these areas and can attack any part of the digestive tract. Crohn disease causes inflammation that extends much deeper into the layers of the intestinal wall than ulcerative colitis does. Crohn disease generally tends to involve the entire bowel wall, whereas ulcerative colitis affects only the lining of the bowel.

What causes it?

Medical research hasn't determined yet what causes inflammatory bowel disease. But researchers believe that a number of factors may be involved, such as the environment, diet, and possibly genetics.

Current evidence suggests that there's likely a genetic defect that affects how our immune system works and how the inflammation is turned on and off in those people with inflammatory bowel disease, in response to an offending agent, like bacteria, a virus, or a protein in food.

The problem in people with the disease is that the inflammation gets turned on, but it doesn't get turned off. Medical evidence also indicates that smoking may enhance the likelihood of developing Crohn disease.

What are the signs and symptoms?

The most common symptoms of both ulcerative colitis and Crohn disease are diarrhea and abdominal pain. Diarrhea can range from mild to severe (as many as 20 or more trips to the bathroom a day). If the diarrhea is extreme, it can lead to dehydration, rapid heartbeat, and a drop in blood pressure. And continued loss of small amounts of blood in the stool can lead to anemia.

At times, those with inflammatory bowel disease may also have constipation. With Crohn disease, this can happen as a result of a partial obstruction (called stricture) in the intestines. In ulcerative colitis, constipation may be a symptom of inflammation of the rectum (also known as proctitis).

Because of the loss of fluid and nutrients from diarrhea and chronic inflammation of the bowel, someone with inflammatory bowel disease may also experience fever, fatigue, weight loss, dehydration, and malnutrition. Pain usually results from the abdominal cramping, which is caused by irritation of the nerves and muscles that control intestinal contractions.

But inflammatory bowel disease can cause other health problems that occur outside the digestive system. Although medical researchers don't know why these complications happen, some people with the disease may show signs of inflammation elsewhere in the body, such as in the joints, eyes, skin, and liver. Skin tags that look like hemorrhoids or abscesses may also develop around the anus.

Inflammatory bowel disease may also cause a delay in puberty or growth problems for some kids and teens with the condition because it can interfere with a person getting nutrients from the foods he or she eats.

How is it diagnosed?

Inflammatory bowel disease can be hard to diagnose because there may be no symptoms, even if the person's bowel has become increasingly damaged for years. Once symptoms do appear, they often resemble those of other conditions, which may make it difficult for doctors to diagnose.

If your child has any of the symptoms of the disease, it's important to see your child's doctor. In addition to doing a physical examination, the doctor will ask you and your child about any concerns and symptoms your child has, your child's past health, your family's health, any medications your child is taking, any allergies your child may have, and other issues. This is called the medical history.

After hearing your child's symptoms, if the doctor suspects inflammatory bowel disease, he or she may suggest certain tests. Blood tests may be done to determine if there are signs of inflammation in your child's body, which are often present with the disease. The doctor may also check for anemia and for other causes of your symptoms, like infection.

The doctor will examine your child's stool for the presence of blood. He or she may look at your child's colon with an instrument called an endoscope. Also called a colonoscope or coloscope, this instrument is a long, thin tube inserted through the anus and attached to a television monitor. This procedure is called a colonoscopy, which allows the doctor to see inflammation, bleeding, or ulcers on the wall of your child's colon.

The doctor may also do a test called an upper endoscopy to check the esophagus, stomach, and upper small intestine for inflammation, bleeding, or ulcers. During the exam, the doctor may perform a biopsy, which involves taking a small sample of tissue from part of the colon so it can be viewed with a microscope or sent to a laboratory for other kinds of analysis.

A doctor may also order a barium study of the intestines. This procedure involves drinking a thick white solution called barium, which shows up white on an x-ray film, allowing a doctor to get a better look at what's going on in a person's intestines.

How is it treated?

Drug treatment is the main method for relieving the symptoms of both ulcerative colitis and Crohn disease. Great progress is being made in the development of medications for treating inflammatory bowel disease. Your child's doctor may prescribe:

- anti-inflammatory drugs (used to decrease the inflammation caused by the disease);

- immunosuppressive agents (which work to restrain the immune system from attacking the body's own tissues and causing further inflammation).

If a child with inflammatory bowel disease doesn't respond to either of these medicines, your child's doctor may suggest surgery. But surgical procedures for ulcerative colitis and Crohn disease are quite different.

With Crohn disease, doctors make every attempt to avoid surgery because of the recurring nature of the disease. There's also a concern that an aggressive surgical approach to Crohn disease will cause further complications, such as short bowel syndrome (which involves growth failure and a reduced ability to absorb nutrients).

In the case of ulcerative colitis, removal of the colon (large intestine) may be necessary, along with a surgical procedure called an ileo-anal anastomosis (also called an ileoanal pull-through) in which doctors form a pouch from the small bowel to collect stool in the pelvis. This allows the stool to pass through the anus.

Caring for Your Child

How can you help your child cope with inflammatory bowel disease? Because of the unpredictable nature of the disease, it's easy to feel helpless. Your child will likely be fatigued, irritable, and anxious—the best way to help your child is to seek treatment as soon as symptoms appear to help relieve as much discomfort as possible.

Although it can be difficult to get any child to eat properly, a balanced diet with adequate calories becomes even more important for kids with inflammatory bowel disease. Diarrhea, loss of nutrients, and the side effects of drug treatment may all lead to malnutrition.

Encourage your child to eat small meals throughout the day to help lessen any symptoms. Pack nutritious snacks and lunches so your child won't be tempted to indulge in junk food that's high in fat and sodium, which can intensify the symptoms of the disease. Eventually, your child may be able to determine which foods provoke symptoms and learn to avoid those foods.

If your child begins to lose weight quickly, has repeated bouts of diarrhea, or complains of abdominal cramping, inflammatory bowel disease may be the cause. Call your child's doctor if you notice any of these symptoms to ensure that your child gets proper evaluation and treatment.

Inflammatory bowel disease is a serious condition, but with proper treatment and medical care, your child can enjoy a productive, normal life.

Chapter 24

Interstitial Cystitis and Painful Bladder Syndrome

Interstitial cystitis (IC) is a condition that results in recurring discomfort or pain in the bladder and the surrounding pelvic region. The symptoms vary from case to case and even in the same individual. People may experience mild discomfort, pressure, tenderness, or intense pain in the bladder and pelvic area. Symptoms may include an urgent need to urinate (urgency), a frequent need to urinate (frequency), or a combination of these symptoms. Pain may change in intensity as the bladder fills with urine or as it empties. Women's symptoms often get worse during menstruation. They may sometimes experience pain with vaginal intercourse.

Because IC varies so much in symptoms and severity, most researchers believe that it is not one, but several diseases. In recent years, scientists have started to use the term painful bladder syndrome (PBS) to describe cases with painful urinary symptoms that may not meet the strictest definition of IC. The term IC/PBS includes all cases of urinary pain that cannot be attributed to other causes, such as infection or urinary stones. The term interstitial cystitis, or IC, is used alone when describing cases that meet all of the IC criteria established by the National Institute of Diabetes and Digestive and Kidney Diseases (NIDDK).

Excerpted from "Interstitial Cystitis/Painful Bladder Syndrome," National Institute of Diabetes and Digestive and Kidney Diseases (NIDDK), NIH Publication No. 05–3220, June 2005. The full text of this document is available at http://kidney.niddk.nih.gov/kudiseases/pubs/interstitialcystitis.

In IC/PBS, the bladder wall may be irritated and become scarred or stiff. Glomerulations (pinpoint bleeding caused by recurrent irritation) often appear on the bladder wall. Hunner's ulcers are present in ten percent of patients with IC. Some people with IC/PBS find that their bladders cannot hold much urine, which increases the frequency of urination. Frequency, however, is not always specifically related to bladder size; many people with severe frequency have normal bladder capacity. People with severe cases of IC/PBS may urinate as many as 60 times a day, including frequent nighttime urination (nocturia). IC/PBS is far more common in women than in men. Of the estimated one million Americans with IC, up to 90 percent are women.

Causes of IC

Some of the symptoms of IC/PBS resemble those of bacterial infection, but medical tests reveal no organisms in the urine of patients with IC/PBS. Furthermore, patients with IC/PBS do not respond to antibiotic therapy. Researchers are working to understand the causes of IC/PBS and to find effective treatments.

In recent years, researchers have isolated a substance found almost exclusively in the urine of people with interstitial cystitis. They have named the substance antiproliferative factor (APF) because it appears to block the normal growth of the cells that line the inside wall of the bladder. Researchers anticipate that learning more about APF will lead to a greater understanding of the causes of IC and to possible treatments. Also, researchers are beginning to explore the possibility that heredity may play a part in some forms of IC. In a few cases, IC has affected a mother and a daughter or two sisters, but it does not commonly run in families.

Diagnosing IC/PBS

Because symptoms are similar to those of other disorders of the urinary bladder and because there is no definitive test to identify IC/PBS, doctors must rule out other treatable conditions before considering a diagnosis of IC/PBS. The most common of these diseases in both genders are urinary tract infections and bladder cancer. IC/PBS is not associated with any increased risk in developing cancer. In men, common diseases include chronic prostatitis or chronic pelvic pain syndrome.

The diagnosis of IC/PBS in the general population is based on the:

- presence of pain related to the bladder, usually accompanied by frequency and urgency; or

- absence of other diseases that could cause the symptoms.

Diagnostic tests that help in ruling out other diseases include urinalysis, urine culture, cystoscopy, biopsy of the bladder wall, distention of the bladder under anesthesia, urine cytology, and laboratory examination of prostate secretions.

Urinalysis and Urine Culture

Examining urine under a microscope and culturing the urine can detect and identify the primary organisms that are known to infect the urinary tract and that may cause symptoms similar to IC/PBS. White and red blood cells and bacteria in the urine may indicate an infection of the urinary tract, which can be treated with an antibiotic. If urine is sterile for weeks or months while symptoms persist, the doctor may consider a diagnosis of IC/PBS.

Culture of Prostate Secretions

Although not commonly done, in men, the doctor might obtain prostatic fluid and examine it for signs of a prostate infection, which can then be treated with antibiotics.

Cystoscopy under Anesthesia with Bladder Distention

The doctor may perform a cystoscopic examination in order to rule out bladder cancer. During cystoscopy, the doctor uses a cystoscope—an instrument made of a hollow tube about the diameter of a drinking straw with several lenses and a light—to see inside the bladder and urethra. The doctor might also distend or stretch the bladder to its capacity by filling it with a liquid or gas. Because bladder distention is painful in patients with IC/PBS, they must be given some form of anesthesia for the procedure.

The doctor may also test the patient's maximum bladder capacity—the maximum amount of liquid or gas the bladder can hold. This procedure must be done under anesthesia since the bladder capacity is limited by either pain or a severe urge to urinate.

Biopsy

A biopsy is a tissue sample that can be examined under a microscope. Samples of the bladder and urethra may be removed during a cystoscopy. A biopsy helps rule out bladder cancer.

Future Diagnostic Tools

Researchers are investigating and validating some promising biomarkers such as anti-proliferative factor (APF), some cytokines, and other growth factors. These might provide more reliable diagnostic markers for IC and lead to more focused treatment for the disease.

Treatments for IC/PBS

Scientists have not yet found a cure for IC/PBS, nor can they predict who will respond best to which treatment. Symptoms may disappear without explanation or coincide with an event such as a change in diet or treatment. Even when symptoms disappear, they may return after days, weeks, months, or years. Scientists do not know why.

Because the causes of IC/PBS are unknown, current treatments are aimed at relieving symptoms. Many people are helped for variable periods by one or a combination of the treatments. As researchers learn more about IC/PBS, the list of potential treatments will change, so patients should discuss their options with a doctor.

Bladder Distention

Many patients have noted an improvement in symptoms after a bladder distention has been done to diagnose IC/PBS. In many cases, the procedure is used as both a diagnostic test and initial therapy. Researchers are not sure why distention helps, but some believe that it may increase capacity and interferes with pain signals transmitted by nerves in the bladder. Symptoms may temporarily worsen 24 to 48 hours after distention, but should return to initial distention levels or improve within 2–4 weeks.

Bladder Instillation

During a bladder instillation, also called a bladder wash or bath, the bladder is filled with a solution that is held for varying periods of time, averaging 10–15 minutes, before being emptied.

The only drug approved by the U.S. Food and Drug Administration (FDA) for bladder instillation is dimethyl sulfoxide (DMSO, RIMSO-50). DMSO treatment involves guiding a narrow tube called a catheter up the urethra into the bladder. A measured amount of DMSO is passed through the catheter into the bladder, where it is retained for about 15 minutes before being expelled. Treatments are given every week or two for 6–8 weeks and repeated as needed. Most people who respond to DMSO notice improvement 3–4 weeks after the first 6- to 8-week cycle of treatments. Highly motivated patients who are willing to catheterize themselves may, after consultation with their doctor, be able to have DMSO treatments at home. Self-administration is less expensive and more convenient than going to the doctor's office.

Doctors think DMSO works in several ways. Because it passes into the bladder wall, it may reach tissue more effectively to reduce inflammation and block pain. It may also prevent muscle contractions that cause pain, frequency, and urgency.

A bothersome but relatively insignificant side effect of DMSO treatments is a garlic-like taste and odor on the breath and skin that may last up to 72 hours after treatment. Blood tests, including a complete blood count and kidney and liver function tests, should be done about every six months.

Oral Drugs

Pentosan polysulfate sodium (Elmiron): This first oral drug developed for IC was approved by the FDA in 1996. In clinical trials, the drug improved symptoms in 30 percent of patients treated. Doctors do not know exactly how it works, but one theory is that it may repair defects that might have developed in the lining of the bladder.

The FDA-recommended oral dosage of Elmiron is 100 mg, three times a day. Patients may not feel relief from IC pain for the first 2–4 months. A decrease in urinary frequency may take up to six months. Patients are urged to continue with therapy for at least six months to give the drug an adequate chance to relieve symptoms.

Other oral medications: Aspirin and ibuprofen may be a first line of defense against mild discomfort. Doctors may recommend other drugs to relieve pain.

Some patients have experienced improvement in their urinary symptoms by taking tricyclic antidepressants (amitriptyline) or antihistamines. Amitriptyline may help to reduce pain, increase bladder capacity, and decrease frequency and nocturia. Some patients may not be able to take it because it makes them too tired during the day. In patients with severe pain, narcotic analgesics such as acetaminophen (Tylenol) with codeine or longer acting narcotics may be necessary.

Note: All drugs—even those sold over the counter—have side effects. Patients should always consult a doctor before using any drug for an extended amount of time.

Transcutaneous Electrical Nerve Stimulation

With transcutaneous electrical nerve stimulation (TENS), mild electric pulses enter the body for minutes to hours, two or more times a day, either through wires placed on the lower back or just above the pubic area between the navel and the pubic hair, or through special devices inserted into the vagina in women or into the rectum in men. Although scientists do not know exactly how TENS relieves pelvic pain, it has been suggested that the electrical pulses may increase blood flow to the bladder, strengthen pelvic muscles that help control the bladder, or trigger the release of substances that block pain.

TENS is relatively inexpensive and allows the patient to take an active part in treatment. Within some guidelines, the patient decides when, how long, and at what intensity TENS will be used. It has been most helpful in relieving pain and decreasing frequency in patients with Hunner's ulcers. Smokers do not respond as well as nonsmokers. If TENS is going to help, improvement is usually apparent in 3–4 months.

Diet

There is no scientific evidence linking diet to IC/PBS, but many doctors and patients find that alcohol, tomatoes, spices, chocolate, caffeinated and citrus beverages, and high-acid foods may contribute to bladder irritation and inflammation. Some patients also note that their symptoms worsen after eating or drinking products containing artificial sweeteners.

Smoking

Many patients feel that smoking makes their symptoms worse. How the by-products of tobacco that are excreted in the urine affect IC/PBS is unknown. Smoking, however, is the major known cause of bladder cancer. Therefore, one of the best things smokers can do for their bladder and their overall health is to quit.

Exercise

Many patients feel that gentle stretching exercises help relieve IC/PBS symptoms.

Bladder Training

People who have found adequate relief from pain may be able to reduce frequency by using bladder training techniques. Methods vary, but basically patients decide to void (empty their bladder) at designated times and use relaxation techniques and distractions to keep to the schedule. Gradually, patients try to lengthen the time between scheduled voids. A diary in which to record voiding times is usually helpful in keeping track of progress.

Surgery

Surgery should be considered only if all available treatments have failed and the pain is disabling. Many approaches and techniques are used, each of which has its own advantages and complications that should be discussed with a surgeon. Your doctor may recommend consulting another surgeon for a second opinion before taking this step. Most doctors are reluctant to operate because the outcome is unpredictable: Some people still have symptoms after surgery.

People considering surgery should discuss the potential risks and benefits, side effects, and long- and short-term complications with a surgeon and with their family, as well as with people who have already had the procedure. Surgery requires anesthesia, hospitalization, and weeks or months of recovery. As the complexity of the procedure increases, so do the chances for complications and for failure. To locate a surgeon experienced in performing specific procedures, check with your doctor.

Are there any special concerns?

Cancer: There is no evidence that IC/PBS increases the risk of bladder cancer.

Pregnancy: Researchers have little information about pregnancy and IC/PBS but believe that the disorder does not affect fertility or the health of the fetus. Some women find that their IC/PBS goes into remission during pregnancy, while others experience a worsening of their symptoms.

Coping: The emotional support of family, friends, and other people with IC/PBS is very important in helping patients cope. Studies have found that patients who learn about the disorder and become involved in their own care do better than patients who do not.

For More Information

Interstitial Cystitis Association of America
110 N. Washington St., Suite 340
Rockville, MD 20850
Toll-Free: 800-435-7422
Fax: 301-610-5308
Website: http://www.ichelp.org
E-mail: icamail@ichelp.org

UruologyHealth.org
http://www.urologyhealth.org

Chapter 25

Irritable Bowel Syndrome

Irritable bowel syndrome is a disorder characterized most commonly by cramping, abdominal pain, bloating, constipation, and diarrhea. IBS causes a great deal of discomfort and distress, but it does not permanently harm the intestines and does not lead to a serious disease, such as cancer. Most people can control their symptoms with diet, stress management, and prescribed medications. For some people, however, IBS can be disabling. They may be unable to work, attend social events, or even travel short distances.

As many as 20 percent of the adult population, or one in five Americans, have symptoms of IBS, making it one of the most common disorders diagnosed by doctors. It occurs more often in women than in men, and it begins before the age of 35 in about 50 percent of people.

What are the symptoms of IBS?

Abdominal pain, bloating, and discomfort are the main symptoms of IBS. However, symptoms can vary from person to person. Some people have constipation, which means hard, difficult-to-pass, or infrequent bowel movements. Often these people report straining and cramping when trying to have a bowel movement but cannot eliminate any stool, or they are able to eliminate only a small amount. If they are able to have a bowel movement, there may be mucus in it,

Excerpted from "Irritable Bowel Syndrome," National Institute of Diabetes and Digestive and Kidney Diseases (NIDDK), NIH Publication No. 07–693, September 2007.

which is a fluid that moistens and protect passages in the digestive system. Some people with IBS experience diarrhea, which is frequent, loose, watery, stools. People with diarrhea frequently feel an urgent and uncontrollable need to have a bowel movement. Other people with IBS alternate between constipation and diarrhea. Sometimes people find that their symptoms subside for a few months and then return, while others report a constant worsening of symptoms over time.

What causes IBS?

Researchers have yet to discover any specific cause for IBS. One theory is that people who suffer from IBS have a colon, or large intestine, that is particularly sensitive and reactive to certain foods and stress. The immune system, which fights infection, may also be involved.

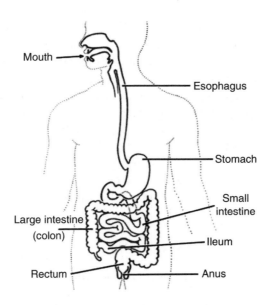

Figure 25.1. *The Digestive System*

- Normal motility, or movement, may not be present in the colon of a person who has IBS. It can be spasmodic or can even stop working temporarily. Spasms are sudden strong muscle contractions that come and go.

- The lining of the colon called the epithelium, which is affected by the immune and nervous systems, regulates the flow of fluids in and out of the colon. In IBS, the epithelium appears to work properly. However, when the contents inside the colon move too quickly, the colon loses its ability to absorb fluids. The result is too much fluid in the stool. In other people, the movement inside the colon is too slow, which causes extra fluid to be absorbed. As a result, a person develops constipation.

- A person's colon may respond strongly to stimuli such as certain foods or stress that would not bother most people.

- Recent research has reported that serotonin is linked with normal gastrointestinal (GI) functioning. Serotonin is a neurotransmitter, or chemical, that delivers messages from one part of your body to another. Ninety-five percent of the serotonin in your body is located in the GI tract, and the other five percent is found in the brain. Cells that line the inside of the bowel work as transporters and carry the serotonin out of the GI tract. People with IBS, however, have diminished receptor activity, causing abnormal levels of serotonin to exist in the GI tract. As a result, they experience problems with bowel movement, motility, and sensation—having more sensitive pain receptors in their GI tract.

- Researchers have reported that IBS may be caused by a bacterial infection in the gastrointestinal tract. Studies show that people who have had gastroenteritis sometimes develop IBS, otherwise called post-infectious IBS.

- Researchers have also found very mild celiac disease in some people with symptoms similar to IBS. People with celiac disease cannot digest gluten, a substance found in wheat, rye, and barley. People with celiac disease cannot eat these foods without becoming very sick because their immune system responds by damaging the small intestine. A blood test can determine whether celiac disease may be present.

How is IBS diagnosed?

If you think you have IBS, seeing your doctor is the first step. IBS is generally diagnosed on the basis of a complete medical history that includes a careful description of symptoms and a physical examination.

There is no specific test for IBS, although diagnostic tests may be performed to rule out other problems. These tests may include stool sample testing, blood tests, and x-rays. Typically, a doctor will perform a sigmoidoscopy, or colonoscopy, which allows the doctor to look inside the colon. This is done by inserting a small, flexible tube with a camera on the end of it through the anus. The camera then transfers the images of your colon onto a large screen for the doctor to see.

If your test results are negative, the doctor may diagnose IBS based on your symptoms, including how often you have had abdominal pain or discomfort during the past year, when the pain starts and stops in relation to bowel function, and how your bowel frequency and stool consistency have changed. Many doctors refer to a list of specific symptoms that must be present to make a diagnosis of IBS.

Symptoms of IBS include:

- Abdominal pain or discomfort for at least 12 weeks out of the previous 12 months. These 12 weeks do not have to be consecutive.

- The abdominal pain or discomfort has two of the following three features:

    - It is relieved by having a bowel movement.

    - When it starts, there is a change in how often you have a bowel movement.

    - When it starts, there is a change in the form of the stool or the way it looks.

- Certain symptoms must also be present, such as

    - a change in frequency of bowel movements;

    - a change in appearance of bowel movements;

    - feelings of uncontrollable urgency to have a bowel movement;

    - difficulty or inability to pass stool;

    - mucus in the stool; or

    - bloating.

- Bleeding, fever, weight loss, and persistent severe pain are not symptoms of IBS and may indicate other problems such as inflammation, or rarely, cancer.

The following have been associated with a worsening of IBS symptoms:

- large meals

- bloating from gas in the colon

- medicines

- wheat, rye, barley, chocolate, milk products, or alcohol

- drinks with caffeine, such as coffee, tea, or colas

- stress, conflict, or emotional upsets

Researchers have found that women with IBS may have more symptoms during their menstrual periods, suggesting that reproductive hormones can worsen IBS problems.

In addition, people with IBS frequently suffer from depression and anxiety, which can worsen symptoms. Similarly, the symptoms associated with IBS can cause a person to feel depressed and anxious.

What is the treatment for IBS?

Unfortunately, many people suffer from IBS for a long time before seeking medical treatment. Up to 70 percent of people suffering from IBS are not receiving medical care for their symptoms. No cure has been found for IBS, but many options are available to treat the symptoms. Your doctor will give you the best treatments for your particular symptoms and encourage you to manage stress and make changes to your diet.

Medications are an important part of relieving symptoms. Your doctor may suggest fiber supplements or laxatives for constipation or medicines to decrease diarrhea, such as Lomotil or loperamide (Imodium). An antispasmodic is commonly prescribed, which helps to control colon muscle spasms and reduce abdominal pain. Antidepressants may relieve some symptoms. However, both antispasmodics and antidepressants can worsen constipation, so some doctors will also prescribe medications that relax muscles in the bladder and intestines, such as Donnapine and Librax. These medications contain a mild sedative, which can be habit forming, so they need to be used under the guidance of a physician.

A medication available specifically to treat IBS is alosetron hydrochloride (Lotronex). Lotronex has been reapproved with significant restrictions by the U.S. Food and Drug Administration (FDA) for women with severe IBS who have not responded to conventional therapy and whose primary symptom is diarrhea. However, even in these patients, Lotronex should be used with great caution because it can have serious side effects such as severe constipation or decreased blood flow to the colon.

With any medication, even over-the-counter medications such as laxatives and fiber supplements, it is important to follow your doctor's instructions. Some people report a worsening in abdominal bloating and gas from increased fiber intake, and laxatives can be habit forming if they are used too frequently.

Medications affect people differently, and no one medication or combination of medications will work for everyone with IBS. You will need to work with your doctor to find the best combination of medicine, diet, counseling, and support to control your symptoms.

How does stress affect IBS?

Stress—feeling mentally or emotionally tense, troubled, angry, or overwhelmed—can stimulate colon spasms in people with IBS. The colon has many nerves that connect it to the brain. Like the heart and the lungs, the colon is partly controlled by the autonomic nervous system, which responds to stress. These nerves control the normal contractions of the colon and cause abdominal discomfort at stressful times. People often experience cramps or "butterflies" when they are nervous or upset. In people with IBS, the colon can be overly responsive to even slight conflict or stress. Stress makes the mind more aware of the sensations that arise in the colon, making the person perceive these sensations as unpleasant.

Some evidence suggests that IBS is affected by the immune system, which fights infection in the body. The immune system is affected by stress. For all these reasons, stress management is an important part of treatment for IBS.

What does the colon do?

The colon, which is about five feet long, connects the small intestine to the rectum and anus. The major function of the colon is to absorb water, nutrients, and salts from the partially digested food that enters from the small intestine. Two pints of liquid matter enter the colon from the small intestine each day. Stool volume is a third of a pint. The difference between the amount of fluid entering the colon from the small intestine and the amount of stool in the colon is what the colon absorbs each day.

Colon motility—the contraction of the colon muscles and the movement of its contents—is controlled by nerves, hormones, and impulses in the colon muscles. These contractions move the contents inside the colon toward the rectum. During this passage, water and nutrients are absorbed into the body, and what is left over is stool. A few times each day contractions push the stool down the colon, resulting in a bowel movement. However, if the muscles of the colon, sphincters, and pelvis do not contract in the right way, the contents inside the colon do not move correctly, resulting in abdominal pain, cramps, constipation, a sense of incomplete stool movement, or diarrhea.

Can changes in diet help IBS?

For many people, careful eating reduces IBS symptoms. Before changing your diet, keep a journal noting the foods that seem to cause distress. Then discuss your findings with your doctor. You may want to consult a registered dietitian who can help you make changes to your diet. For instance, if dairy products cause your symptoms to flare up, you can try eating less of those foods. You might be able to tolerate yogurt better than other dairy products because it contains bacteria that supply the enzyme needed to digest lactose, the sugar found in milk products. Dairy products are an important source of calcium and other nutrients. If you need to avoid dairy products, be sure to get adequate nutrients in the foods you substitute, or take supplements.

In many cases, dietary fiber may lessen IBS symptoms, particularly constipation. However, it may not help with lowering pain or decreasing diarrhea. Whole grain breads and cereals, fruits, and vegetables are good sources of fiber. High-fiber diets keep the colon mildly distended, which may help prevent spasms. Some forms of fiber keep water in the stool, thereby preventing hard stools that are difficult to pass. Doctors usually recommend a diet with enough fiber to produce soft, painless bowel movements. High-fiber diets may cause gas and bloating, although some people report that these symptoms go away within a few weeks. Increasing fiber intake by 2–3 grams per day will help reduce the risk of increased gas and bloating.

Drinking six to eight glasses of plain water a day is important, especially if you have diarrhea. Drinking carbonated beverages, such as sodas, may result in gas and cause discomfort. Chewing gum and eating too quickly can lead to swallowing air, which also leads to gas.

Large meals can cause cramping and diarrhea, so eating smaller meals more often, or eating smaller portions, may help IBS symptoms. Eating meals that are low in fat and high in carbohydrates such as pasta, rice, whole-grain breads and cereals (unless you have celiac disease), fruits, and vegetables may help.

Is IBS linked to other health problems?

As its name indicates, IBS is a syndrome—a combination of signs and symptoms. IBS has not been shown to lead to a serious disease, including cancer. Through the years, IBS has been called by many names, among them colitis, mucous colitis, spastic colon, or spastic bowel. However, no link has been established between IBS and inflammatory bowel diseases such as Crohn disease or ulcerative colitis.

Chapter 26

Kidney Stones

When should I call a doctor?

If you have a kidney stone, you may already know how painful it can be. Most kidney stones pass out of the body without help from a doctor. But sometimes a stone will not pass. It may even get larger. Your doctor can help.

You should call a doctor if you have any of the following signs:

- extreme pain in your back or side that will not go away
- blood in your urine
- fever and chills
- vomiting
- urine that smells bad or looks cloudy
- a burning feeling when you urinate

These may be signs of a kidney stone that needs a doctor's care.

What do my kidneys do?

Your kidneys are bean-shaped organs, each about the size of your fist. They are located near the middle of your back, just below the rib

Excerpted from "What I Need to Know about Kidney Stones," National Institute of Diabetes and Digestive and Kidney Diseases (NIDDK), NIH Publication No. 07–4154, April 2007.

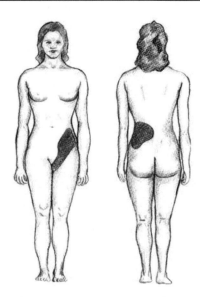

Figure 26.1. Pain in the shaded areas may be caused by a kidney stone.

cage, one on each side of the spine. The kidneys are sophisticated trash collectors. Every day, your kidneys process about 200 quarts of blood to sift out about two quarts of waste products and extra water. The wastes and extra water become urine, which flows to your bladder through tubes called ureters. Your bladder stores urine until you go to the bathroom.

The wastes in your blood come from the normal breakdown of active muscle and from the food you eat. Your body uses the food for energy and self-repair. After your body has taken what it needs from the food, wastes are sent to the blood. If your kidneys did not remove these wastes, they would build up in the blood and damage your body.

In addition to removing wastes, your kidneys help control blood pressure. They also help make red blood cells and keep your bones strong.

What is a kidney stone?

A kidney stone is a solid piece of material that forms in a kidney out of substances in the urine. A stone may stay in the kidney or break loose and travel down the urinary tract. A small stone may pass all the way out of the body without causing too much pain. A larger stone may get stuck in a ureter, the bladder, or the urethra. A problem stone can block the flow of urine and cause great pain.

188

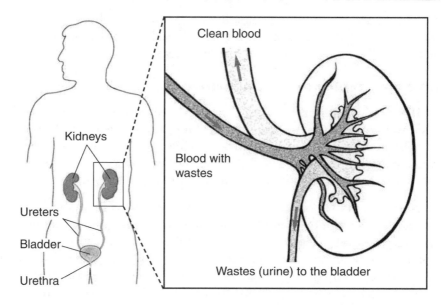

Figure 26.2. *Wastes removed from the blood go to the bladder.*

Doctors have found four major types of kidney stones.

1. The most common type of stone contains calcium. Calcium is a normal part of a healthy diet. Calcium that is not used by the bones and muscles goes to the kidneys. In most people, the kidneys flush out the extra calcium with the rest of the urine. People who have calcium stones keep the calcium in their kidneys. The calcium that stays behind joins with other waste products to form a stone. The most common combination is called calcium oxalate.

2. A struvite stone may form after an infection in the urinary system. These stones contain the mineral magnesium and the waste product ammonia.

3. A uric acid stone may form when the urine contains too much acid. If you tend to form uric acid stones, you may need to cut back on the amount of meat you eat.

4. Cystine stones are rare. Cystine is one of the building blocks that make up muscles, nerves, and other parts of the body. Cystine can build up in the urine to form a stone. The disease that causes cystine stones runs in families.

Kidney stones may be as small as a grain of sand or as large as a pearl. Some stones are even as big as golf balls. Stones may be smooth or jagged. They are usually yellow or brown.

How are problematic kidney stones treated?

If you have a stone that will not pass by itself, your doctor may need to take steps to get rid of it. In the past, the only way to remove a problem stone was through surgery. Now, doctors have new ways to remove problem stones. The following sections describe a few of these methods. Ask your doctor which method is right for you.

Shock waves: Your doctor can use a machine to send shock waves directly to the kidney stone. The shock waves break a large stone into small stones that will pass through your urinary system with your urine. The full name for this method is extracorporeal shock wave lithotripsy (ESWL). Lithotripsy is a Greek word that means stone crushing.

Two types of shock wave machines exist. With one machine, you sit in a tub of water. With most newer machines, you lie on a table. A health technician will use ultrasound or x-ray images to direct the sound waves to the stone.

Tunnel surgery: In tunnel surgery, the doctor makes a small cut into the patient's back and makes a narrow tunnel through the skin to the stone inside the kidney. With a special instrument that goes

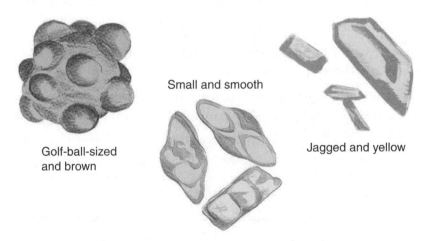

Golf-ball-sized and brown

Small and smooth

Jagged and yellow

Figure 26.3. Kidney stones vary is size and shape. These are not actual size.

through the tunnel, the doctor can find the stone and remove it. The technical name for this method is percutaneous nephrolithotomy.

Ureteroscope: A ureteroscope looks like a long wire. The doctor inserts it into the patient's urethra, passes it up through the bladder, and directs it to the ureter where the stone is located. The ureteroscope has a camera that allows the doctor to see the stone. A cage is used to catch the stone and pull it out, or the doctor may destroy it with a device inserted through the ureteroscope.

How will my doctor find out what kind of stone I have?

The best way for your doctor to find out what kind of stone you have is to test the stone itself. If you know that you are passing a stone, try to catch it in a strainer.

Your doctor may ask for a urine sample or take blood to find out what caused your stone. You may need to collect your urine for a 24-hour period. These tests will help your doctor find ways for you to avoid stones in the future.

Why do I need to know the kind of stone?

The therapy your doctor gives you depends on the type of stone you have. For example, a medicine that helps prevent calcium stones will not work if you have a struvite stone. The diet changes that help prevent uric acid stones may not work to prevent calcium stones. Therefore, careful analysis of the stone will help guide your treatment.

What can I do to avoid more stones?

Drink more water. Try to drink 12 full glasses of water a day. Drinking lots of water helps to flush away the substances that form stones in the kidneys.

You can also drink ginger ale, lemon-lime sodas, and fruit juices. But water is best. Limit your coffee, tea, and cola to one or two cups a day because the caffeine may cause you to lose fluid too quickly.

Your doctor may ask you to eat more of some foods and to cut back on other foods. For example, if you have a uric acid stone, your doctor may ask you to eat less meat, because meat breaks down to make uric acid.

If you are prone to forming calcium oxalate stones, you may need to limit foods that are high in oxalate. These foods include rhubarb, beets, spinach, and chocolate.

The doctor may give you medicines to prevent calcium and uric acid stones.

For More Information

American Urological Association Foundation
1000 Corporate Blvd., Suite 410
Linthicum, MD 21090
Toll-Free: 866-746-4282
Phone: 410-689-3700
Fax: 410-689-3800
Website: http://www.auafoundation.org
E-mail: patienteducation@auafoundation.org

National Kidney and Urologic Diseases Information Clearinghouse
3 Information Way
Bethesda, MD 20892-3580
Toll-Free: 800-891-5390
Fax: 703-738-4929
Website: http://www.kidney.niddk.nih.gov
E-mail: nkudic@info.niddk.nih.gov

National Kidney Foundation, Inc.
30 East 33rd St.
New York, NY 10016
Toll-Free: 800-622-9010
Phone: 212-889-2210
Fax: 212-689-9261
Website: http://www.kidney.org

Oxalosis and Hyperoxaluria Foundation
201 East 19th St., Suite 12E
New York, NY 10003
Toll-Free: 800-643-8699
Phone: 212-777-0470
Fax: 212-777-0471
Website: http://www.ohf.org

Chapter 27

Knee Problems

The knees provide stable support for the body. They also allow the legs to bend and straighten. Both flexibility and stability are needed to stand, walk, run, crouch, jump, and turn. Other parts of the body help the knees do their job including: bones, cartilage, muscles, ligaments, and tendons. If any of these parts are injured, the knee may hurt and not be able to do its job.

Who gets knee problems?

Men, women, and children can have knee problems. They occur in people of all races and ethnic backgrounds.

What causes knee problems?

Mechanical knee problems can be caused by:

- A direct blow or sudden movements that strain the knee.
- Osteoarthritis in the knee, resulting from wear and tear on its parts.

Inflammatory knee problems can be caused by certain rheumatic diseases, such as rheumatoid arthritis and systemic lupus erythematosus (lupus). These diseases cause swelling which can damage the knees permanently.

"What Are Knee Problems?" National Institute of Arthritis and Musculoskeletal and Skin Diseases (NIAMS), March 2006.

How are knee problems diagnosed?

Doctors diagnose knee problems by using the following:

- Medical history
- Physical examination
- Diagnostic tests (such as x-rays, bone scan, computed tomography (CT) scan, magnetic resonance imaging (MRI), arthroscopy, and biopsy)

How does arthritis affect the knees?

The most common type of arthritis of the knee is osteoarthritis. In this disease, the cartilage in the knee gradually wears away. Treatments for osteoarthritis include the following:

- Medicines to reduce pain, such as aspirin and acetaminophen
- Medicines to reduce swelling and inflammation, such as ibuprofen and nonsteroidal anti-inflammatory drugs (NSAIDs)
- Exercises to improve movement and strength
- Weight loss

Rheumatoid arthritis is another type of arthritis that affects the knee. In rheumatoid arthritis, the knee becomes inflamed and cartilage may be destroyed. The following treatments may be prescribed:

- Physical therapy
- Medications
- Knee replacement surgery (for a seriously damaged knee)

How do cartilage injuries and disorders affect the knees?

Chondromalacia occurs when the cartilage of the knee cap softens. This can be caused by injury, overuse, or muscle weakness, or if parts of the knee are out of alignment. Chondromalacia can develop if a blow to the knee cap tears off a piece of cartilage or a piece of cartilage containing a bone fragment.

The meniscus is a C-shaped piece of cartilage that acts like a pad between the femur (thigh bone) and tibia (shin bone). It is easily injured if the knee is twisted while bearing weight. A partial or total tear may occur. If the tear is tiny, the meniscus stays connected to the front and back of the knee. If the tear is large, the meniscus may be left hanging by a thread of cartilage. The seriousness of the injury depends on the location and the size of the tear.

Treatment for cartilage injuries includes the following:

- Exercises to strengthen muscles

- Electrical stimulation to strengthen muscles

- Surgery for severe injuries

How do ligament injuries affect the knees?

Two commonly injured ligaments in the knee are the anterior cruciate ligament (ACL) and the posterior cruciate ligament (PCL). An injury to these ligaments is sometimes called a "sprain." The ACL is most often stretched or torn (or both) by a sudden twisting motion. The PCL is usually injured by a direct impact, such as in an automobile accident or football tackle.

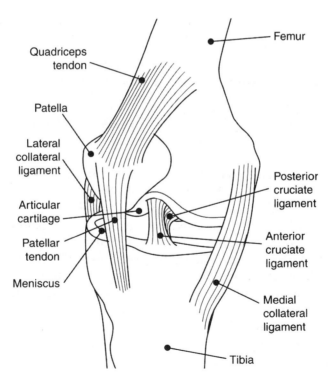

Figure 27.1. *Lateral View of the Knee*

The medial and lateral collateral ligaments are usually injured by a blow to the outer side of the knee. This can stretch and tear a ligament. These blows frequently occur in sports such as football or hockey.

Ligament injuries are treated with the following:

- Ice packs (right after the injury) to reduce swelling

- Exercises to strengthen muscles

- A brace

- Surgery (for more severe injuries)

How do tendon injuries and disorders affect the knees?

The three main types of tendon injuries and disorders are:

- tendonitis and ruptured tendons,

- Osgood-Schlatter disease, and

- iliotibial band syndrome.

Tendon injuries range from tendonitis (inflammation of a tendon) to a ruptured (torn) tendon. Torn tendons most often occur from:

- Overusing a tendon (particularly in some sports). The tendon stretches like a worn-out rubber band and becomes inflamed.

- Trying to break a fall. If thigh muscles contract, the tendon can tear. This is most likely to happen in older people with weak tendons.

One type of tendonitis of the knee is called jumper's knee. In sports that require jumping, such as basketball, the tendon can become inflamed or can tear.

Osgood-Schlatter disease is caused by stress or tension on part of the growth area of the upper shin bone. It causes swelling in the knee and upper part of the shin bone. It can happen if a person's tendon tears away from the bone, taking a piece of bone with it. Young people who run and jump while playing sports can have this type of injury.

Iliotibial band syndrome occurs when a tendon rubs over the outer bone of the knee causing swelling. It happens if the knee is overused for a long time. This sometimes occurs in sports training.

Treatment for tendon injuries and disorders includes the following:

- Rest

- Ice

- Elevation

- Medicines such as aspirin or ibuprofen to relieve pain and reduce swelling

- Limiting sports activity

- Exercise for stretching and strengthening

- A cast if there is a partial tear

- Surgery for complete tears or very severe injuries

What other injuries cause knee problems?

Osteochondritis dissecans occurs when not enough blood goes to part of the bone under a joint surface. The bone and cartilage gradually loosen and cause pain. Some cartilage may break off and cause sharp pain, weakness, and locking of the joint. A person with this condition may develop osteoarthritis. Surgery is the main treatment.

- If cartilage fragments have not broken loose, a surgeon may pin or screw them in place. This can stimulate new blood flow to the cartilage.

- If fragments are loose, the surgeon may scrape the cavity to reach fresh bone and add a bone graft to fix the fragments in position.

- Research is being done to investigate cartilage and tissue transplants.

Plica syndrome occurs when bands of tissue in the knee called plicae swell from overuse or injury. Following are treatments for this syndrome:

- Medicines such as aspirin or ibuprofen to reduce swelling

- Rest

- Ice

- Elastic bandage on the knee

- Exercises to strengthen muscles

- Cortisone injection into the plicae

- Surgery to remove the plicae if the first treatments do not fix the problem

197

What kinds of doctors treat knee problems?

Injuries and diseases of the knees are usually treated by an orthopaedist (a doctor who treats problems with bones, joints, ligaments, tendons, and muscles).

How can knee problems be prevented?

Some knee problems (such as those resulting from an accident) cannot be prevented. But many knee problems can be prevented by doing the following:

- Warm up before playing sports. Walking and stretching are good warm-up exercises. Stretching the muscles in the front and the back of the thighs is a good way to warm up the knees.

- Make the leg muscles strong by doing certain exercises (for example, walking up stairs, riding a stationary bicycle, or working out with weights).

- Avoid sudden changes in the intensity of exercise.

- Increase the force or duration of activity slowly.

- Wear shoes that fit and are in good condition.

- Maintain a healthy weight. Extra weight puts pressure on the knees.

What types of exercise are best for someone with knee problems?

Three types of exercise are best for people with arthritis:

- Range-of-motion exercises: These exercises help maintain or increase flexibility. They also help relieve stiffness in the knee.

- Strengthening exercises: These exercises help maintain or increase muscle strength. Strong muscles help support and protect joints with arthritis.

- Aerobic or endurance exercises: These exercises improve heart function and blood circulation. They also help control weight. Some studies show that aerobic exercise can reduce swelling in some joints.

Chapter 28

Muscle Pain

Definition

Muscle aches and pains are common and can involve more than one muscle. Muscle pain also can involve ligaments, tendons, and fascia, the soft tissues that connect muscles, bones, and organs.

Considerations

Muscle pain is most frequently related to tension, overuse, or muscle injury from exercise or physically-demanding work. In these situations, the pain tends to involve specific muscles and starts during or just after the activity. It is usually obvious which activity is causing the pain.

Muscle pain also can be a sign of conditions affecting your whole body, like some infections (including the flu) and disorders that affect connective tissues throughout the body (such as lupus).

One common cause of muscle aches and pain is fibromyalgia, a condition that includes tenderness in your muscles and surrounding soft tissue, sleep difficulties, fatigue, and headaches.

Causes

The most common causes are:

- Injury or trauma including sprains and strains

"Muscle Aches," © 2008 A.D.A.M., Inc. Reprinted with permission.

- Overuse: using a muscle too much, too soon, too often
- Tension or stress

Muscle pain may also be due to:

- Certain drugs, including:
  - ACE inhibitors for lowering blood pressure
  - Cocaine
  - Statins for lowering cholesterol
- Dermatomyositis
- Electrolyte imbalances like too little potassium or calcium
- Fibromyalgia
- Infections, including:
  - Influenza (the flu)
  - Lyme disease
  - Malaria
  - Muscle abscess
  - Polio
  - Rocky Mountain spotted fever
  - Trichinosis (roundworm)
- Lupus
- Polymyalgia rheumatica
- Polymyositis
- Rhabdomyolysis

Home Care

For muscle pain from overuse or injury, rest that body part and take acetaminophen or ibuprofen. Apply ice for the first 24–72 hours of an injury to reduce pain and inflammation. After that, heat often feels more soothing.

Muscle aches from overuse and fibromyalgia often respond well to massage. Gentle stretching exercises after a long rest period are also helpful.

Regular exercise can help restore proper muscle tone. Walking, cycling, and swimming are good aerobic activities to try. A physical therapist can teach you stretching, toning, and aerobic exercises to feel better and stay pain-free. Begin slowly and increase workouts gradually. Avoid high-impact aerobic activities and weight lifting when injured or while in pain.

Be sure to get plenty of sleep and try to reduce stress. Yoga and meditation are excellent ways to help you sleep and relax.

If home measures aren't working, call your doctor, who will consider prescription medication, physical therapy referral, or referral to a specialized pain clinic.

If your muscle aches are due to a specific disease, follow the instructions of your doctor to treat the primary illness.

When to Contact a Medical Professional

Call your doctor if:

- Your muscle pain persists beyond three days.

- You have severe, unexplained pain.

- You have any sign of infection, like swelling or redness around the tender muscle.

- You have poor circulation in the area where you have muscles aches (for example, in your legs).

- You have a tick bite or a rash.

- Your muscle pain has been associated with starting or changing doses of a medicine, such as a statin.

Call 911 if:

- You have sudden weight gain, water retention, or you are urinating less than usual.

- You are short of breath or have difficulty swallowing.

- You have muscle weakness or cannot move any part of your body.

- You have vomiting, a very stiff neck, or high fever.

What to Expect at Your Office Visit

Your doctor will perform a physical examination and ask questions about your muscle pain, such as:

- When did it start? How long did it last?

- Where is it exactly? Is it all over or only in a specific area?
- Is it always in the same location?
- What makes it better or worse?
- Do other symptoms occur at the same time, like joint pain, fever, vomiting, weakness, malaise, or difficulty using the affected muscle?
- Is there a pattern to the muscle aches?
- Have you taken any new medications lately?

Tests that may be done include:

- Complete blood count (CBC)
- Other blood tests to look at muscle enzymes (creatine kinase) and possibly a test for Lyme disease or a connective tissue disorder

Physical therapy may be helpful.

Prevention

- Warm up before exercising and cool down afterward.
- Stretch before and after exercising.
- Drink lots of fluids before, during, and after exercise.
- If you work in the same position most of the day (like sitting at a computer), stretch at least every hour.

References

Dannecker EA. Self-care behaviors for muscle pain. *J Pain*. 2004; 5(9): 521–527.

Goldenberg DL, Burckhardt C, Crofford L. Management of fibromyalgia syndrome. *JAMA*. 2004 Nov 17; 292(19): 2388–95.

Chapter 29

Neck Pain

Fast Facts

- Neck pain affects 10% of the population each year.

- Whiplash from motor vehicle accidents is a common cause of neck pain.

- The diagnosis of neck pain is determined by a medical history and physical examination, and rarely requires expensive or uncomfortable tests.

What Neck Pain Is

Neck pain is just that—pain in the neck. Pain can be localized to the cervical spine or may radiate down an arm (radiculopathy).

What Causes Neck Pain

Most episodes of neck pain are caused by mechanical disorders associated with gradual changes associated with aging, or with overuse of the neck or arms. About 10% of instances of neck pain are associated with systemic illnesses, such as polymyalgia rheumatica.

- Muscle strains usually related to sustained physical activity such as sitting at computer terminals for prolonged periods of time. Acute strain may occur after sleeping in an awkward position.

- Osteoarthritis resulting from the narrowing of the intervertebral discs located between the vertebrae of the spine. The adjacent vertebrae grow spurs in response to the increasing pressure placed on them. The bony growths can cause localized pain in the neck or arm related to nerve compression.

- Herniated intervertebral discs, which cause arm pain more frequently than neck pain. The pinching of a nerve in the neck causes severe arm pain (brachialgia). Disc herniations can cause a loss of function of the nerve including loss of reflex, sensation, or muscle strength.

- Spinal stenosis which is a narrowing of the spinal canal that causes compression of the spinal cord (cervical myelopathy). The narrowing is caused by disc bulging, bony spurs, and thickening of spinal ligaments. The squeezing of the spinal cord may not cause neck pain in all cases but is associated with leg numbness, weakness, and incontinence.

- Whiplash, an acceleration-deceleration injury to the soft tissues of the neck, most commonly caused by rear-impact motor vehicle accidents. The pain and stiffness associated with these accidents generally develop 24 to 48 hours after the injury.

Systemic disorders that can lead to neck pain include ankylosing spondylitis, rheumatoid arthritis, polymyalgia rheumatica, tumors, and infections.

Who Gets Neck Pain

About 10% of the population has an episode of neck pain each year. Neck pain may occur slightly more frequently in women than in men.

How Neck Pain Is Diagnosed

In most circumstances, a medical history and physical examination are the essential components of an evaluation required for diagnosis of neck disorders. On occasion, individuals who do not respond to initial therapy may undergo specialized radiographic tests, such as plain x-rays, magnetic resonance imaging (MRI) or computerized tomography (CT) to screen for additional involvement of soft tissues, ruptured discs, spinal stenosis, tumors, or nerve injuries.

How Neck Pain Is Treated

Maintaining motion is an important component of therapy for neck pain. The use of neck braces should be kept to a minimum.

While regular exercise should be discontinued until the neck pain is improved, movement of the neck is encouraged. Gradual movement in all planes of motion of the neck stretch muscles that may be excessively contracted.

Applying ice massages for 5–10 minutes at a time to a painful area within the first 48 hours of pain onset can help relieve pain as can heat, which relaxes the muscles. Heat should be applied for pains lasting greater than 48 hours. Over-the-counter pain relievers such as acetaminophen and non-steroidal anti-inflammatory drugs (NSAIDs), including aspirin, are frequently adequate to control episodes of neck pain, and muscle relaxants may help those with limited motion secondary to muscle tightness.

Individuals with increased stress may have contracted neck muscles. Massage therapy has proven helpful for those with chronic muscular neck pain.

A small minority of neck pain patients, particularly those with arm pain or signs of spinal cord compression, require cervical spine surgery.

Living with Neck Pain

The best way of living with neck pain is trying to prevent it. Do not sit at the computer for hours without getting up frequently to stretch the neck and back. Take the stress of the day out of your neck muscles and do your exercise routine. If you smoke, stop. Smoking is a predisposing factor for neck pain. If you are overweight, get into shape. Bottom line: pay attention to your body and exercise, eat right, and maintain a healthy lifestyle.

Points to Remember

- Neck pain is a common problem and is rarely associated with a systemic illness.

- The vast majority of individuals improve by taking over-the-counter medications and remaining active.

- Most individuals are better in one to two weeks; over 90 percent are healed in eight weeks.

For More Information

American College of Rheumatology
1800 Century Place, Suite 250
Atlanta, GA 30345
Phone: 404-633-3777
Fax: 404-633-1870
Website: http://www.rheumatology.org

Chapter 30

Nerve Pain

Chapter Contents

Section 30.1

Peripheral Neuropathy

Excerpted from "Peripheral Neuropathy Fact Sheet," National Institute of Neurological Disorders and Stroke (NINDS), NIH Publication No. 04–4853, January 10, 2008.

Peripheral neuropathy describes damage to the peripheral nervous system, the vast communications network that transmits information from the brain and spinal cord (the central nervous system) to every other part of the body. Peripheral nerves also send sensory information back to the brain and spinal cord, such as a message that the feet are cold or a finger is burned. Damage to the peripheral nervous system interferes with these vital connections. Like static on a telephone line, peripheral neuropathy distorts and sometimes interrupts messages between the brain and the rest of the body.

Because every peripheral nerve has a highly specialized function in a specific part of the body, a wide array of symptoms can occur when nerves are damaged. Some people may experience temporary numbness, tingling, and pricking sensations (paresthesia), sensitivity to touch, or muscle weakness. Others may suffer more extreme symptoms, including burning pain (especially at night), muscle wasting, paralysis, or organ or gland dysfunction. People may become unable to digest food easily, maintain safe levels of blood pressure, sweat normally, or experience normal sexual function. In the most extreme cases, breathing may become difficult or organ failure may occur.

Some forms of neuropathy involve damage to only one nerve and are called mononeuropathies. More often though, multiple nerves affecting all limbs are affected—called polyneuropathy. Occasionally, two or more isolated nerves in separate areas of the body are affected—called mononeuritis multiplex.

In acute neuropathies, such as Guillain-Barré syndrome, symptoms appear suddenly, progress rapidly, and resolve slowly as damaged nerves heal. In chronic forms, symptoms begin subtly and progress slowly. Some people may have periods of relief followed by relapse. Others may reach a plateau stage where symptoms stay the same for many months or years. Some chronic neuropathies worsen over time, but very few forms prove fatal unless complicated by other diseases. Occasionally the neuropathy is a symptom of another disorder.

In the most common forms of polyneuropathy, the nerve fibers (individual cells that make up the nerve) most distant from the brain and the spinal cord malfunction first. Pain and other symptoms often appear symmetrically, for example, in both feet followed by a gradual progression up both legs. Next, the fingers, hands, and arms may become affected, and symptoms can progress into the central part of the body. Many people with diabetic neuropathy experience this pattern of ascending nerve damage.

How are the peripheral neuropathies classified?

More than 100 types of peripheral neuropathy have been identified, each with its own characteristic set of symptoms, pattern of development, and prognosis. Impaired function and symptoms depend on the type of nerves—motor, sensory, or autonomic—which are damaged. Motor nerves control movements of all muscles under conscious control, such as those used for walking, grasping things, or talking. Sensory nerves transmit information about sensory experiences, such as the feeling of a light touch or the pain resulting from a cut. Autonomic nerves regulate biological activities that people do not control consciously, such as breathing, digesting food, and heart and gland functions. Although some neuropathies may affect all three types of nerves, others primarily affect one or two types. Therefore, doctors may use terms such as predominately motor neuropathy, predominately sensory neuropathy, sensory-motor neuropathy, or autonomic neuropathy to describe a patient's condition.

What are the symptoms of peripheral nerve damage?

Symptoms are related to the type of affected nerve and may be seen over a period of days, weeks, or years. Muscle weakness is the most common symptom of motor nerve damage. Other symptoms may include painful cramps and fasciculations (uncontrolled muscle twitching visible under the skin), muscle loss, bone degeneration, and changes in the skin, hair, and nails. These more general degenerative changes also can result from sensory or autonomic nerve fiber loss.

Sensory nerve damage causes a more complex range of symptoms because sensory nerves have a wider, more highly specialized range of functions. Larger sensory fibers enclosed in myelin (a fatty protein that coats and insulates many nerves) register vibration, light touch, and position sense. Damage to large sensory fibers lessens the ability to feel vibrations and touch, resulting in a general sense of numbness, especially in the hands and feet. People may feel as if they are wearing gloves and stockings even when they are not. Many patients cannot recognize by touch alone the shapes of small objects or distinguish between different shapes. This damage to sensory fibers may contribute to the loss of reflexes (as can motor nerve damage). Loss of position sense often makes people unable to coordinate complex movements like walking or fastening buttons, or to maintain their balance when their eyes are shut. Neuropathic pain is difficult to control and can seriously affect emotional well-being and overall quality of life. Neuropathic pain is often worse at night, seriously disrupting sleep and adding to the emotional burden of sensory nerve damage.

Smaller sensory fibers without myelin sheaths transmit pain and temperature sensations. Damage to these fibers can interfere with the ability to feel pain or changes in temperature. People may fail to sense that they have been injured from a cut or that a wound is becoming infected. Others may not detect pains that warn of impending heart attack or other acute conditions. (Loss of pain sensation is a particularly serious problem for people with diabetes, contributing to the high rate of lower limb amputations among this population.) Pain receptors in the skin can also become over-sensitized, so that people may feel severe pain (allodynia) from stimuli that are normally painless (for example, some may experience pain from bed sheets draped lightly over the body).

Symptoms of autonomic nerve damage are diverse and depend upon which organs or glands are affected. Autonomic nerve dysfunction can become life threatening and may require emergency medical care in cases when breathing becomes impaired or when the heart begins beating irregularly. Common symptoms of autonomic nerve damage include an inability to sweat normally, which may lead to heat intolerance; a loss of bladder control, which may cause infection or incontinence; and an inability to control muscles that expand or contract blood vessels to maintain safe blood pressure levels. A loss of control over blood pressure can cause dizziness, lightheadedness, or even fainting when a person moves suddenly from a seated to a standing position (a condition known as postural or orthostatic hypotension).

Gastrointestinal symptoms frequently accompany autonomic neuropathy. Nerves controlling intestinal muscle contractions often malfunction, leading to diarrhea, constipation, or incontinence. Many people also have problems eating or swallowing if certain autonomic nerves are affected.

What causes peripheral neuropathy?

Peripheral neuropathy may be either inherited or acquired. Causes of acquired peripheral neuropathy include physical injury (trauma) to a nerve, tumors, toxins, autoimmune responses, nutritional deficiencies, alcoholism, and vascular and metabolic disorders. Acquired peripheral neuropathies are grouped into three broad categories: those caused by systemic disease, those caused by trauma from external agents, and those caused by infections or autoimmune disorders affecting nerve tissue. One example of an acquired peripheral neuropathy is trigeminal neuralgia (also known as tic douloureux), in which damage to the trigeminal nerve (the large nerve of the head and face) causes episodic attacks of excruciating, lightning-like pain on one side of the face. In some cases, the cause is an earlier viral infection, pressure on the nerve from a tumor or swollen blood vessel, or, infrequently, multiple sclerosis. In many cases, however, a specific cause cannot be identified. Doctors usually refer to neuropathies with no known cause as idiopathic neuropathies.

Physical injury (trauma) is the most common cause of injury to a nerve. Injury or sudden trauma, such as from automobile accidents, falls, and sports-related activities, can cause nerves to be partially or completely severed, crushed, compressed, or stretched, sometimes so forcefully that they are partially or completely detached from the spinal cord. Less dramatic traumas also can cause serious nerve damage. Broken or dislocated bones can exert damaging pressure on neighboring nerves, and slipped disks between vertebrae can compress nerve fibers where they emerge from the spinal cord.

Systemic diseases—disorders that affect the entire body—often cause peripheral neuropathy. These disorders may include:

Metabolic and endocrine disorders. Nerve tissues are highly vulnerable to damage from diseases that impair the body's ability to transform nutrients into energy, process waste products, or manufacture the substances that make up living tissue. Diabetes mellitus, characterized by chronically high blood glucose levels, is a leading cause of peripheral neuropathy in the United States. About 60 percent to 70 percent of people with diabetes have mild to severe forms of nervous system damage.

Kidney disorders can lead to abnormally high amounts of toxic substances in the blood that can severely damage nerve tissue. A majority of patients who require dialysis because of kidney failure develop poly-neuropathy. Some liver diseases also lead to neuropathies as a result of chemical imbalances.

Hormonal imbalances can disturb normal metabolic processes and cause neuropathies. For example, an underproduction of thyroid hormones slows metabolism, leading to fluid retention and swollen tissues that can exert pressure on peripheral nerves. Overproduction of growth hormone can lead to acromegaly, a condition characterized by the abnormal enlargement of many parts of the skeleton, including the joints. Nerves running through these affected joints often become entrapped.

Vitamin deficiencies and alcoholism can cause widespread damage to nerve tissue. Vitamins E, B_1, B_6, B_{12}, and niacin are essential to healthy nerve function. Thiamine deficiency, in particular, is common among people with alcoholism because they often also have poor dietary habits. Thiamine deficiency can cause a painful neuropathy of the extremities. Some researchers believe that excessive alcohol consumption may, in itself, contribute directly to nerve damage, a condition referred to as alcoholic neuropathy.

Vascular damage and blood diseases can decrease oxygen supply to the peripheral nerves and quickly lead to serious damage to, or death of, nerve tissues, much as a sudden lack of oxygen to the brain can cause a stroke. Diabetes frequently leads to blood vessel constriction. Various forms of vasculitis (blood vessel inflammation) frequently cause vessel walls to harden, thicken, and develop scar tissue, decreasing their diameter and impeding blood flow. This category of nerve damage, in which isolated nerves in different areas are damaged, is called mononeuropathy multiplex or multifocal mononeuropathy.

Connective tissue disorders and chronic inflammation can cause direct and indirect nerve damage. When the multiple layers of protective tissue surrounding nerves become inflamed, the inflammation can spread directly into nerve fibers. Chronic inflammation also leads to the progressive destruction of connective tissue, making nerve fibers more vulnerable to compression injuries and infections. Joints can become inflamed and swollen and entrap nerves, causing pain.

Cancers and benign tumors can infiltrate or exert damaging pressure on nerve fibers. Tumors also can arise directly from nerve tissue cells. Widespread polyneuropathy is often associated with the neurofi-bromatoses, genetic diseases in which multiple benign tumors grow on nerve tissue. Neuromas, benign masses of overgrown nerve tissue that can develop after any penetrating injury that severs nerve fibers, generate very intense pain signals and sometimes engulf neighboring nerves, leading to further damage and even greater pain. Neuroma formation can be one element of a more widespread neuropathic pain condition called complex regional pain syndrome or reflex sympathetic dystrophy syndrome, which can be caused by traumatic injuries or surgical trauma. Paraneoplastic syndromes, a group of rare degenerative disorders that are triggered by a person's immune system response to a cancerous tumor, also can indirectly cause widespread nerve damage.

Repetitive stress frequently leads to entrapment neuropathies, a special category of compression injury. Cumulative damage can result from repetitive, forceful, awkward activities that require flexing of any group of joints for prolonged periods. The resulting irritation may cause ligaments, tendons, and muscles to become inflamed and swollen, constricting the narrow passageways through which some nerves pass. These injuries become more frequent during pregnancy, probably because weight gain and fluid retention also constrict nerve passageways.

Toxins can also cause peripheral nerve damage. People who are exposed to heavy metals (for example, arsenic, lead, mercury, thallium), industrial drugs, or environmental toxins frequently develop neuropathy. Certain anticancer drugs, anticonvulsants, antiviral agents, and antibiotics have side effects that can include peripheral nerve damage, thus limiting their long-term use.

Infections and autoimmune disorders can cause peripheral neuropathy. Viruses and bacteria that can attack nerve tissues include herpes varicella-zoster (shingles), Epstein-Barr virus, cytomegalovirus, and herpes simplex-members of the large family of human herpes viruses. These viruses severely damage sensory nerves, causing attacks of sharp, lightning-like pain. Postherpetic neuralgia often occurs after an attack of shingles and can be particularly painful.

The human immunodeficiency virus (HIV), which causes acquired immunodeficiency syndrome (AIDS), also causes extensive damage to the central and peripheral nervous systems. The virus can cause several different forms of neuropathy, each strongly associated with a specific stage of active immunodeficiency disease. A rapidly progressive, painful polyneuropathy affecting the feet and hands is often the first clinically apparent sign of HIV infection.

Lyme disease, diphtheria, and leprosy are bacterial diseases characterized by extensive peripheral nerve damage. Diphtheria and leprosy are now rare in the United States, but Lyme disease is on the rise. It can cause a wide range of neuropathic disorders, including a rapidly developing, painful polyneuropathy, often within a few weeks after initial infection by a tick bite.

Viral and bacterial infections can also cause indirect nerve damage by provoking conditions referred to as autoimmune disorders, in which specialized cells and antibodies of the immune system attack the body's own tissues. These attacks typically cause destruction of the nerve's myelin sheath or axon (the long fiber that extends out from the main nerve cell body).

Some neuropathies are caused by inflammation resulting from immune system activities rather than from direct damage by infectious organisms. Inflammatory neuropathies can develop quickly or slowly, and chronic forms can exhibit a pattern of alternating remission and relapse. Acute inflammatory demyelinating neuropathy, better known as Guillain-Barré syndrome, can damage motor, sensory, and autonomic nerve fibers. Most people recover from this syndrome although severe cases can be life threatening. Chronic inflammatory demyelinating polyneuropathy (CIDP), generally less dangerous, usually damages sensory and motor nerves, leaving autonomic nerves intact. Multifocal motor neuropathy is a form of inflammatory neuropathy that affects motor nerves exclusively; it may be chronic or acute.

Inherited forms of peripheral neuropathy are caused by inborn mistakes in the genetic code or by new genetic mutations. Some genetic errors lead to mild neuropathies with symptoms that begin in early adulthood and result in little, if any, significant impairment. More severe hereditary neuropathies often appear in infancy or childhood.

The most common inherited neuropathies are a group of disorders collectively referred to as Charcot-Marie-Tooth disease. These neuropathies result from flaws in genes responsible for manufacturing neurons or the myelin sheath. Hallmarks of typical Charcot-Marie-Tooth disease include extreme weakening and wasting of muscles in the lower legs and feet, gait abnormalities, loss of tendon reflexes, and numbness in the lower limbs.

How is peripheral neuropathy diagnosed?

Diagnosing peripheral neuropathy is often difficult because the symptoms are highly variable. A thorough neurological examination is usually required and involves taking an extensive patient history (including the patient's symptoms, work environment, social habits, exposure to any toxins, history of alcoholism, risk of HIV or other infectious disease, and family history of neurological disease), performing tests that may identify the cause of the neuropathic disorder, and conducting tests to determine the extent and type of nerve damage.

A general physical examination and related tests may reveal the presence of a systemic disease causing nerve damage. Blood tests can detect diabetes, vitamin deficiencies, liver or kidney dysfunction, other metabolic disorders, and signs of abnormal immune system activity. An examination of cerebrospinal fluid that surrounds the brain and spinal cord can reveal abnormal antibodies associated with neuropathy. More specialized tests may reveal other blood or cardiovascular diseases, connective tissue disorders, or malignancies. Tests of muscle strength, as well as evidence of cramps or fasciculations, indicate motor fiber involvement. Evaluation of a patient's ability to register vibration, light touch, body position, temperature, and pain reveals sensory nerve damage and may indicate whether small or large sensory nerve fibers are affected.

Based on the results of the neurological exam, physical exam, patient history, and any previous screening or testing, additional testing may be ordered to help determine the nature and extent of the neuropathy.

Computed tomography, or CT scan, is a noninvasive, painless process used to produce rapid, clear two-dimensional images of organs, bones, and tissues. X-rays are passed through the body at various angles and are detected by a computerized scanner. The data is processed and displayed as cross-sectional images, or "slices," of the internal structure of the body or organ. Neurological CT scans can detect bone and vascular irregularities, certain brain tumors and cysts, herniated disks, encephalitis, spinal stenosis (narrowing of the spinal canal), and other disorders.

Magnetic resonance imaging (MRI) can examine muscle quality and size, detect any fatty replacement of muscle tissue, and determine whether a nerve fiber has sustained compression damage. The MRI equipment creates a strong magnetic field around the body. Radio waves are then passed through the body to trigger a resonance signal that can be detected at different angles within the body. A computer processes this resonance into either a three-dimensional picture or a two-dimensional "slice" of the scanned area.

Electromyography (EMG) involves inserting a fine needle into a muscle to compare the amount of electrical activity present when muscles are at rest and when they contract. EMG tests can help differentiate between muscle and nerve disorders.

Nerve conduction velocity (NCV) tests can precisely measure the degree of damage in larger nerve fibers, revealing whether symptoms are being caused by degeneration of the myelin sheath or the axon. During this test, a probe electrically stimulates a nerve fiber which responds by generating its own electrical impulse. An electrode placed further along the nerve's pathway measures the speed of impulse transmission along the axon. Slow transmission rates and impulse blockage tend to indicate damage to the myelin sheath, while a reduction in the strength of impulses is a sign of axonal degeneration.

Nerve biopsy involves removing and examining a sample of nerve tissue, most often from the lower leg. Although this test can provide valuable information about the degree of nerve damage, it is an invasive procedure that is difficult to perform and the procedure may cause neuropathic side effects. Many experts do not believe that a biopsy is always needed for diagnosis.

Skin biopsy is a test in which doctors remove a thin skin sample and examine nerve fiber endings. This test offers some unique advantages over NCV tests and nerve biopsy. Unlike NCV, it can reveal damage present in smaller fibers; in contrast to conventional nerve biopsy, skin biopsy is less invasive, has fewer side effects, and is easier to perform.

What treatments are available?

No medical treatments now exist that can cure inherited peripheral neuropathy. However, there are therapies for many other forms. Any underlying condition is treated first, followed by symptomatic treatment. Peripheral nerves have the ability to regenerate, as long as the nerve cell itself has not been killed. Symptoms often can be controlled, and eliminating the causes of specific forms of neuropathy often can prevent new damage.

In general, adopting healthy habits—such as maintaining optimal weight, avoiding exposure to toxins, following a physician-supervised exercise program, eating a balanced diet, correcting vitamin deficiencies, and limiting or avoiding alcohol consumption—can reduce the physical and emotional effects of peripheral neuropathy. Active and passive forms of exercise can reduce cramps, improve muscle strength, and prevent muscle wasting in paralyzed limbs. Various dietary strategies can improve gastrointestinal symptoms. Timely treatment of injury can help prevent permanent damage. Quitting smoking is particularly important because smoking constricts the blood vessels that supply nutrients to the peripheral nerves and can worsen neuropathic symptoms. Self-care skills such as meticulous foot care and careful wound treatment in people with diabetes and others who have an impaired ability to feel pain can alleviate symptoms and improve quality of life. Such changes often create conditions that encourage nerve regeneration.

Systemic diseases frequently require more complex treatments. Strict control of blood glucose levels has been shown to reduce neuropathic symptoms and help people with diabetic neuropathy avoid further nerve damage. Inflammatory and autoimmune conditions leading to neuropathy can be controlled in several ways. Immunosuppressive drugs such as prednisone, cyclosporine, or azathioprine may be beneficial. Plasmapheresis—a procedure in which blood is removed, cleansed of immune system cells and antibodies, and then returned to the body—can limit inflammation or suppress immune system activity. High doses of immunoglobulins, proteins that function as antibodies, also can suppress abnormal immune system activity.

Neuropathic pain is often difficult to control. Mild pain may sometimes be alleviated by analgesics sold over the counter. Several classes of drugs have recently proved helpful to many patients suffering from more severe forms of chronic neuropathic pain. These include mexiletine, a drug developed to correct irregular heart rhythms (sometimes associated with severe side effects); several antiepileptic drugs, including gabapentin, phenytoin, and carbamazepine; and some classes of antidepressants, including tricyclics such as amitriptyline. Injections of local anesthetics such as lidocaine or topical patches containing lidocaine may relieve more intractable pain. In the most severe cases, doctors can surgically destroy nerves; however, the results are often temporary and the procedure can lead to complications.

Mechanical aids can help reduce pain and lessen the impact of physical disability. Hand or foot braces can compensate for muscle weakness or alleviate nerve compression. Orthopedic shoes can improve gait disturbances and help prevent foot injuries in people with a loss of pain sensation. If breathing becomes severely impaired, mechanical ventilation can provide essential life support.

Surgical intervention often can provide immediate relief from mononeuropathies caused by compression or entrapment injuries. Repair of a slipped disk can reduce pressure on nerves where they emerge from the spinal cord; the removal of benign or malignant tumors can also alleviate damaging pressure on nerves. Nerve entrapment often can be corrected by the surgical release of ligaments or tendons.

Section 30.2

Diabetic Neuropathy.

Excerpted from "Diabetic Neuropathies: The Nerve Damage of Diabetes," National Institute of Diabetes and Digestive and Kidney Diseases (NIDDK), NIH Publication No. 08–3185, February 2008.

Diabetic neuropathies are a family of nerve disorders caused by diabetes. People with diabetes can, over time, develop nerve damage throughout the body. Some people with nerve damage have no symptoms. Others may have symptoms such as pain, tingling, or numbness—loss of feeling—in the hands, arms, feet, and legs. Nerve problems can occur in every organ system, including the digestive tract, heart, and sex organs.

About 60 to 70 percent of people with diabetes have some form of neuropathy. People with diabetes can develop nerve problems at any time, but risk rises with age and longer duration of diabetes. The highest rates of neuropathy are among people who have had diabetes for at least 25 years. Diabetic neuropathies also appear to be more common in people who have problems controlling their blood glucose, also called blood sugar, as well as those with high levels of blood fat and blood pressure and those who are overweight.

Symptoms of Diabetic Neuropathies

Symptoms depend on the type of neuropathy and which nerves are affected. Some people with nerve damage have no symptoms at all. For others, the first symptom is often numbness, tingling, or pain in the feet. Symptoms are often minor at first, and because most nerve damage occurs over several years, mild cases may go unnoticed for a long time. Symptoms can involve the sensory, motor, and autonomic— or involuntary—nervous systems. In some people, mainly those with focal neuropathy, the onset of pain may be sudden and severe.

Symptoms of nerve damage may include the following:

- numbness, tingling, or pain in the toes, feet, legs, hands, arms, and fingers
- wasting of the muscles of the feet or hands
- indigestion, nausea, or vomiting
- diarrhea or constipation
- dizziness or faintness due to a drop in blood pressure after standing or sitting up
- problems with urination
- erectile dysfunction in men or vaginal dryness in women
- weakness

Symptoms that are not due to neuropathy, but often accompany it, include weight loss and depression.

Types of Diabetic Neuropathy

Diabetic neuropathy can be classified as peripheral, autonomic, proximal, or focal. Each affects different parts of the body in various ways.

- Peripheral neuropathy, the most common type of diabetic neuropathy, causes pain or loss of feeling in the toes, feet, legs, hands, and arms.

- Autonomic neuropathy causes changes in digestion, bowel and bladder function, sexual response, and perspiration. It can also affect the nerves that serve the heart and control blood pressure, as well as nerves in the lungs and eyes. Autonomic neuropathy can also cause hypoglycemia unawareness, a condition in which people no longer experience the warning symptoms of low blood glucose levels.

- Proximal neuropathy causes pain in the thighs, hips, or buttocks and leads to weakness in the legs.

- Focal neuropathy results in the sudden weakness of one nerve or a group of nerves, causing muscle weakness or pain. Any nerve in the body can be affected.

Peripheral Neuropathy

Peripheral neuropathy, also called distal symmetric neuropathy or sensorimotor neuropathy, is nerve damage in the arms and legs. Your feet and legs are likely to be affected before your hands and arms. Many people with diabetes have signs of neuropathy that a doctor could note but feel no symptoms themselves. Symptoms of peripheral neuropathy may include the following:

- numbness or insensitivity to pain or temperature
- a tingling, burning, or prickling sensation
- sharp pains or cramps
- extreme sensitivity to touch, even light touch
- loss of balance and coordination

These symptoms are often worse at night.

Peripheral neuropathy may also cause muscle weakness and loss of reflexes, especially at the ankle, leading to changes in the way a person walks. Foot deformities, such as hammertoes and the collapse of the midfoot, may occur. Blisters and sores may appear on numb areas of the foot because pressure or injury goes unnoticed. If foot injuries are not treated promptly, the infection may spread to the bone, and the foot may then have to be amputated. Some experts estimate that half of all such amputations are preventable if minor problems are caught and treated in time.

Autonomic Neuropathy

Autonomic neuropathy affects the nerves that control the heart, regulate blood pressure, and control blood glucose levels. Autonomic neuropathy also affects other internal organs, causing problems with digestion, respiratory function, urination, sexual response, and vision. In addition, the system that restores blood glucose levels to normal after a hypoglycemic episode may be affected, resulting in loss of the warning symptoms of hypoglycemia.

Hypoglycemia unawareness: Normally, symptoms such as shakiness, sweating, and palpitations occur when blood glucose levels drop below 70 milligrams (mg)/deciliter (dL). In people with autonomic neuropathy, symptoms may not occur, making hypoglycemia difficult to recognize. Problems other than neuropathy can also cause hypoglycemia unawareness.

Heart and blood vessels: The heart and blood vessels are part of the cardiovascular system, which controls blood circulation. Damage to nerves in the cardiovascular system interferes with the body's ability to adjust blood pressure and heart rate. As a result, blood pressure may drop sharply after sitting or standing, causing a person to feel light-headed or even to faint. Damage to the nerves that control heart rate can mean that your heart rate stays high, instead of rising and falling in response to normal body functions and physical activity.

Digestive system: Nerve damage to the digestive system most commonly causes constipation. Damage can also cause the stomach to empty too slowly, a condition called gastroparesis. Severe gastroparesis can lead to persistent nausea and vomiting, bloating, and loss of appetite. Gastroparesis can also make blood glucose levels fluctuate widely, due to abnormal food digestion.

Nerve damage to the esophagus may make swallowing difficult, while nerve damage to the bowels can cause constipation alternating with frequent, uncontrolled diarrhea, especially at night. Problems with the digestive system can lead to weight loss.

Urinary tract and sex organs: Autonomic neuropathy often affects the organs that control urination and sexual function. Nerve damage can prevent the bladder from emptying completely, allowing bacteria to grow in the bladder and kidneys and causing urinary tract infections. When the nerves of the bladder are damaged, urinary incontinence may result because a person may not be able to sense when the bladder is full or control the muscles that release urine.

Autonomic neuropathy can also gradually decrease sexual response in men and women, although the sex drive may be unchanged. A man may be unable to have erections or may reach sexual climax without ejaculating normally. A woman may have difficulty with arousal, lubrication, or orgasm.

Sweat glands: Autonomic neuropathy can affect the nerves that control sweating. When nerve damage prevents the sweat glands from working properly, the body cannot regulate its temperature as it should. Nerve damage can also cause profuse sweating at night or while eating.

Eyes: Finally, autonomic neuropathy can affect the pupils of the eyes, making them less responsive to changes in light. As a result, a person may not be able to see well when a light is turned on in a dark room or may have trouble driving at night.

Proximal Neuropathy

Proximal neuropathy, sometimes called lumbosacral plexus neuropathy, femoral neuropathy, or diabetic amyotrophy, starts with pain in the thighs, hips, buttocks, or legs, usually on one side of the body. This type of neuropathy is more common in those with type 2 diabetes and in older adults with diabetes. Proximal neuropathy causes weakness in the legs and the inability to go from a sitting to a standing position without help. Treatment for weakness or pain is usually needed. The length of the recovery period varies, depending on the type of nerve damage.

Focal Neuropathy

Focal neuropathy appears suddenly and affects specific nerves, most often in the head, torso, or leg. Focal neuropathy may cause the following:

- inability to focus the eye
- double vision
- aching behind one eye
- paralysis on one side of the face, called Bell's palsy
- severe pain in the lower back or pelvis
- pain in the front of a thigh
- pain in the chest, stomach, or side
- pain on the outside of the shin or inside of the foot

- chest or abdominal pain that is sometimes mistaken for heart disease, a heart attack, or appendicitis

Focal neuropathy is painful and unpredictable and occurs most often in older adults with diabetes. However, it tends to improve by itself over weeks or months and does not cause long-term damage.

People with diabetes also tend to develop nerve compressions, also called entrapment syndromes. One of the most common is carpal tunnel syndrome, which causes numbness and tingling of the hand and sometimes muscle weakness or pain. Other nerves susceptible to entrapment may cause pain on the outside of the shin or the inside of the foot.

Preventing Diabetic Neuropathies

The best way to prevent neuropathy is to keep your blood glucose levels as close to the normal range as possible. Maintaining safe blood glucose levels protects nerves throughout your body.

Diagnosing Diabetic Neuropathies

Doctors diagnose neuropathy on the basis of symptoms and a physical exam. During the exam, your doctor may check blood pressure, heart rate, muscle strength, reflexes, and sensitivity to position changes, vibration, temperature, or light touch.

Foot Exams

Experts recommend that people with diabetes have a comprehensive foot exam each year to check for peripheral neuropathy. People diagnosed with peripheral neuropathy need more frequent foot exams. A comprehensive foot exam assesses the skin, muscles, bones, circulation, and sensation of the feet. Your doctor may assess protective sensation or feeling in your feet by touching your foot with a nylon monofilament—similar to a bristle on a hairbrush—attached to a wand or by pricking your foot with a pin. People who cannot sense pressure from a pinprick or monofilament have lost protective sensation and are at risk for developing foot sores that may not heal properly. The doctor may also check temperature perception or use a tuning fork, which is more sensitive than touch pressure, to assess vibration perception.

Other Tests

The doctor may perform other tests as part of your diagnosis.

- **Nerve conduction studies or electromyography** are sometimes used to help determine the type and extent of nerve damage. Nerve conduction studies check the transmission of electrical current through a nerve. Electromyography shows how well muscles respond to electrical signals transmitted by nearby nerves. These tests are rarely needed to diagnose neuropathy.

- **A check of heart rate variability** shows how the heart responds to deep breathing and to changes in blood pressure and posture.

- **Ultrasound** uses sound waves to produce an image of internal organs. An ultrasound of the bladder and other parts of the urinary tract, for example, can show how these organs preserve a normal structure and whether the bladder empties completely after urination.

Treatment of Diabetic Neuropathies

The first treatment step is to bring blood glucose levels within the normal range to help prevent further nerve damage. Blood glucose monitoring, meal planning, physical activity, and diabetes medicines or insulin will help control blood glucose levels. Symptoms may get worse when blood glucose is first brought under control, but over time, maintaining lower blood glucose levels helps lessen symptoms. Good blood glucose control may also help prevent or delay the onset of further problems. As scientists learn more about the underlying causes of neuropathy, new treatments may become available to help slow, prevent, or even reverse nerve damage.

As described in the following sections, additional treatment depends on the type of nerve problem and symptom. If you have problems with your feet, your doctor may refer you to a foot care specialist.

Pain Relief

Doctors usually treat painful diabetic neuropathy with oral medications, although other types of treatments may help some people. People with severe nerve pain may benefit from a combination of medications or treatments. Talk with your health care provider about options for treating your neuropathy.

Medications used to help relieve diabetic nerve pain include the following:

- Tricyclic antidepressants, such as amitriptyline, imipramine, and desipramine (Norpramin, Pertofrane)

- Other types of antidepressants, such as duloxetine (Cymbalta), venlafaxine, bupropion (Wellbutrin), paroxetine (Paxil), and citalopram (Celexa)

- Anticonvulsants, such as pregabalin (Lyrica), gabapentin (Gabarone, Neurontin), carbamazepine, and lamotrigine (Lamictal)

- Opioids and opioid-like drugs, such as controlled-release oxycodone, an opioid; and tramadol (Ultram), an opioid that also acts as an antidepressant

Duloxetine and pregabalin are approved by the U.S. Food and Drug Administration specifically for treating painful diabetic peripheral neuropathy.

You do not have to be depressed for an antidepressant to help relieve your nerve pain. All medications have side effects, and some are not recommended for use in older adults or those with heart disease. Because over-the-counter pain medicines such as acetaminophen and ibuprofen may not work well for treating most nerve pain and can have serious side effects, some experts recommend avoiding these medications.

Treatments that are applied to the skin—typically to the feet—include capsaicin cream and lidocaine patches. Studies suggest that nitrate sprays or patches for the feet may relieve pain. Studies of alpha-lipoic acid, an antioxidant, and evening primrose oil have shown that they can help relieve symptoms and may improve nerve function.

A device called a bed cradle can keep sheets and blankets from touching sensitive feet and legs. Acupuncture, biofeedback, or physical therapy may help relieve pain in some people. Treatments that involve electrical nerve stimulation, magnetic therapy, and laser or light therapy may be helpful but need further study. Researchers are also studying several new therapies in clinical trials.

Gastrointestinal Problems

To relieve mild symptoms of gastroparesis—indigestion, belching, nausea, or vomiting—doctors suggest eating small, frequent meals; avoiding fats; and eating less fiber. When symptoms are severe, doctors may prescribe erythromycin to speed digestion, metoclopramide to speed digestion and help relieve nausea, or other medications to help regulate digestion or reduce stomach acid secretion.

To relieve diarrhea or other bowel problems, doctors may prescribe an antibiotic such as tetracycline, or other medications as appropriate.

Dizziness and Weakness

Sitting or standing slowly may help prevent the lightheadedness, dizziness, or fainting associated with blood pressure and circulation problems. Raising the head of the bed or wearing elastic stockings may also help. Some people benefit from increased salt in the diet and treatment with salt-retaining hormones. Others benefit from high blood pressure medications. Physical therapy can help when muscle weakness or loss of coordination is a problem.

Urinary and Sexual Problems

To clear up a urinary tract infection, the doctor will probably prescribe an antibiotic. Drinking plenty of fluids will help prevent another infection. People who have incontinence should try to urinate at regular intervals—every three hours, for example—since they may not be able to tell when the bladder is full.

To treat erectile dysfunction in men, the doctor will first do tests to rule out a hormonal cause. Several methods are available to treat erectile dysfunction caused by neuropathy. Medicines are available to help men have and maintain erections by increasing blood flow to the penis. Some are oral medications and others are injected into the penis or inserted into the urethra at the tip of the penis. Mechanical vacuum devices can also increase blood flow to the penis. Another option is to surgically implant an inflatable or semirigid device in the penis.

Vaginal lubricants may be useful for women when neuropathy causes vaginal dryness. To treat problems with arousal and orgasm, the doctor may refer women to a gynecologist.

Foot Care

People with neuropathy need to take special care of their feet. The nerves to the feet are the longest in the body and are the ones most often affected by neuropathy. Loss of sensation in the feet means that sores or injuries may not be noticed and may become ulcerated or infected. Circulation problems also increase the risk of foot ulcers.

More than half of all lower-limb amputations in the United States occur in people with diabetes—86,000 amputations per year. Doctors estimate that nearly half of the amputations caused by neuropathy and poor circulation could have been prevented by careful foot care.

Follow these steps to take care of your feet:

- Clean your feet daily, using warm—not hot—water and a mild soap. Avoid soaking your feet. Dry them with a soft towel and dry carefully between your toes.

- Inspect your feet and toes every day for cuts, blisters, redness, swelling, calluses, or other problems. Use a mirror—laying a mirror on the floor works well—or get help from someone else if you cannot see the bottoms of your feet. Notify your health care provider of any problems.

- Moisturize your feet with lotion, but avoid getting the lotion between your toes.

- After a bath or shower, file corns and calluses gently with a pumice stone.

- Each week or when needed, cut your toenails to the shape of your toes and file the edges with an emery board.

- Always wear shoes or slippers to protect your feet from injuries. Prevent skin irritation by wearing thick, soft, seamless socks.

- Wear shoes that fit well and allow your toes to move. Break in new shoes gradually by first wearing them for only an hour at a time.

- Before putting your shoes on, look them over carefully and feel the insides with your hand to make sure they have no tears, sharp edges, or objects in them that might injure your feet.

- If you need help taking care of your feet, make an appointment to see a foot doctor, also called a podiatrist.

Points to Remember

- Diabetic neuropathies are nerve disorders caused by many of the abnormalities common to diabetes, such as high blood glucose.

- Neuropathy can affect nerves throughout the body, causing numbness and sometimes pain in the hands, arms, feet, or legs, and problems with the digestive tract, heart, sex organs, and other body systems.

- Treatment first involves bringing blood glucose levels within the normal range. Good blood glucose control may help prevent or delay the onset of further problems.

- Foot care is an important part of treatment. People with neuropathy need to inspect their feet daily for any injuries. Untreated injuries increase the risk of infected foot sores and amputation.

- Treatment also includes pain relief and other medications as needed, depending on the type of nerve damage.

- Smoking significantly increases the risk of foot problems and amputation. If you smoke, ask your health care provider for help with quitting.

Section 30.3

Glossopharyngeal Neuralgia

"Glossopharyngeal Neuralgia Information Page," National Institute of Neurological Disorders and Stroke (NINDS), January 10, 2008.

What is glossopharyngeal neuralgia?

Glossopharyngeal neuralgia (GN) is a rare pain syndrome that affects the glossopharyngeal nerve (the ninth cranial nerve that lies deep within the neck) and causes sharp, stabbing pulses of pain in the back of the throat and tongue, the tonsils, and the middle ear. The excruciating pain of GN can last for a few seconds to a few minutes, and may return multiple times in a day or once every few weeks. Many individuals with GN relate the attacks of pain to specific trigger factors such as swallowing, drinking cold liquids, sneezing, coughing, talking, clearing the throat, and touching the gums or inside the mouth. GN can be caused by compression of the glossopharyngeal nerve, but in some cases, no cause is evident. Like trigeminal neuralgia, it is associated with multiple sclerosis. GN primarily affects the elderly.

Is there any treatment?

Most doctors will attempt to treat the pain first with drugs. Some individuals respond well to anticonvulsant drugs, such as carbamazepine and gabapentin. Surgical options, including nerve resection, tractotomy, or microvascular decompression, should be considered when individuals either do not respond to, or stop responding to, drug therapy. Surgery is usually successful at ending the cycles of pain, although there may be some sensory loss in the mouth, throat, or tongue.

What is the prognosis?

Some individuals recover from an initial attack and never have another. Others will experience clusters of attacks followed by periods of short or long remission. Individuals may lose weight if they fear that chewing, drinking, or eating will cause an attack.

Section 30.4

Paresthesia

"Paresthesia Information Page," National Institute of Neurological Disorders and Stroke (NINDS), April 12, 2007.

What is paresthesia?

Paresthesia refers to a burning or prickling sensation that is usually felt in the hands, arms, legs, or feet, but can also occur in other parts of the body. The sensation, which happens without warning, is usually painless and described as tingling or numbness, skin crawling, or itching.

Most people have experienced temporary paresthesia—a feeling of "pins and needles"—at some time in their lives when they have sat with legs crossed for too long, or fallen asleep with an arm crooked under their head. It happens when sustained pressure is placed on a nerve. The feeling quickly goes away once the pressure is relieved.

Chronic paresthesia is often a symptom of an underlying neurological disease or traumatic nerve damage. Paresthesia can be caused by disorders affecting the central nervous system, such as stroke and transient ischemic attacks (mini-strokes), multiple sclerosis, transverse myelitis, and encephalitis. A tumor or vascular lesion pressed up against the brain or spinal cord can also cause paresthesia. Nerve entrapment syndromes, such as carpal tunnel syndrome, can damage peripheral nerves and cause paresthesia accompanied by pain. Diagnostic evaluation is based on determining the underlying condition causing the paresthetic sensations. An individual's medical history, physical examination, and laboratory tests are essential for the diagnosis. Physicians may order additional tests depending on the suspected cause of the paresthesia.

Is there any treatment?

The appropriate treatment for paresthesia depends on accurate diagnosis of the underlying cause.

What is the prognosis?

The prognosis for those with paresthesia depends on the severity of the sensations and the associated disorders.

What research is being done?

The National Institute of Neurological disorders and Stroke (NINDS) supports research on disorders of the brain, spinal cord, and peripheral nerves that can cause paresthesia. The goals of this research are to increase scientific understanding of these disorders and to find ways to prevent, treat, and cure them.

Chapter 31

Osteonecrosis (Avascular Necrosis)

Osteonecrosis is a disease resulting from the temporary or permanent loss of blood supply to the bones. Without blood, the bone tissue dies, and ultimately the bone may collapse. If the process involves the bones near a joint, it often leads to collapse of the joint surface. Osteonecrosis is also known as avascular necrosis, aseptic necrosis, and ischemic necrosis. Osteonecrosis affects both men and women. It can occur in people of any age, from children to the elderly. However, it is most common in people in their thirties, forties, and fifties.

Although it can happen in any bone, osteonecrosis most commonly affects the ends (epiphysis) of the femur, the bone extending from the knee joint to the hip joint. Other common sites include the upper arm bone, knees, shoulders, and ankles. The disease may affect just one bone, more than one bone at the same time, or more than one bone at different times. According to the American Academy of Orthopaedic Surgeons, 10,000 to 20,000 people develop osteonecrosis each year, and most of them are between 20 and 50 years of age. Osteonecrosis is the underlying diagnosis in approximately ten percent of hip replacements.

Causes of Osteonecrosis

Osteonecrosis is caused by impaired blood supply to the bone, but it is not always clear what causes that impairment. Osteonecrosis

Excerpted from "Questions and Answers about Osteonecrosis (Avascular Necrosis)," National Institute of Arthritis and Musculoskeletal and Skin Diseases (NIAMS), NIH Publication No. 06–4857, March 2006.

often occurs in people with certain risk factors (such as high-dose corticosteroid use and excessive alcohol intake) and medical conditions. However, it also affects people with no health problems and for no known reason. Following are some potential causes of osteonecrosis and other health conditions associated with its development.

Steroid Medications

Aside from injury, one of the most common causes of osteonecrosis is the use of corticosteroid medications such as prednisone. Studies suggest that long-term use of oral or intravenous (IV) corticosteroids is associated with nontraumatic osteonecrosis. Patients should discuss concerns about steroid use with their doctor.

Alcohol Use

Excessive alcohol use is another common cause of osteonecrosis. People who drink alcohol in excess can develop fatty substances that may block blood vessels, causing a decreased blood supply to the bones.

Injury

When a fracture, a dislocation, or some other joint injury occurs, the blood vessels may be damaged. This can interfere with the blood circulation to the bone and lead to trauma-related osteonecrosis. In fact, studies suggest that hip dislocation and hip fractures are major risk factors for osteonecrosis.

Increased pressure within the bone may be another cause of osteonecrosis. When there is too much pressure within the bone, the blood vessels narrow, making it hard for them to deliver enough blood to the bone cells. The cause of increased pressure is not fully understood.

Other Risk Factors

Other risk factors for osteonecrosis include radiation therapy, chemotherapy, and organ transplantation (particularly kidney transplantation). Osteonecrosis is also associated with a number of medical conditions, including cancer, lupus, blood disorders, Gaucher disease, Caisson disease, gout, vasculitis, osteoarthritis, and osteoporosis.

Symptoms

In the early stages of osteonecrosis, people may not have any symptoms. As the disease progresses, however, most experience joint pain.

At first, the pain occurs only when putting weight on the affected joint. Later, it occurs even when resting. Pain usually develops gradually, and may be mild or severe. If osteonecrosis progresses and the bone and surrounding joint surface collapse, pain may develop or increase dramatically. Pain may be severe enough to limit range of motion in the affected joint. In some cases, particularly those involving the hip, disabling osteoarthritis may develop. The period of time between the first symptoms and loss of joint function is different for each person, but it typically ranges from several months to more than a year.

Diagnosing Osteonecrosis

After performing a complete physical examination and asking about the patient's medical history, the doctor may use one or more bone imaging techniques to diagnose osteonecrosis. As with many other diseases, early diagnosis increases the chances of treatment success. The tests described below may be used to determine the amount of bone affected and how far the disease has progressed.

X-Ray

A radiograph, or x-ray, is probably the first test the doctor will recommend. A simple way to produce pictures of bones, an x-ray is often useful in diagnosing the cause of joint pain. For osteonecrosis, however, x-rays are not sensitive enough to detect bone changes in the early stages of the disease. So if the x-ray is normal, the doctor may order more tests. In later stages of osteonecrosis, x-rays may show bone damage, and once the diagnosis is made, they are often used to monitor disease progression.

Magnetic Resonance Imaging (MRI)

Research studies have shown that MRI is the most sensitive method for diagnosing osteonecrosis in the early stages. Unlike x-rays, bone scans, and CT (computed/computerized tomography) scans, MRI detects chemical changes in the bone marrow. MRI provides the doctor with a picture of the affected area and the bone-rebuilding process. In addition, MRI may show diseased areas that are not yet causing any symptoms. Some doctors caution against aggressive treatment of osteonecrosis that has been detected by MRI but is not causing symptoms. One study has shown evidence that for a select group of patients in the early stages of osteonecrosis, the disease may improve spontaneously.

Computed/Computerized Tomography (CT scan)

A CT scan is an imaging technique that provides the doctor with a three-dimensional picture of the bone. It also shows slices of the bone, making the picture much clearer than x-rays and bone scans. Some doctors disagree about the usefulness of this test to diagnose osteonecrosis. Although a diagnosis usually can be made without a CT scan, the technique may be useful in determining the extent of bone damage. CT scans are less sensitive than MRIs.

Bone Scan

A type of test called technetium-99m bone scanning is used most commonly in patients who have normal x-rays and no risk factors for osteonecrosis. In this test, a harmless radioactive material is injected through an intravenous line, and a picture of the bone is taken with a special camera. The picture shows how the injected material travels through blood vessels in bone. A single bone scan finds all areas in the body that are affected, thus reducing the need to expose the patient to more radiation.

Biopsy

A biopsy is a surgical procedure in which a tissue sample from the affected bone is removed and studied. Although a biopsy is a conclusive way to diagnose osteonecrosis, it is rarely used because it requires surgery.

Functional Evaluation of Bone

Tests to measure the pressure inside a bone may be used when the doctor strongly suspects that a patient has osteonecrosis, despite normal results of x-rays, bone scans, and MRI. These tests are very sensitive for detecting increased pressure within the bone, but they require surgery.

Treatments for Osteonecrosis

Appropriate treatment for osteonecrosis is necessary to keep joints from breaking down. Without treatment, most people with the disease will experience severe pain and limitation in movement within two years. To determine the most appropriate treatment, the doctor considers the following:

- the age of the patient
- the stage of the disease (early or late)

- the location and whether bone is affected over a small or large area

- the underlying cause of osteonecrosis (With an ongoing cause such as corticosteroid or alcohol use, treatment may not work unless use of the substance is stopped.)

The goal in treating osteonecrosis is to improve the patient's use of the affected joint, stop further damage to the bone, and ensure bone and joint survival. To reach these goals, the doctor may use one or more of the following surgical or nonsurgical treatments.

Nonsurgical Treatments

Usually, doctors will begin with nonsurgical treatments, alone or in combination. Unfortunately, although these treatments may relieve pain or help in the short term, for most people they do not bring lasting improvement.

- **Medications:** Nonsteroidal anti-inflammatory drugs (NSAIDs) are often prescribed to reduce pain. People with clotting disorders may be given blood thinners to reduce clots that block the blood supply to the bone. Cholesterol-lowering medications may be used to reduce fatty substances (lipids) that increase with corticosteroid treatment (a major risk factor for osteonecrosis). In one study, people who took cholesterol-lowering medications called statins along with corticosteroids significantly reduced the risk of developing osteonecrosis in the first place.

- **Reduced weightbearing:** If osteonecrosis is diagnosed early, the doctor may begin treatment by having the patient remove weight from the affected joint. The doctor may recommend limiting activities or using crutches. In some cases, reduced weightbearing can slow the damage caused by osteonecrosis and permit natural healing. When combined with pain medication, reduced weightbearing can be an effective way to avoid or delay surgery for some patients.

- **Range-of-motion exercises:** An exercise program involving the affected joints may help keep them mobile and increase their range of motion.

- **Electrical stimulation:** This treatment has been used in several centers to induce bone growth, and in some studies has been helpful when used prior to femoral head collapse.

Surgical Treatment

A number of different surgical procedures are used to treat osteonecrosis. Most people with osteonecrosis will eventually need surgery.

- **Core decompression:** This surgical procedure removes the inner cylinder of bone, which reduces pressure within the bone, increases blood flow to the bone, and allows more blood vessels to form. Core decompression works best in people who are in the earliest stages of osteonecrosis, often before the collapse of the joint. This procedure sometimes reduces pain and slows the progression of bone and joint destruction.

- **Osteotomy:** This treatment involves reshaping the bone to reduce stress on the affected area. Recovery can be a lengthy process, requiring 3–12 months of very limited activities. This procedure is most effective for patients with early-stage osteonecrosis and those with a small area of affected bone.

- **Bone graft:** This is the transplantation of healthy bone from another part of the body. It is often used to support a joint after core decompression. In many cases, the surgeon will use what is called a vascular graft—which includes an artery and vein—to increase the blood supply to the affected area. Recovery from a bone graft can take from 6–12 months. The procedure is complex and its effectiveness is unproven. Clinical studies are underway to determine its effectiveness.

- **Arthroplasty/total joint replacement:** Total joint replacement is the treatment of choice in late-stage osteonecrosis and when the joint is destroyed. In this surgery, the diseased joint is replaced with artificial parts. Total joint replacement, or sometimes femoral head resurfacing, is often recommended for people for whom other efforts to preserve the joint have failed. Various types of replacements are available, and people should discuss specific needs with their doctor.

For most people with osteonecrosis, treatment is an ongoing process. Depending upon the stage of the disease, doctors may first recommend the least complex or nonoperative treatment plans, such as medication or reduced weightbearing. If these modalities are unsuccessful, surgical treatments may be needed. It is important that patients carefully follow instructions about activity limitations and work closely with their doctors to ensure that appropriate treatments are used.

Chapter 32

Paget Disease of Bone

Facts to Know about Paget Disease

Paget disease of bone causes bones to grow larger and weaker than normal. The disease may affect one or more bones but does not spread from affected bones to other bones in the body. You can have Paget disease in any bone in your body, but most people have it in their pelvis, skull, spine, or leg bones. These bones may become misshapen, and they can break more easily because they are weaker than normal bones. Some people with Paget disease feel pain in these bones, too.

An estimated one million people in the U.S. have Paget disease, or about 1.3 people per 100 men and women age 45–74. The disease is more common in older people and those of Northern European heritage. Men are about twice as likely as women to have the disease.

Is Paget disease of bone a form of arthritis?

People with Paget disease often have arthritis at the same time, but they are different diseases. Sometimes Paget disease is confused with arthritis because the pain from Paget disease may be located on

This chapter includes text from "Facts a New Patient Needs to Know about Paget's Disease of Bone," National Institute of Arthritis and Musculoskeletal and Skin Diseases (NIAMS), January 2008; and "Pain and Paget's Disease of Bone," NIAMS, January 2008.

the part of the bone closest to a joint. So, it may feel a lot like the joint pain of arthritis. Paget disease can cause arthritis over time when enlarged and misshapen bones put extra stress on nearby joints. Your doctor may use several tests to help tell if you have Paget disease or not.

How did I get Paget disease?

Doctors are not sure what causes the disease. Some people have hereditary Paget disease, which means it runs in their family and was passed down by their parents. But most people do not have any relatives with Paget disease. Doctors think a virus also may be the cause of Paget disease in some cases. They are studying different kinds of viruses to try to find ones that may cause the disease.

Will my Paget disease get worse? What should I expect?

Paget disease does not affect everyone in the same way. Some people have a very mild case with few or no symptoms. Other people have symptoms and complications. Pain is the most common symptom. Depending on which of your bones are affected by Paget disease, you might have other symptoms and complications, such as those listed in Table 32.1.

Although it is rare, the most serious complication of Paget disease is bone cancer.

Table 32.1. Paget Disease Location and Possible Symptoms

If you have Paget disease here:	You may have some of these symptoms and complications:
Pelvis	Pain, arthritis in the hip joint
Skull	Enlarged head, hearing loss, headaches
Spine	Curved spine, back pain, damage to nerves causing such problems as tingling and numbness
Leg	Bowed legs, pain, arthritis in the hip and knee joints

Will my children get this disease?

Although Paget disease does not always run in families, research suggests that a close relative of someone with Paget disease is seven times more likely to develop the disease than someone without an affected relative. Finding and treating Paget disease early is important, so some doctors recommend that children, brothers, and sisters of a person with Paget disease be tested for the disease every two to three years after the age of 40.

To screen for Paget disease, a doctor uses the serum alkaline phosphatase (SAP) test. If the SAP level is high, suggesting that there might be Paget disease, the doctor can do a test called a bone scan to learn which bones may be affected. The doctor will then order an x-ray of the affected bones to make sure the diagnosis of Paget disease is correct.

Pain and Paget Disease of Bone

Types of Pain

Paget disease can cause several different kinds of pain.

Bone pain: Small breaks called microfractures can occur in pagetic bone. These breaks can cause pain, especially in weight-bearing bone such as the spine, pelvis, or leg.

Joint pain: Cartilage (a hard but slippery tissue that cushions the joints) can be damaged when Paget disease reaches the end of a long bone or changes the shape of bones located near joints. This can result in osteoarthritis and joint pain.

Muscle pain: When bone is changed by Paget disease, the muscles that support the bone may have to work harder and at different angles, causing muscle pain.

Nervous system pain: Bones enlarged by Paget disease can put pressure on the brain, spinal cord, or nerves. This can cause headache; pain in the neck, back, and legs; and sciatica—a shooting pain that travels down the sciatic nerve from the lower back to the leg.

Available Treatments

It is important for most people with Paget disease to receive medical treatment as soon as possible. Today's treatments can help reduce pain and possibly prevent the development of further complications.

- **Medicines:** Several types of medicines are used to address the pain caused by Paget disease. A doctor may recommend drugs designed to control the Paget disease or to relieve pain. The doctor also may recommend drugs to address painful complications of Paget disease, such as arthritis.

- **Surgery:** When severe pain cannot be controlled with medicine, surgery on the affected bone or joint may be needed.

- **Exercise:** An appropriate program of regular exercise also can help people with Paget disease reduce or eliminate pain.

Table 32.2. Prescription Drugs Used to Treat Paget Disease

Therapies of choice

Drug	Brand Name[1]	How Given
Bisphosphonates		
risedronate sodium	Actonel	Tablet
alendronate sodium	Fosamax	Tablet
pamidronate disodium	Aredia	Intravenous (through a vein)
pamidronate disodium	generic only	Injection (with a needle)
zoledronic acid2	Reclast	Intravenous (through a vein)
tiludronate disodium	Skelid	Tablet
etidronate disodium	Didronel	Tablet

Recommended for certain patients

Drug	Brand Name[1]	How Given
Calcitonin	Miacalcin	Injection (with a needle)

[1] Brand names included in this chapter are provided as examples only, and their inclusion does not mean that these products are endorsed by the National Institutes of Health or any other government agency. Also, if a particular brand name is not mentioned, this does not mean or imply that the product is unsatisfactory.

[2] Zoledronic acid used for treating Paget disease outside the U.S. is known as Aclasta; when used for certain cancer treatments, it is called Zometa.

Prescription Drugs Used to Treat Paget Disease

Medicines used to treat Paget disease help slow the rate at which affected bone is changed, thereby reducing pain. The U.S. Food and Drug Administration (FDA) has approved the prescription drugs in Table 32.2 for the treatment of Paget disease.

Over-the-Counter Drugs to Treat the Pain Caused by Paget Disease

Several over-the-counter (nonprescription) drugs can be used to reduce the pain associated with Paget disease. Each of these medicines is taken orally (by mouth), usually in tablet form. Although there are many brand names for these drugs, they can be purchased on the basis of their key ingredient: ibuprofen, naproxen, aspirin, or acetaminophen.

In some cases physicians will recommend the use of pain-relieving medicine that requires a prescription.

Surgery to Manage Pain

Although surgery is rarely required for Paget disease, it should be considered in certain circumstances. Hip or knee replacement surgery may help people with severe pain from Paget disease-related arthritis. Surgery can also realign affected leg bones to reduce the stress and pain at knee and ankle joints or help broken bones heal in a better position.

The Value of Exercise

Physical exercise is an important tool for persons with Paget disease. Regular exercise can help patients to:

- maintain bone strength,
- avoid weight gain (and the pressure added weight puts on weakened bone), and
- keep weight-bearing joints mobile and free of pain.

To make sure that pagetic bone is not harmed, patients should discuss their plans with a doctor before beginning any exercise program.

There Is No Need to Be in Pain

Although there is no cure for Paget disease, people with the disorder do not have to live with constant pain. As this chapter describes, available therapies—especially when started early—can greatly reduce or, in some cases, eliminate the pain associated with the disease.

Chapter 33

Pancreatitis

Pancreatitis is an inflammation of the pancreas. The pancreas is a large gland behind the stomach and close to the duodenum. The duodenum is the upper part of the small intestine. The pancreas secretes digestive enzymes into the small intestine through a tube called the pancreatic duct. These enzymes help digest fats, proteins, and carbohydrates in food. The pancreas also releases the hormones insulin and glucagon into the bloodstream. These hormones help the body use the glucose it takes from food for energy.

Normally, digestive enzymes do not become active until they reach the small intestine, where they begin digesting food. But if these enzymes become active inside the pancreas, they start "digesting" the pancreas itself.

Acute pancreatitis occurs suddenly and lasts for a short period of time and usually resolves. Chronic pancreatitis does not resolve itself and results in a slow destruction of the pancreas. Either form can cause serious complications. In severe cases, bleeding, tissue damage, and infection may occur. Pseudocysts, accumulations of fluid and tissue debris, may also develop. And enzymes and toxins may enter the bloodstream, injuring the heart, lungs, and kidneys, or other organs.

Text in this chapter is from "Pancreatitis," National Institute of Diabetes and Digestive and Kidney Diseases (NIDDK), NIH Publication No. 04–1596, February 2004.

Acute Pancreatitis

Some people have more than one attack and recover completely after each, but acute pancreatitis can be a severe, life-threatening illness with many complications. About 80,000 cases occur in the United States each year; some 20 percent of them are severe. Acute pancreatitis occurs more often in men than women.

Acute pancreatitis is usually caused by gallstones or by drinking too much alcohol, but these are not the only causes. If alcohol use and gallstones are ruled out, other possible causes of pancreatitis should be carefully examined so that appropriate treatment—if available—can begin.

Symptoms

Acute pancreatitis usually begins with pain in the upper abdomen that may last for a few days. The pain may be severe and may become constant—just in the abdomen—or it may reach to the back and other areas. It may be sudden and intense or begin as a mild pain that gets worse when food is eaten. Someone with acute pancreatitis often looks and feels very sick. Other symptoms may include the following:

- swollen and tender abdomen

- nausea

- vomiting

- fever

- rapid pulse

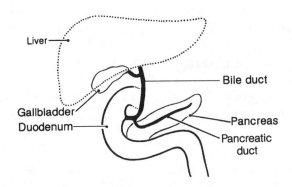

Figure 33.1. *Pancreas, Liver, and Gallbladder*

Severe cases may cause dehydration and low blood pressure. The heart, lungs, or kidneys may fail. Shock, and sometimes even death, may follow if bleeding occurs in the pancreatis.

Diagnosis

Besides asking about a person's medical history and doing a physical exam, a doctor will order a blood test to diagnose acute pancreatitis. During acute attacks, the blood contains at least three times more amylase and lipase than usual. Amylase and lipase are digestive enzymes formed in the pancreas. Changes may also occur in blood levels of glucose, calcium, magnesium, sodium, potassium, and bicarbonate. After the pancreas improves, these levels usually return to normal.

A doctor may also order an abdominal ultrasound to look for gallstones and a computed tomography (CT) scan to look for inflammation or destruction of the pancreas. CT scans are also useful in locating pseudocysts.

Treatment

Treatment depends on the severity of the attack. If no kidney or lung complications occur, acute pancreatitis usually improves on its own. Treatment, in general, is designed to support vital bodily functions and prevent complications. A hospital stay will be necessary so that fluids can be replaced intravenously.

If pancreatic pseudocysts occur and are considered large enough to interfere with the pancreas's healing, your doctor may drain or surgically remove them.

Unless the pancreatic duct or bile duct is blocked by gallstones, an acute attack usually lasts only a few days. In severe cases, a person may require intravenous feeding for 3–6 weeks while the pancreas slowly heals. This process is called total parenteral nutrition. However, for mild cases of the disease, total parenteral nutrition offers no benefit.

Before leaving the hospital, a person will be advised not to drink alcohol and not to eat large meals. After all signs of acute pancreatitis are gone, the doctor will try to decide what caused it in order to prevent future attacks. In some people, the cause of the attack is clear, but in others, more tests are needed.

Complications

Acute pancreatitis can cause breathing problems. Many people develop hypoxia, which means that cells and tissues are not receiving enough oxygen. Doctors treat hypoxia by giving oxygen through a face mask. Despite receiving oxygen, some people still experience lung failure and require a ventilator.

Sometimes a person cannot stop vomiting and needs to have a tube placed in the stomach to remove fluid and air. In mild cases, a person may not eat for 3–4 days and instead may receive fluids and pain relievers through an intravenous line.

If an infection develops, the doctor may prescribe antibiotics. Surgery may be needed for extensive infections. Surgery may also be necessary to find the source of bleeding, to rule out problems that resemble pancreatitis, or to remove severely damaged pancreatic tissue.

Acute pancreatitis can sometimes cause kidney failure. If your kidneys fail, you will need dialysis to help your kidneys remove wastes from your blood.

Gallstones and Pancreatitis

Gallstones can cause pancreatitis and they usually require surgical removal. Ultrasound or a CT scan can detect gallstones and can sometimes give an idea of the severity of the pancreatitis. When gallstone surgery can be scheduled depends on how severe the pancreatitis is. If the pancreatitis is mild, gallstone surgery may proceed within about a week. More severe cases may mean gallstone surgery is delayed for a month or more. After the gallstones are removed and inflammation goes away, the pancreas usually returns to normal.

Chronic Pancreatitis

If injury to the pancreas continues, chronic pancreatitis may develop. Chronic pancreatitis occurs when digestive enzymes attack and destroy the pancreas and nearby tissues, causing scarring and pain. The usual cause of chronic pancreatitis is many years of alcohol abuse, but the chronic form may also be triggered by only one acute attack, especially if the pancreatic ducts are damaged. The damaged ducts cause the pancreas to become inflamed, tissue to be destroyed, and scar tissue to develop.

While common, alcoholism is not the only cause of chronic pancreatitis. The main causes of chronic pancreatitis are:

- alcoholism,

- blocked or narrowed pancreatic duct because of trauma or pseudocysts have formed,

- heredity, or

- idiopathic (unknown cause).

Damage from alcohol abuse may not appear for many years, and then a person may have a sudden attack of pancreatitis. In up to 70 percent of adult patients, chronic pancreatitis appears to be caused by alcoholism. This form is more common in men than in women and often develops between the ages of 30 and 40.

Hereditary pancreatitis usually begins in childhood but may not be diagnosed for several years. A person with hereditary pancreatitis usually has the typical symptoms that come and go over time. Episodes last from two days to two weeks. A determining factor in the diagnosis of hereditary pancreatitis is two or more family members with pancreatitis in more than one generation.

Other causes of chronic pancreatitis are:

- congenital conditions such as pancreas divisum,

- cystic fibrosis,

- high levels of calcium in the blood (hypercalcemia),

- high levels of blood fats (hyperlipidemia or hypertriglyceridemia),

- some drugs, and

- certain autoimmune conditions.

Symptoms

Most people with chronic pancreatitis have abdominal pain, although some people have no pain at all. The pain may get worse when eating or drinking, spread to the back, or become constant and disabling. In certain cases, abdominal pain goes away as the condition advances, probably because the pancreas is no longer making digestive enzymes. Other symptoms include nausea, vomiting, weight loss, and fatty stools.

People with chronic disease often lose weight, even when their appetite and eating habits are normal. The weight loss occurs because the body does not secrete enough pancreatic enzymes to break down food, so nutrients are not absorbed normally. Poor digestion leads to excretion of fat, protein, and sugar into the stool. If the insulin-producing cells of the pancreas (islet cells) have been damaged, diabetes may also develop at this stage.

Diagnosis

Diagnosis may be difficult, but new techniques can help. Pancreatic function tests help a doctor decide whether the pancreas is still making enough digestive enzymes. Using ultrasonic imaging, endoscopic retrograde cholangiopancreatography (ERCP), and CT scans, a doctor can see problems indicating chronic pancreatitis.

Treatment

Relieving pain is the first step in treating chronic pancreatitis. The next step is to plan a diet that is high in carbohydrates and low in fat.

A doctor may prescribe pancreatic enzymes to take with meals if the pancreas does not secrete enough of its own. The enzymes should be taken with every meal to help the body digest food and regain some weight. Sometimes insulin or other drugs are needed to control blood glucose.

In some cases, surgery is needed to relieve pain. The surgery may involve draining an enlarged pancreatic duct or removing part of the pancreas.

For fewer and milder attacks, people with pancreatitis must stop drinking alcohol, stick to their prescribed diet, and take the proper medications.

Pancreatitis in Children

Chronic pancreatitis is rare in children. Trauma to the pancreas and hereditary pancreatitis are two known causes of childhood pancreatitis. Children with cystic fibrosis may also have pancreatitis. But more often the cause is not known.

Chapter 34

Pediatric Pain

Chapter Contents

Section 34.1

Growing Pains

If you can read this on your own, you can probably turn on the faucet to brush your teeth. And if you can reach the faucet, it's a good bet you can get your own drinking glass from a kitchen cabinet.

These are all signs that you're getting bigger and growing up. But for some kids, growing up comes with something doctors call growing pains.

What Are Growing Pains?

Growing pains aren't a disease. You probably won't have to go to the doctor for them. But they can hurt. Usually they happen when kids are between the ages of three and five or eight and twelve. Doctors don't believe that growing actually causes pain, but growing pains stop when kids stop growing. By the teen years, most kids don't get growing pains anymore.

Kids get growing pains in their legs. Most of the time they hurt in the front of the thighs (the upper part of your legs), in the calves (the back part of your legs below your knees), or behind the knees. Usually, both legs hurt.

Growing pains often start to ache right before bedtime. Sometimes you go to bed without any pain, but you might wake up in the middle of the night with your legs hurting. The best news about growing pains is that they go away by morning.

What Causes Growing Pains?

Growing pains don't hurt around the bones or joints (the flexible parts that connect bones and let them move)—only in the muscles.

For this reason, some doctors believe that kids might get growing pains because they've tired out their muscles. When you run, climb, or jump a lot during the day, you might have aches and pains in your legs at night.

What Can I Do to Feel Better?

Your parent can help your growing pains feel better by giving you an over-the-counter pain medicine like acetaminophen or ibuprofen. Kids should not take aspirin because it can cause a rare but serious illness called Reye syndrome.

Here are three other things that might help you feel better:

- placing a heating pad on the spot where your legs hurt
- stretching your legs like you do in gym class
- having your parent massage your legs

When to Go to the Doctor

If you have a fever, you're limping when you walk, or your leg looks red or is swollen (puffed up), your parent should take you to the doctor. Growing pains should not keep you from running, playing, and doing what you normally do. If the pain is bothering you during the day, talk to your parent about it.

You might never feel any growing pains, but if you do, remember that before you know it, you will outgrow them.

Section 34.2

Abdominal Pain

Stomachaches

The pain may come in waves: sharp enough that you catch your breath, then gone as quickly as it came. Or perhaps it's a dull, constant ache. Maybe you're spending what seems like hours in the bathroom—or just wish you could.

What Causes Belly Pain?

Pain is the body's way of signaling that something is going on. Stomach pain alerts us to something that's happening inside us that we might not know about otherwise.

Some reasons for stomach pain are obvious—like when someone gets hit in the gut, or a toddler accidentally eats something poisonous. A lot of the time, though, belly pain might be hard to figure out. With so many organs in the abdomen, different problems can have similar symptoms.

Here are some of the things that cause tummy troubles:

Infection: When bacteria or viruses get into a person's system, the body reacts by trying to rid itself of the infection—often through vomiting or diarrhea.

- Bacterial infections cause what we call food poisoning. Bacteria are also responsible for other conditions that may give a person belly pain, such as pneumonia, urinary tract infections, strep throat, sexually transmitted diseases (STDs), or the rare condition toxic shock syndrome.

- Viruses, another type of infection, are behind what we call stomach flu. Both bacteria and viruses can be easily passed from person to person. The good news is you can often avoid them simply by washing your hands properly and not sharing cups, straws, or utensils with other people.

Constipation: Being constipated is one of the most common reasons for frequent belly pain. People usually become constipated because their diet doesn't include enough fluids and fiber.

Irritation and inflammation: When one of the body's internal organs becomes irritated or swollen, that can bring on belly pain. Pain from problems like appendicitis, ulcers, irritable bowel syndrome, and inflammatory bowel disease (IBD) is the body's way of telling us to get medical help.

Food reactions: Food reactions can be more than eating too much or basic indigestion. When people are unable to digest certain foods, doctors say they have a food intolerance. Conditions like lactose intolerance often cause belly pain when a person eats the food (milk products in the case of lactose intolerance). If you notice a reaction after eating certain foods, make an appointment with your doctor.

Conditions like celiac disease (a reaction to proteins in certain grains) or food allergies (like peanut allergy) are different from food intolerance. They involve immune system reactions that can actually harm the body beyond just producing a temporary reaction. When someone has a true food allergy, they must always avoid that food—even a small amount could be deadly.

Reproductive problems: The digestive system isn't the only cause of bellyaches. Menstrual cramps are probably the most common example of pain in the reproductive organs. Infections in the reproductive system, such as pelvic inflammatory disease (PID) or other STDs, also can cause abdominal pain in girls.

Testicular injuries can make a guy feel sick or even throw up if they are particularly severe.

Women often feel nausea during pregnancy. Ectopic pregnancies (when the pregnancy implants in the wrong place) can cause abdominal pain. Because problems like ectopic pregnancy need to be treated immediately, girls who have belly pain and think they might be pregnant should call a doctor right away.

Anatomical problems: Some diseases or defects can interfere with the way the organs do their jobs, causing pain. Crohn disease can cause the wall of the intestine to swell and scar enough that it may block the intestine. Hernias can also block a person's intestines, as can growths like tumors. Torsion is a medical term that means twisting. Torsion can affect the intestine, ovaries, and testicles, cutting off blood supply or blocking their functions.

Emotional distress: When people get too stressed out, anxious, or depressed, their emotions can trigger physical symptoms, such as headaches or stomach pain.

In addition to these causes, belly pain also may be a result of problems that can happen when people have certain illnesses, such as sickle cell disease or diabetes.

When to See a Doctor

Sometimes, what seems like one problem—food poisoning, for example—can turn out to be something more serious, like appendicitis. So it's a good idea to see a doctor if pain is very strong, you're vomiting a lot, you already have another health condition, or the discomfort gets worse over time or doesn't go away. A parent or other adult can help you decide if you need to see a doctor.

What Doctors Do

Your doctor will ask about your symptoms and what's going on. He or she may also ask about illnesses you may have had in the past, or any health conditions that other family members have.

Your doctor will probably also give you a physical exam and might order tests, such as an x-ray, ultrasound, or blood test. It all depends on what the doctor thinks is causing the problem.

If stress or anxiety seems to be behind the pain, the doctor may recommend talking to a counselor or therapist to resolve the problem. As medical experts, they're trained to help people figure out what's behind their stress—and then provide advice on how to fix problems or handle them better.

What You Can Do

The good news is belly pain isn't usually serious in teens. Although there are lots of different reasons why people get it, most are easy to treat. You can even lessen your chances of getting belly pain by taking a few simple precautions:

- Wash your hands before eating.

- Don't overeat, and try not to eat right before going to sleep.

- Eat fiber-rich foods, such as fruits and vegetables, to keep food moving through your digestive system.

- If you have a food allergy or intolerance, avoid eating foods that make you sick.

- Always use a condom when having sex to protect against STDs and pregnancy.

Chronic Abdominal Pain Puts a Cramp in Kids' Quality of Life

"Chronic Abdominal Pain Puts a Cramp in Kids' Quality of Life," January 2006, reprinted with permission from www.kidshealth.org. Copyright © 2006 The Nemours Foundation. This information was provided by KidsHealth, one of the largest resources online for medically reviewed health information written for parents, kids, and teens. For more articles like this one, visit www.KidsHealth .org., or www.TeensHealth.org.

According to the International Foundation for Functional Gastrointestinal Disorders, chronic abdominal pain, sometimes referred to as functional abdominal pain(FAP), occurs because of sensitivity to nerve impulses in the gut. But kids with this disorder tend to experience more than just belly pain—they may also miss more schooldays, suffer social withdrawal, and feel anxious and depressed about their condition. Researchers from Goryeb Children's Hospital/ Atlantic Health System in Morristown, New Jersey, examined the extent to which functional abdominal pain affects kids and families.

Sixty-five 5- to 18-year-old children answered questions about how FAP affected their physical, emotional, and social life, and their ability to function at school. Their parents also answered questions about how functional abdominal pain affected their child's quality of life. Later researchers compared the results of children with FAP with the survey results of healthy children and children with other types of gastrointestinal disorders, such as inflammatory bowel disease (IBD) and gastroesophageal reflux disease (GERD).

Kids with FAP reported having a quality of life similar to those of kids with other chronic gastrointestinal conditions, such as IBD and

GERD. Children with FAP scored lower on the quality of life index compared with healthy kids. Parents rated the quality of life of their children with FAP even lower that the children themselves did.

In addition, about 44% of parents noted that they too experienced bowel problems. The study authors suggest that in some cases, children may pick up on their parent's experiences, which could contribute to their anxiety about belly pain or their reports of a lower quality of life.

What This Means to You

The results of this study suggest that both children and parents feel that functional abdominal pain worsens a child's overall quality of life. Other studies have indicated that kids with FAP may be less likely to participate in sports and school activities and are more likely to consider their lives a failure, compared with kids with no abdominal pain.

If your child has chronic abdominal pain, talk to your child's doctor about how the condition has affected your child's life. The doctor may be able to make suggestions about treatments or strategies for helping your child feel more comfortable at home and at school.

Chapter 35

Podiatric Pain

Chapter Contents

Section 35.1

Foot Pain

Definition

Pain or discomfort can be felt anywhere in the foot, including the heel, toes, arch, instep, sole, or ankles.

Causes

Foot pain can be caused by:

- Bunions—a protrusion at the base of the big toe, which can become inflamed. Bunions often develop over time from wearing narrow-toed shoes.

- Hammer toes—toes that curl downward into a claw-like position.

- Calluses and corns—thickened skin from friction or pressure. Calluses are on the balls of the feet or heels. Corns appear on your toes.

- Plantar warts—from pressure on the soles of your feet.

- Fallen arches—also called flat feet.

Ill-fitting shoes often cause these problems. Aging and being overweight also increase your chances of having foot problems.

Morton's neuroma is a type of foot pain that is usually centered between the third and fourth toes. It results from thickening and swelling of tissue around a nerve in the area. Symptoms include tingling and sharp, shooting, or burning pains in the ball of your foot (and sometimes toes), especially when wearing shoes or pressing on the area. Pain gradually gets worse over time. Morton's neuroma is more common in women than men.

Other common causes of foot pain include:

- Broken bones

- Stress fracture
- Arthritis
- Gout
- Plantar fasciitis
- Bone spur
- Sprains
- Bursitis of the heel
- Tendonitis

Home Care

- Apply ice to reduce pain and swelling. Do this just after an activity that aggravates your pain.
- Elevate your painful foot as much as possible.
- Reduce activity until the problem improves.
- Wear foot pads in areas of friction or pressure. This will prevent rubbing and irritation.
- Take over-the-counter pain medicine, like ibuprofen or acetaminophen. Try this for 2–3 weeks (unless you have a history of an ulcer, liver disease, or other condition that does not allow you to take one of these drugs).

For plantar warts, try an over-the-counter wart removal preparation.

For calluses, soak in warm water and then rub them down with a pumice stone. Do not cut or burn corns or calluses.

For foot pain caused by a stress fracture, an extended rest period is often necessary. Crutches may be used for a week or so to take the pressure off, if your foot is particularly painful.

For foot pain due to plantar fasciitis, shoe inserts may help.

When to Contact a Medical Professional

Call your doctor if:

- You have sudden, severe pain.
- Your pain began following an injury—especially if there is bleeding, bruising, deformity, or you cannot bear weight.

- You have redness or swelling of the joint, an open sore or ulcer on your foot, or a fever.

- You have diabetes or peripheral vascular disease—a condition characterized by poor circulation.

- You do not respond to self-care within 1–2 weeks.

What to Expect at Your Office Visit

Your doctor will perform a physical examination, paying particular attention to your feet, legs, and back, and your stance, posture, and gait.

To help diagnose the cause of the problem, your doctor will ask medical history questions, such as:

- Are both of your feet affected? If only one, which one?

- Exactly what part of your foot is affected?

- Does the pain move from joint to joint or does it always occur in the same location?

- Did your pain begin suddenly and severely or slowly and mildly, gradually getting worse?

- How long have you had the pain?

- Is it worse at night or when you first wake up in the morning?

- Is it getting better?

- Does anything make your pain feel better or worse?

- Do you have any other symptoms?

X-rays may be useful in making a diagnosis.

For bunions, plantar fasciitis, bone spurs, Morton's neuroma, or other conditions, your doctor may inject cortisone. This will be considered if oral medication, changing your shoes, and other measures have not helped. No more than three injections in a year should be attempted in most cases.

A broken foot will be casted. Broken toes will be taped.

Orthotics fit by a podiatrist or other specialist can help many structurally related problems. Physical therapy is also quite helpful for conditions related to overuse or tight muscles, like plantar fasciitis or Achilles tendinitis.

Removal of plantar warts, corns, or calluses may be necessary. This is generally performed by a podiatrist.

Surgery may be considered for certain conditions like bunions or hammer toes if the pain interferes with walking or other activities.

Prevention

The following steps can prevent foot problems and foot pain:

- Wear comfortable, properly fitting shoes. They should have good arch support and cushioning.

- Wear shoes with adequate room around the ball of your foot and toe.

- Wear sneakers as often as possible, especially when walking.

- Avoid narrow-toed shoes and high heels.

- Replace running shoes frequently.

- Warm up before exercise, cool down after exercise, and stretch adequately.

- Increase your amount of exercise slowly over time to avoid putting excessive strain on your feet.

- Lose weight if you need to.

- Learn exercises to strengthen your feet and avoid pain. This can help flat feet and other potential foot problems.

- Keep feet dry to avoid friction. This may help prevent corns and calluses.

- Avoid alcohol to prevent attacks of gout.

Section 35.2

Heel Pain

Heel Pain Has Many Causes

In our pursuit of healthy bodies, pain can be an enemy. In some instances, however, it is of biological benefit. Pain that occurs right after an injury or early in an illness may play a protective role, often warning us about the damage we've suffered.

When we sprain an ankle, for example, the pain warns us that the ligament and soft tissues may be frayed and bruised, and that further activity may cause additional injury.

Pain, such as may occur in our heels, also alerts us to seek medical attention. This alert is of utmost importance because of the many afflictions that contribute to heel pain.

Heel Pain

Heel pain is generally the result of faulty biomechanics (walking gait abnormalities) that place too much stress on the heel bone and the soft tissues that attach to it. The stress may also result from injury, or a bruise incurred while walking, running, or jumping on hard surfaces; wearing poorly constructed footwear; or being overweight.

The heel bone is the largest of the 26 bones in the human foot, which also has 33 joints and a network of more than 100 tendons, muscles, and ligaments. Like all bones, it is subject to outside influences that can affect its integrity and its ability to keep us on our feet. Heel pain, sometimes disabling, can occur in the front, back, or bottom of the heel.

Heel Spurs

A common cause of heel pain is the heel spur, a bony growth on the underside of the heel bone. The spur, visible by x-ray, appears as a protrusion that can extend forward as much as half an inch. When there is no indication of bone enlargement, the condition is sometimes referred to as "heel spur syndrome."

Heel spurs result from strain on the muscles and ligaments of the foot, by stretching of the long band of tissue that connects the heel and the ball of the foot, and by repeated tearing away of the lining or membrane that covers the heel bone. These conditions may result from biomechanical imbalance, running or jogging, improperly fitted or excessively worn shoes, or obesity.

Plantar Fasciitis

Both heel pain and heel spurs are frequently associated with an inflammation of the band of fibrous connective tissue (fascia) running along the bottom (plantar surface) of the foot, from the heel to the ball of the foot. The inflammation is called plantar fasciitis. It is common among athletes who run and jump a lot, and it can be quite painful.

The condition occurs when the plantar fascia is strained over time beyond its normal extension, causing the soft tissue fibers of the fascia to tear or stretch at points along its length; this leads to inflammation, pain, and possibly the growth of a bone spur where it attaches to the heel bone.

The inflammation may be aggravated by shoes that lack appropriate support, especially in the arch area, and by the chronic irritation that sometimes accompanies an athletic lifestyle.

Resting provides only temporary relief. When you resume walking, particularly after a night's sleep, you may experience a sudden elongation of the fascia band, which stretches and pulls on the heel. As you walk, the heel pain may lessen or even disappear, but that may be just a false sense of relief. The pain often returns after prolonged rest or extensive walking.

Excessive Pronation

Heel pain sometimes results from excessive pronation. Pronation is the normal flexible motion and flattening of the arch of the foot that allows it to adapt to ground surfaces and absorb shock in the normal walking pattern.

As you walk, the heel contacts the ground first; the weight shifts first to the outside of the foot, then moves toward the big toe. The arch rises, the foot generally rolls upward and outward, becoming rigid and stable in order to lift the body and move it forward. Excessive pronation—excessive inward motion—can create an abnormal amount of stretching and pulling on the ligaments and tendons attaching to the bottom back of the heel bone. Excessive pronation may also contribute to injury to the hip, knee, and lower back.

Disease and Heel Pain

Some general health conditions can also bring about heel pain.

- Rheumatoid arthritis and other forms of arthritis, including gout, which usually manifests itself in the big toe joint, can cause heel discomfort in some cases.

- Heel pain may also be the result of an inflamed bursa (bursitis), a small, irritated sack of fluid; a neuroma (a nerve growth); or other soft-tissue growth. Such heel pain may be associated with a heel spur or may mimic the pain of a heel spur.

- Haglund's deformity (pump bump) is a bone enlargement at the back of the heel bone, in the area where the Achilles tendon attaches to the bone. This sometimes painful deformity generally is the result of bursitis caused by pressure against the shoe and can be aggravated by the height or stitching of a heel counter of a particular shoe.

- Pain at the back of the heel is associated with inflammation of the Achilles tendon as it runs behind the ankle and inserts on the back surface of the heel bone. The inflammation is called Achilles tendonitis. It is common among people who run and walk a lot and have tight tendons. The condition occurs when the tendon is strained over time, causing the fibers to tear or stretch along its length, or at its insertion onto the heel bone. This leads to inflammation, pain, and the possible growth of a bone spur on the back of the heel bone. The inflammation is aggravated by the chronic irritation that sometimes accompanies an active lifestyle and certain activities that strain an already tight tendon.

- Bone bruises are common heel injuries. A bone bruise or contusion is an inflammation of the tissues that cover the heel bone. A bone bruise is a sharply painful injury caused by the direct impact of a hard object or surface on the foot.

- Stress fractures of the heel bone also can occur, although infrequently.

Children's Heel Pain

Heel pain can also occur in children, most commonly between ages eight and thirteen, as they become increasingly active in sports activity in and out of school. This physical activity, particularly jumping, inflames the growth centers of the heels; the more active the child, the more likely the condition will occur. When the bones mature, the problems disappear and are not likely to recur. If heel pain occurs in this age group, podiatric care is necessary to protect the growing bone and to provide pain relief. Other good news is that heel spurs do not often develop in children.

Prevention

A variety of steps can be taken to avoid heel pain and accompanying afflictions:

- Wear shoes that fit well—front, back, and sides—and have shock-absorbent soles, rigid shanks, and supportive heel counters.

- Wear the proper shoes for each activity.

- Do not wear shoes with excessive wear on heels or soles.

- Prepare properly before exercising. Warm up and do stretching exercises before and after running.

- Pace yourself when you participate in athletic activities.

- Don't underestimate your body's need for rest and good nutrition.

- If obese, lose weight.

Podiatric Medical Care

If pain and other symptoms of inflammation—redness, swelling, heat—persist, you should limit normal daily activities and contact a doctor of podiatric medicine. The podiatric physician will examine the area and may perform diagnostic x-rays to rule out problems of the bone.

Early treatment might involve oral or injectable anti-inflammatory medication, exercise and shoe recommendations, taping or strapping, or use of shoe inserts or orthotic devices. Taping or strapping supports the foot, placing stressed muscles and tendons in a physiologically restful state. Physical therapy may be used in conjunction with such treatments.

A functional orthotic device may be prescribed for correcting biomechanical imbalance, controlling excessive pronation, and supporting of the ligaments and tendons attaching to the heel bone. It will effectively treat the majority of heel and arch pain without the need for surgery.

Only a relatively few cases of heel pain require more advanced treatments or surgery. If surgery is necessary, it may involve the release of the plantar fascia, removal of a spur, removal of a bursa, or removal of a neuroma or other soft-tissue growth.

Heel Pain Tips

- If you have experienced painful heels try wearing your shoes around your house in the evening. Don't wear slippers or socks or go barefoot. You may also try gentle calf stretches for 20 to 30 seconds on each leg. This is best done barefoot, leaning forward towards a wall with one foot forward and one foot back.

- If the pain persists longer than one month, you should visit a podiatrist for evaluation and treatment. Your feet should not hurt, and professional podiatric care may be required to help relieve your discomfort.

- If you have not exercised in a long time, consult your podiatric physician before starting a new exercise program.

- Begin an exercise program slowly. Don't go too far or too fast.

- Purchase and maintain good shoes and replace them regularly.

- Stretch each foot and Achilles tendon before and after exercise.

- Avoid uneven walking surfaces or stepping on rocks as much as possible.

- Avoid going barefoot on hard surfaces.

- Vary the incline on a treadmill during exercise. Nobody walks uphill all the time.

- If it hurts, stop. Don't try to work through the pain.

Your podiatric physician/surgeon has been trained specifically and extensively in the diagnosis and treatment of all manner of foot conditions. This training encompasses all of the intricately related systems and structures of the foot and lower leg including neurological, circulatory, skin, and the musculoskeletal system, which includes bones, joints, ligaments, tendons, muscles, and nerves.

Chapter 36

Polymyalgia Rheumatica and Giant Cell Arteritis

What is polymyalgia rheumatica?

Polymyalgia rheumatica is a rheumatic disorder associated with moderate-to-severe musculoskeletal pain and stiffness in the neck, shoulder, and hip area. Stiffness is most noticeable in the morning or after a period of inactivity, and typically lasts longer than 30 minutes. This disorder may develop rapidly; in some people, it comes on literally overnight. But for most people, polymyalgia rheumatica develops more gradually.

The cause of polymyalgia rheumatica is not known. But it is associated with immune system problems, genetic factors, and an event, such as an infection, that triggers symptoms. The fact that polymyalgia rheumatica is rare in people under the age of 50 and becomes more common as age increases suggests that it may be linked to the aging process.

Polymyalgia rheumatica usually resolves within one to two years. The symptoms of polymyalgia rheumatica are quickly controlled by treatment with corticosteroids, but symptoms return if treatment is stopped too early. Corticosteroid treatment does not appear to influence the length of the disease.

"Questions and Answers about Polymyalgia Rheumatica and Giant Cell Arteritis," National Institute of Arthritis and Musculoskeletal and Skin Diseases (NIAMS), NIH Publication No. 07–4908, December 2006.

What is giant cell arteritis?

Giant cell arteritis, also known as temporal arteritis and cranial arteritis, is a disorder that results in inflammation of arteries of the scalp (most apparent in the temporal arteries, which are located on the temples on each side of the head), neck, and arms. This inflammation causes the arteries to narrow, impeding adequate blood flow. For a good prognosis, it is critical to receive early treatment, before irreversible tissue damage occurs.

How are polymyalgia rheumatica and giant cell arteritis related?

It is unclear how or why polymyalgia rheumatica and giant cell arteritis frequently occur together. But some people with polymyalgia rheumatica also develop giant cell arteritis either simultaneously, or after the musculoskeletal symptoms have disappeared. Other people with giant cell arteritis also have polymyalgia rheumatica at some time while the arteries are inflamed.

When undiagnosed or untreated, giant cell arteritis can cause potentially serious problems, including permanent vision loss and stroke. So regardless of why giant cell arteritis might occur along with polymyalgia rheumatica, it is important that doctors look for symptoms of the arteritis in anyone diagnosed with polymyalgia rheumatica.

Patients, too, must learn and watch for symptoms of giant cell arteritis, because early detection and proper treatment are key to preventing complications. Any symptoms should be reported to your doctor immediately.

What are the symptoms of polymyalgia rheumatica?

In addition to the musculoskeletal stiffness mentioned earlier, people with polymyalgia rheumatica also may have flu-like symptoms, including fever, weakness, and weight loss.

What are the symptoms of giant cell arteritis?

Early symptoms of giant cell arteritis may resemble flu symptoms such as fatigue, loss of appetite, and fever. Symptoms specifically related to the inflamed arteries of the head include headaches, pain and tenderness over the temples, double vision or visual loss, dizziness or problems with coordination, and balance. Pain may also affect the jaw and tongue, especially when eating, and opening the mouth wide may become difficult. In rare cases, giant cell arteritis causes ulceration of the scalp.

Who is at risk for these conditions?

Caucasian women over the age of 50 have the highest risk of developing polymyalgia rheumatica and giant cell arteritis. While women are more likely than men to develop the conditions, research suggests that men with giant cell arteritis are more likely to suffer potentially blinding eye involvement. Both conditions almost exclusively affect people over the age of 50, with the incidence of both peaking between 70 and 80 years of age.

Polymyalgia rheumatica and giant cell arteritis are quite common according to the National Arthritis Data Work Group. In the United States, it is estimated that 700 per 100,000 people in the general population over 50 years of age develop polymyalgia rheumatica. An estimated 200 per 100,000 people over 50 years of age develop giant cell arteritis.

How are polymyalgia rheumatica and giant cell arteritis diagnosed?

A diagnosis of polymyalgia rheumatica is based primarily on the patient's medical history and symptoms, and on a physical examination. No single test is available to definitively diagnose polymyalgia rheumatica. However, doctors often use lab tests to confirm a diagnosis or rule out other diagnoses or possible reasons for the patient's symptoms.

The most typical laboratory finding in people with polymyalgia rheumatica is an elevated erythrocyte sedimentation (sed) rate. This test measures inflammation by determining how quickly red blood cells fall to the bottom of a test tube of blood. Rapidly descending cells (an elevated sed rate) indicate inflammation in the body. While the sed rate measurement is a helpful diagnostic tool, it alone does not confirm polymyalgia rheumatica. An abnormal result indicates only that tissue is inflamed, but this is also a symptom of many forms of arthritis and other rheumatic diseases.

Before making a diagnosis of polymyalgia rheumatica, the doctor may order additional tests. For example, the C-reactive protein test is another common means of measuring inflammation. There is also a common test for rheumatoid factor, an antibody (a protein made by the immune system) that is sometimes found in the blood of people with rheumatoid arthritis. While polymyalgia rheumatica and rheumatoid arthritis share many symptoms, those with polymyalgia rheumatica rarely test positive for rheumatoid factor. Therefore, a positive rheumatoid factor might suggest a diagnosis of rheumatoid arthritis instead of polymyalgia rheumatica.

As with polymyalgia rheumatica, a diagnosis of giant cell arteritis is based largely on symptoms and a physical examination. The exam may reveal that the temporal artery is inflamed and tender to the touch, and that it has a reduced pulse.

Any doctor who suspects giant cell arteritis should order a temporal artery biopsy. In this procedure, a small section of the artery is removed through an incision in the skin over the temple area and examined under a microscope. A biopsy that is positive for giant cell arteritis will show abnormal cells in the artery walls. Some patients showing symptoms of giant cell arteritis will have negative biopsy results. In such cases, the doctor may suggest a second biopsy.

How are polymyalgia rheumatica and giant cell arteritis treated?

The treatment of choice for both polymyalgia rheumatica and giant cell arteritis is corticosteroid medication, usually prednisone. Polymyalgia rheumatica responds to a low daily dose of prednisone that is increased as needed until symptoms disappear. At this point, the doctor may gradually reduce the dosage to determine the lowest amount needed to alleviate symptoms. Most patients can discontinue medication after six months to two years. If symptoms recur, prednisone treatment is required again.

Nonsteroidal anti-inflammatory drugs (NSAIDs), such as aspirin and ibuprofen (Advil, Motrin), also may be used to treat polymyalgia rheumatica. The medication must be taken daily, and long-term use may cause stomach irritation. For most patients, NSAIDs alone are not enough to relieve symptoms. Even without treatment, polymyalgia rheumatica usually disappears in one to several years. With treatment, however, symptoms disappear quickly, usually in 24 to 48 hours. If prednisone does not bring improvement, the doctor is likely to consider other possible diagnoses.

Giant cell arteritis is treated with high doses of prednisone. If not treated promptly, the condition carries a small but definite risk of blindness, so prednisone should be started as soon as possible, perhaps even before confirming the diagnosis with a temporal artery biopsy. As with polymyalgia rheumatica, the symptoms of giant cell arteritis quickly disappear with treatment; however, high doses of prednisone are typically maintained for one month. Once symptoms disappear and the sed rate is normal, there is much less risk of blindness. At that point, the doctor can begin to gradually reduce the prednisone dose.

In both polymyalgia rheumatica and giant cell arteritis, an increase in symptoms may develop when the prednisone dose is reduced to lower levels. The physician may need to hold the lower dose for a longer period of time or even modestly increase it again, temporarily, to control the symptoms. Once the symptoms are in remission and the prednisone has been discontinued for several months, recurrence is less common.

Whether taken on a long-term basis for polymyalgia rheumatica or for a shorter period for giant cell arteritis, prednisone carries a risk of side effects. While long-term use or higher doses carry the greatest risk, people taking the drug at any dose or for any length of time should be aware of the potential side effects, which include the following:

- fluid retention and weight gain

- rounding of the face

- delayed wound healing

- bruising easily

- diabetes

- myopathy (muscle wasting)

- glaucoma

- increased blood pressure

- decreased calcium absorption in the bones which can lead to osteoporosis

- irritation of the stomach

- increase in infections

People taking corticosteroids may have some side effects or none at all. Anyone who experiences side effects should report them to his or her doctor. When the medication is stopped, the side effects disappear. Because prednisone and other corticosteroid drugs reduce the body's natural production of corticosteroid hormones, which are necessary for the body to function properly, it is important not to stop taking the medication unless instructed by a doctor to do so. The patient and doctor must work together to gradually reduce the medication.

What is the outlook?

Most people with polymyalgia rheumatica and giant cell arteritis lead productive, active lives. The duration of drug treatment differs by patient. Once treatment is discontinued, polymyalgia may recur; but once again, symptoms respond rapidly to prednisone. When properly treated, giant cell arteritis rarely recurs.

Chapter 37

Post-Amputation Pain

Silas Weir Mitchell, a prominent 19th century Philadelphia physician, first coined the phrase "phantom limb" following the Civil War. Gangrene was a common result of battle injuries, and without antibiotics, surgeons sawed infected limbs off thousands of soldiers. These men returned home from war with phantom pain, setting off speculation among doctors as to its cause. Weir Mitchell published the first article on the topic under a pseudonym so as to not risk facing ridicule from his colleagues.

Since Weir Mitchell's time, all types of conjecture regarding phantom pain, ranging from the sublime to the ridiculous, has been printed. As recently as 15 years ago, a paper in a Canadian psychiatry journal stated that phantom limb sensation is merely the result of wishful thinking. The authors argued that patients desperately want their limbs back, so therefore, experience the phantom.

A more popular explanation for phantom sensation is that the frayed and curled-up nerve endings in the residual area tend to become inflamed and irritated, thereby fooling higher brain centers into thinking that the missing limb is still there. Though there are far too many problems with this nerve irritation theory, because it's a simple and convenient explanation, many physicians cling to it today.

"Capturing the Phantom," by Christina DiMartino. This article originally appeared in the September/October 2000 issue of *inMotion*, © Amputee Coalition of America. Reprinted with permission. This information is deemed pertinent and is available with other current information for amputees on the Amputee Coalition of America website at http://www.amputee-coalition.org.

A Patient's Perspective

Despite what is said about phantom pain and sensation, patients who suffer adamantly argue that it's not in their head. It's real pain—often so severe that even morphine-laden drugs don't offer relief. For some, years pass without a solid night's sleep.

Some patients say the pain they felt in their limbs immediately before amputation persists as a kind of pain memory. For example, soldiers who have grenades explode in their hands reported that their phantom hand is in a fixed position, clenching the grenade, ready to toss it. The pain in the hand is excruciating—the same they felt the instant the grenade exploded.

One woman in England suffered severe frostbite on her thumb as a child. Gangrene developed and the thumb had to be amputated. Now, 50 years later, she reports having chilblains (a frost-like pain due to cold weather) in her thumb when the weather turns cold.

A girl born without forearms experienced phantom hands six inches below her residual arms. She reported using her phantom fingers to calculate arithmetic problems.

Today, thousands of such stories have the medical profession, unlike in Weir Mitchell's day, acknowledging what these people feel is real—and often debilitating. A large group of doctors even specialize in phantom pain and sensation. Their hope is that research will help thousands of people around the world to enjoy pain-free lives.

What Physicians Know Now

David R. Del Toro, M.D., is a specialist who works in the Department of Physical Medicine and Rehabilitation at the Medical College of Wisconsin in Milwaukee, Wisconsin. He has researched, studied, and treated patients with phantom pain for more than 20 years and is credited with dozens of articles published in medical and consumer journals. "The basis of my expertise with phantom pain is taking care of patients with all types of amputations," he says. "Approximately ten percent of patients I see have had upper limb, and ninety percent have lower limb amputations."

Del Toro says from a research basis, the etiology of the mechanism of phantom pain causes aren't known. "We feel it's multi-factorial," he says. "As clinical research continues, we in the field continue testing treatments to help relieve the pain patients experience."

Some medications, according to Del Toro, offer promise. "One, generically named gabapentin, was marketed in the mid-1990s as an anti-seizure medication," he continues. "However, it's found helpful in offering relief for phantom pain. It's believed effective because it works on nerves, and consequently neuropathic pain. Today, more than 40 percent of prescriptions for the drug are for pain control, rather than seizure. It's also well-accepted because it has less side effects than other pain drugs."

Del Toro acknowledges the widespread use of antidepressants for phantom pain today, but says he'd rather see an effective short-term drug developed. "Antidepressants have to be taken daily and over a long time period," he says. "Anytime patients are put on medicine indefinitely they must be monitored constantly to ensure the patient doesn't suffer with severe side effects or toxicity. A short-term treatment that's effective in offering relief is truly the preferred goal for phantom pain sufferers."

Educating the Patient Is Imperative

Del Toro says he looks for two keys in determining preferred treatment. "Those who have a sleep disturbance caused by the pain, and those whose pain impairs their ability to wear their prosthesis," he says. "A prosthesis seems to help relieve pain for most patients, and we find a definite correlation between the amount of time it's worn and the intensity of pain. Time also is a great healer. Many patients report their pain dissipated over time, while others become accustomed to it."

Preoperative consultation, Del Toro says, also is imperative to the best possible results regarding pain. "I tell them exactly what to expect," he says. "They'll have two kinds of pain following the amputation procedure—residual limb and phantom pain. Therapy begins as soon as possible following surgery, including massage desensitization. An elastic shrinker, a sock that applies gradient pressure, is placed on the residual limb to help overload the sensory input to the brain."

Although a radical difference exists between the level of pain patients feel, Del Toro says most need a low dose of medication to help them sleep for at least a short time following surgery. "Because we tell them everything that can happen, their anxiety level is lessened before surgery," he says. "Studies show that stress adds to the level of pain, and educating the patient helps reduce it," he says. "It's also important to let them know that the pain they feel is real—not in their head. For now, and until research offers us improved treatment techniques, it's a matter of managing the problem rather than curing it. We just don't understand phantom pain enough to put an end to it.

The first goal, therefore, is to help patients restore their functions and reach a gainful quality of life."

Not in Your Head

Richard A. Sherman, Ph.D., is the chief consultant for Orthopedic Research at Madigan Army Medical Center in Tacoma, Washington. He has researched and evaluated phantom pain causes and treatments for more than 30 years, and has written several books on the topic. His research reveals approximately 80 percent of people with amputations feel phantom pain—but a small majority of this group has it severely and on a continual basis. Most suffer slight pain, and only some of the time. He says it's crucial that people understand why they experience this pain. "If they believe they're having psychological problems, rather than real pain, it increases their level of distress," he says. "This, in turn, intensifies their pain. Phantom pain is a very normal sensation, and patients must be made to realize it."

Sherman offers an example of how our brains are wired: "The brain has a picture of all the body parts," he says. "Every sensation that occurs in the body is carried to that image in the brain. This is how your conscious knows what part of you has been touched. If you touch your big toe—the image of the toe in the brain lights up. The conscious part of the mind, however, has no idea where the signals are coming from. Let's say you hit your funny bone. You feel pain at the elbow, but also down the arm and in your hand—but you didn't hurt those parts. The nerve gathering the information from the arm, forearm, and hand has passed to the brain. In short, those parts of the brain light up so you feel you've been touched in those areas. If your arm was amputated somewhere between the forearm and elbow, then you hit your elbow, you'd still feel pain in your hand—even though it's missing—because the image in your brain is still there."

The level and intensity of phantom pain does change somewhat after amputation, according to Sherman, but for many people it never dissipates completely. "Anytime the nerves are used that stimulate those pictures in the brain, some level of sensation will occur," he says. "However, phantom pain is indeed different for everyone. We've conducted research using more than 12,000 people with amputations, and find there is no pattern to whether phantom pain will fade or not—or to what level. Some people don't even have it until many years after their amputation procedure."

276

More Than One Type of Pain

Sherman says people with amputations report two typical types of phantom pain. "A burning and tingling sensation is common and attributed to decreased blood flow in the residual limb," he continues. "As circulation decreases due to age, medicines, inactivity, or other reasons, these sensations tend to increase. We generally treat this with medications or biofeedback.

"Muscle tension causes the other type of pain. If spasms occur, people experience cramping type pain. Generally, the more severe the cramps, the more severe the pain. The cramps are usually very fast and spasmodic—a high frequency muscle spasm, unlike a Charlie horse. Treatment includes cramp-reducing drugs, or muscle tension biofeedback."

Depression, Sherman agrees, increases phantom pain, and he, too, recommends antidepressants be used only until alternative treatments are found. "Phantom pain is a 'referred pain' phenomena," he says. "You can give the patient a surface 'fix', or you can attack the mechanism. Once the mechanism is destroyed, the phantom pain is eliminated and the need for daily medication stops."

Sherman treats about 50 people with amputations annually. "We help most people to at least some extent," he reports. "About 90 percent report that following therapy they no longer have the severe pain they once did. However, only 50 to 60 percent are cured completely. It's important to know that if medications and biofeedback don't help, it's likely because of a severely decreased blood flow caused by a condition, such as hardening of the arteries. We have little success with these patients. Nor do we understand the mechanisms of shocking treatments—like electric charges, and find there's little success in that area. One problem that continues to impede the progress in this area is that no two people experience the same type or intensity of pain—so there isn't a pill that works for all. Each patient requires treatment based on what they experience."

Levels of Therapy for Severe Cases

Todd Kuiken, M.D., Ph.D., works in biomedical engineering at the Rehabilitation Institute of Chicago (RIC), and is the director of amputee services for the institute. He also is an assistant professor at Northwestern University Medical School in Chicago, Illinois. Kuiken sees an average of 150 new patients with amputations annually. He says almost everyone who has an amputation has phantom limb sensation. "Some patients wake up after surgery and report that their missing toes and fingers are moving," Kuiken says. "Some tell us they like the sensation because it helps them walk with their prosthesis. Other times they say it's annoying. Some even report radically unusual feelings—like their foot is on backwards. In one case, a woman's arm was laid across her chest as she was rushed to the emergency room. After the amputation she felt the arm still lying on her chest. It's important to use caution when asking the patient if they're having sensation after surgery. We don't want to put the idea of pain in their mind if it's not already there."

Despite what literature says about phantom pain, Kuiken says an extensive difference exists in the percentage of people who feel it, and its severity. "We find between ten and twenty percent of patients request medication for their pain," he says. "They sometimes feel shooting, stabbing, or cramping, and often it's the same as what they felt prior to amputation. With most patients, the level of pain decreases over time, usually after the first few months, but a percentage suffer long-term pain."

For this reason, Kuiken changes treatment over time. "For the first few months treatments include desensitization techniques; tapping, rubbing, friction, and massaging the residual limb," he says. "Contrast baths—alternating from hot to cold water, is another treatment that works well. I prefer to try alternatives to medication first—but when the pain is intense enough to interfere with sleep or functioning, it's often required. Pain is subjective. Some people have higher pain tolerance levels than others—so each case must be evaluated individually. The patient must be told that the side effects of some medications can be worse than the pain itself. Neuropathic remedies, like antidepressants, are also effective, and tricyclic antidepressants are the best studied. They tend to make people sleepy, which can be good when taken at night; however, they also can cause palpitations, dry mouth, and weight gain."

Kuiken says more difficult cases require tougher treatment. He works closely with Dr. Norman Harden, at the Center for Pain Studies at RIC, in many of these cases. "We use a comprehensive multidisciplinary approach," he says. It includes psychotherapy, biofeedback, and physical and occupational therapy to their maximum potential. This is done on a daily basis as an outpatient service. The length of treatment varies depending on the patient's severity of pain—and until results are reached. This program teaches people how to live with their pain and get on with life."

Physical Therapists Staying Abreast

Cathie Szemere, a physical therapist at HealthSouth Sunrise Rehab Hospital, in Sunrise, Florida, treats patients with all types of ailments, but she specializes in pain management for people with amputations. Szemere says most people with amputations come to the inpatient facility from acute care hospitals in south Florida.

"It's important to distinguish between phantom pain and sensation," Szemere says. "Phantom pain is difficult to manage because there's no clear-cut definition or cause. Some patients report cramping or burning, and others say they feel their missing limb is in an awkward position—such as twisted underneath their body. These sensations usually are experienced shortly after surgery. People who experience these sensations generally say it dissipates within weeks. Other's report their pain is constant or intermittent—from mildly annoying to intolerable."

Szemere says gait training—learning to walk—is beneficial because it enhances the perception and provides a sense of the limb's normal position in space. "This helps give the patient a sense of when the knee should be bent to take a step," she says. "It reduces phantom pain for some. Desensitizing by rubbing a terry cloth on the residual limb, tapping gently on body parts, and hand-held massage units all help to decrease sensitivity. Residual limb swelling is another cause of pain. We apply compression with a shrinker, but in cases of severe swelling doctors sometimes use a rigid cast dressing. Swelling often continues unless a form of therapy reduces it. Using a prosthesis also helps eliminate swelling. Visualization techniques also help. We teach patients to close their eyes and visualize the missing limb is there—then pump the limb up and down."

Szemere also uses transcutaneous electrical nerve stimulation (TENS) for phantom pain treatment. "These are little electrodes that are moved over the skin," she continues. "Through trial and error we find where the slight current they provide offers the most relief. TENS helps to block the pain pathway to the brain so patients don't perceive it. It's a harmless apparatus, and patients can use it on their own. We like this treatment because it reduces the need for drugs. Trends in treatment today are moving away from medications—and we advocate as little use of drugs as possible, especially addictive pain pills. The key is to work with each patient individually to determine what works best for them."

Finally, Szemere says it's important to use caution in distinguishing between phantom pain and neuroma. "When the surgeon operates, a small ball forms on the end of the nerves," she says. "This causes pain in the residual limb that feels like an electrical current. We use an ultrasound treatment to decrease the inflammation in the area. Doctors sometimes inject analgesics with steroids into the residual. In severe cases, the surgeon has to go in and resect the nerve to another area to relieve the swelling responsible for the pain. If pain persists beyond these treatments, and before more aggressive treatment is tried, it's important to ensure that scar tissue, joint contractions, poor circulation, and other physiological conditions aren't the cause of the pain. Above all, Szemere says it's imperative for patients to get as much psychological support as possible."

Looking into a Future of Phantom Pain Relief

In recent years, Farabloc Development Corporation in British Columbia, Canada, has reported success with its proprietary fabric of woven nylon and fine metal fibers to help reduce phantom limb pain. In November 1993, the *Canadian Journal of Rehabilitation* reported that in a double-blind study using 34 sequentially randomized participants those using the Farabloc intervention reported complete, or near complete pain relief when using the garment, as compared to when they weren't wearing it. The study demonstrated that Farabloc does work for many amputees experiencing phantom limb pain, but not for every person—and it provides varying levels of pain relief.

Another treatment considered by some to be in the future investigation arena is Botox. This agent is derived from the bacterium, *Clostridium botulinum*, and is known as botulinus toxin type A. Botox is produced in controlled laboratory conditions and given in extremely small doses. Azad Bhatt, M.D., in Toms River, New Jersey, works in rehabilitation medicine, disability evaluations, electromyography, and pain management. He explains that the brain sends electrical messages to the muscles so they can contract and move. "The electrical message is transmitted to the muscle by a substance called acetylcholine," he says. "Botox works to block the release of acetylcholine and, as a result, the muscle doesn't receive the message to contract. This means the muscle spasms stop, or are greatly reduced, thereby providing pain relief."

Botox hasn't been tested in controlled environments or in studies on phantom pain, but Bhatt says it's reasonable to assume it will work with amputees the same way it works on others. "By injecting it into the residual area, the cramping and shooting pain would be alleviated although the limb is missing," he says.

Dr. Del Toro says he prefers to stick with medically proven treatments. "We're looking at pregabalin, a local anesthetic steroid, for future hope," he says. Studies currently underway indicate this medication, now used preoperatively, may hold hope for phantom pain sufferers. Results, however, have been mixed. I am using it in cases where the patient doesn't respond to other techniques, but I'd like to see more research in this field before it's used as a common pain-relief agent."

Dr. Sherman says because most people find relief with today's treatments, he too will stick to proven applications. "It's important to help the patient find relief—regardless of how many techniques the doctor or therapist has to try," he says. "One thing is sure, pain is pain, and people who suffer with intense amounts of it will ultimately go elsewhere and try just about anything they think will offer them relief. The danger is that they may subject themselves to something that damages their body in another way."

Chapter 38

Sciatica

Definition

Sciatica is a condition involving pain, weakness, numbness, or tingling in the leg. It is caused by injury to or compression of the sciatic nerve.

Causes

Sciatica is a form of peripheral neuropathy. It occurs when there is damage to the sciatic nerve, located in the back of the leg. This nerve controls the muscles of the back of the knee and lower leg and provides sensation to the back of the thigh, part of the lower leg and the sole of the foot. Incomplete damage to the sciatic nerve may appear identical to damage to one of the branches of the sciatic nerve (tibial nerve dysfunction or common peroneal nerve dysfunction).

A problem in a single nerve group, such as the sciatic nerve, is classified as a mononeuropathy. The usual causes are direct trauma (often due to an injection into the buttocks), prolonged external pressure on the nerve, and pressure on the nerve from nearby body structures. It can also be caused by entrapment—pressure on the nerve where it passes through a narrow structure. The damage slows or prevents conduction of impulses through the nerve.

The sciatic nerve is commonly injured by fractures of the pelvis, gunshot wounds, or other trauma to the buttocks or thigh. Prolonged

---

sitting or lying with pressure on the buttocks may also injure it. Systemic diseases, such as diabetes, can typically damage many different nerves, including the sciatic nerve. The sciatic nerve may also be harmed by pressure from masses such as a tumor or abscess, or by bleeding in the pelvis. In many cases, no cause can be identified.

Note: A ruptured lumbar disk in the spine may cause symptoms that simulate the symptoms of sciatic nerve dysfunction.

Symptoms

- Sensation changes
  - Of the back of the calf or the sole of the foot
  - Numbness, decreased sensation
  - Tingling, burning sensation
  - Pain, may be severe
  - Abnormal sensations

- Weakness of the knee or foot
  - Difficulty walking
  - Inability to move the foot (in severe cases)
  - Inability to bend the knee (in severe cases)

Exams and Tests

Sciatica might be revealed by a neuromuscular examination of the legs by a physician. There may be weakness of knee bending or foot movement, or difficulty bending the foot inward or down. Reflexes may be abnormal, with weak or absent ankle-jerk reflex. Pain down the leg can be reproduced by lifting the leg straight up off the examining table.

Tests that reveal sciatic nerve dysfunction may include:

- Electromyogram (EMG)—a recording of electrical activity in muscles;

- Nerve conduction tests.

Tests are guided by the suspected cause of the dysfunction, as suggested by the history, symptoms, and pattern of symptom development. They may include various blood tests, x-rays, magnetic resonance imaging (MRI), or other tests and procedures.

Treatment

Treatment is aimed at maximizing mobility and independence. The cause of the nerve dysfunction should be identified and treated as appropriate. In some cases, no treatment is required and recovery is spontaneous.

Conservative treatment is usually appropriate if there was sudden onset, minimal sensation changes, no difficulty in movement, no history of trauma to the area, and no evidence of degeneration of the nerve axon.

Surgical removal of lesions that press on the nerve, such as a herniated disk, may relieve symptoms. In cases of severe injury to the nerve, such as laceration, recovery may be not possible or may be limited.

Injections can be used to reduce inflammation around the nerve. Over-the-counter or prescription analgesics may be needed to control nerve pain.

Various other medications may reduce the stabbing pains that some people experience, including phenytoin, carbamazepine, or tricyclic antidepressants such as amitriptyline. Steroids may help with nerve inflammation related to a herniated disk. Whenever possible, their use should be avoided or minimized to reduce the risk of medication side effects.

Physical therapy exercises may be appropriate for some people to maintain muscle strength. The use of braces, splints, orthopedic shoes, or other appliances may help compensate for lost or impaired function. Vocational counseling, occupational therapy, occupational changes, job retraining, or similar interventions may be recommended.

Outlook (Prognosis)

If the cause of the sciatic nerve dysfunction can be identified and successfully treated, full recovery is possible. The extent of disability varies from no disability to partial or complete loss of movement or sensation. Nerve pain may be severe and persist for a prolonged period of time.

Possible Complications

- Partial or complete loss of leg movement
- Partial or complete loss of sensation in the leg

- Recurrent or unnoticed injury to the leg

- Side effects of medications

When to Contact a Medical Professional

Call your health care provider if you have symptoms of this disorder. Nerve pain is very difficult to treat. If you have ongoing problems with pain, you may want to see a pain specialist to ensure that you have access to the widest range of treatment options.

Prevention

Prevention varies depending on the cause of the nerve damage. Avoid prolonged sitting or lying with pressure on the buttocks.

Chapter 39

Shingles and Postherpetic Neuralgia

When the itchy red spots of childhood chickenpox disappear and life returns to normal, the battle with the virus that causes chickenpox seems won. But for too many of us this triumph of immune system over virus is temporary. The virus has not been destroyed but remains dormant in our nerve cells, ready to strike again later in life. This second eruption of the chickenpox virus is the disease called shingles or herpes zoster.

While young people do develop shingles, the disease most often strikes after age forty. But since shingles is so common, affecting an estimated one-quarter of Americans at some point during their lifetimes, cases in young people are not rare.

What is shingles?

Scientists call the virus that causes chickenpox and shingles varicella-zoster virus or VZV. VZV belongs to a group of viruses called herpesviruses. This group includes the herpes simplex virus that causes cold sores, fever blisters, mononucleosis, genital herpes (a sexually transmitted disease), and Epstein-Barr virus involved in infectious mononucleosis. Like VZV, other herpesviruses can hide in the nervous system after an initial infection and then travel down nerve cell fibers to cause a renewed infection. Repeated episodes of cold sores on the lips are the most common example.

Excerpted from "Shingles: Hope through Research," National Institute of Neurological Disorders and Stroke (NINDS), NIH Publication No. 06–307, July 2006, updated January 10, 2008.

As early as 1909, scientists suspected that the viruses causing chickenpox and shingles were one and the same. In 1958, detailed analyses of the viruses taken from patients with either chickenpox or shingles confirmed that the viruses were identical.

Virtually all adults in the United States have had chickenpox, even if it was so mild as to pass unnoticed, and thus may develop shingles later in life. In the original exposure to VZV (chickenpox), some of the virus particles leave the blood and settle into clusters of nerve cells (neurons) called sensory ganglia, where they remain for many years in an inactive (latent) form. The sensory ganglia, which are adjacent to the spinal cord and brain, relay information to the brain about what the body is sensing—heat, cold, touch, pain.

When the VZV reactivates, it spreads down the long nerve fibers (axons) that extend from the sensory cell bodies to the skin. The viruses multiply, the telltale rash erupts, and the person now has herpes zoster, or shingles. With shingles, the nervous system is more deeply involved than it was during the bout with chickenpox, and the symptoms are often more complex and severe.

Who is at risk for shingles?

About 25 percent of all adults, mostly otherwise healthy, will get shingles during their lifetimes, usually after age forty. The incidence increases with age so that shingles is ten times more likely to occur in adults over sixty than in children under ten. People with compromised immune systems—from use of immunosuppressive medications such as prednisone, from serious illnesses such as cancer, or from infection with human immunodeficiency virus (HIV)—are at special risk of developing shingles. These individuals also can have re-eruptions and some may have shingles that never heals. Most people who get shingles re-boost their immunity to VZV and will not get the disease for another few decades.

Youngsters whose mothers had chickenpox late in pregnancy—five to twenty-one days before giving birth—or who had chickenpox in infancy, have an increased risk of pediatric shingles. Sometimes these children are born with chickenpox or develop a typical case within a few days.

What are the symptoms of shingles?

The first sign of shingles is often burning or tingling pain, or itch, in one particular location on only one side of the body. After several days or a week, a rash of fluid-filled blisters, similar to chickenpox, appears in one area on one side of the body. Recent studies have shown that subtle cases of shingles with only a few lesions, or none, are more common than previously thought. These cases will usually remain unrecognized. Cases without any known lesions are known as *zoster sine herpete*.

Shingles pain can be mild or intense. Some people have mostly itching; some feel pain from the gentlest touch or breeze. The most common location for shingles is a band, called a dermatome, spanning one side of the trunk around the waistline. The second most common location is on one side of the face around the eye and on the forehead. However, shingles can involve any part of the body. The number of lesions is variable. Some rashes merge and produce an area that looks like a severe burn. Other patients may have just a few scattered lesions that don't cause severe symptoms.

For most healthy people, shingles rashes heal within a few weeks, the pain and itch that accompany the lesions subside, and the blisters leave no scars. Other people may have sensory symptoms that linger for a few months.

How should shingles be treated?

Shingles attacks can be made less severe and shorter by using prescription antiviral drugs: acyclovir, valacyclovir, or famciclovir. Acyclovir is available in a generic form, but the pills must be taken five times a day, whereas valacyclovir and famciclovir pills are taken three times a day. It is important not to miss any doses and not to stop taking the medication early. Antiviral drugs can reduce by about half the risk of being left with postherpetic neuralgia which is chronic pain that can last for months or years after the shingles rash clears. Doctors recommend starting antiviral drugs at the first sign of the shingles rash, or even if the telltale symptoms indicate that a rash is about to erupt. Even if a patient is not seen by a doctor at the beginning of the illness, it may still be useful to start antiviral medications if new lesions are still forming. Other treatments to consider are anti-inflammatory corticosteroids such as prednisone. These are routinely used when the eye or other facial nerves are affected.

Is shingles contagious?

A person with a shingles rash can pass the virus to someone, usually a child, who has never had chickenpox, but the child will develop chickenpox, not shingles. The child must come into direct contact with the open sores of the shingles rash. Merely being in the same room with a shingles patient will not cause the child to catch chickenpox because during a shingles infection the virus is not normally in the lungs and therefore can't be spread through the air.

People with chickenpox cannot communicate shingles to someone else although they can pass the chickenpox on to someone who has never had chickenpox. In cases of chickenpox, the virus can become airborne because it is found in the upper respiratory tract. Shingles occurs when an unknown trigger causes the virus hiding inside the person's body to become activated. Unlike chickenpox, shingles can't be caught from someone else.

How can shingles be prevented?

Chickenpox vaccine: Immunization with the varicella vaccine (or chickenpox vaccine)—now recommended in the United States for all children between 18 months and adolescence—can protect children from getting chickenpox. People who have been vaccinated against chickenpox are less likely to get shingles because the weak, attenuated strain of virus used in the chickenpox vaccine is less likely to survive in the body over decades. A definitive answer to the question of whether shingles can occur later in life in a person vaccinated against chickenpox will only be provided when enough data have been gathered over the next several decades.

Some scientists believe that immunizing children against chickenpox increases the risk of shingles in adults who were not themselves immunized during childhood. This is because when adults care for children sick with chickenpox, it boosts their own immunity that keeps the virus in their nerve cells from reactivating as shingles. With fewer children coming down with chickenpox, there are fewer opportunities for this boosting of adult immunity, and so there may be more shingles cases for the next 40–50 years.

Shingles vaccine: In May 2006, the U.S. Food and Drug Administration (FDA) approved a VZV vaccine (Zostavax) for use in people age sixty and older who have had chickenpox. When the vaccine becomes more widely available, many older adults will for the first time have a means of preventing shingles.

Researchers have found that giving older adults the vaccine reduced the expected number of cases of shingles by half. And in people who still got the disease despite immunization, the severity and complications of shingles were dramatically reduced. The shingles vaccine is only a preventive therapy and not a treatment for those who already have shingles or postherpetic neuralgia.

What is postherpetic neuralgia?

Sometimes, particularly in older people, shingles pain persists long after the rash has healed. This postherpetic neuralgia can be mild or severe—the most severe cases can lead to insomnia, weight loss, depression, and disability. Postherpetic neuralgia is not directly life-threatening. About a dozen medications in four categories have been shown in clinical trials to provide some pain relief. These include:

- *Tricyclic antidepressants (TCAs):* TCAs are often the first type of drug given to patients suffering from postherpetic neuralgia.

- *Anticonvulsants:* Some drugs that reduce seizures can also treat postherpetic neuralgia because seizures and pain both involve abnormally increased firing of nerve cells. An antiseizure medication, carbamazepine, is effective for postherpetic neuralgia but has rare, potentially dangerous side effects so a newer anticonvulsant, gabapentin, is far more often prescribed.

- *Opioids:* Opioids are strong pain medications used for all types of pain. They include oxycodone, morphine, tramadol, and methadone. Opioids can have side effects—including drowsiness, mental dulling, and constipation—and can be addictive, so their use must be monitored carefully in those with a history of addiction.

- *Topical local anesthetics:* Local anesthetics applied directly to the skin of the painful area affected by postherpetic neuralgia are also effective. Lidocaine, the most commonly prescribed, is available in cream, gel, or spray form. It is also available in a patch that has been approved by the FDA for use specifically in postherpetic neuralgia. With topical local anesthetics, the drug stays in the skin and therefore does not cause problems such as drowsiness or constipation. Capsaicin cream may be somewhat effective and is available over the counter, but most people find that it causes severe burning pain during application.

Postherpetic itch: The itch that sometimes occurs during or after shingles can be quite severe and painful. Clinical experience suggests that postherpetic itch is harder to treat than postherpetic neuralgia.

Topical local anesthetics (which numb the skin) provide substantial relief to some patients. Since postherpetic itch typically develops in skin that has severe sensory loss, it is particularly important to avoid scratching. Scratching numb skin too long or too hard can cause injury.

What are other complication of shingles?

People with ophthalmic shingles—lesions in or around the eye and forehead—can suffer painful eye infections, and in some cases immediate or delayed vision loss. People with shingles in or near the eye should see an ophthalmologist immediately. Shingles infections within or near the ear (Ramsay-Hunt syndrome) can cause hearing or balance problems as well as weakness of the muscles on the affected side of the face. In rare cases, shingles can spread into the brain or spinal cord and cause serious complications such as stroke or meningitis (an infection of the membranes outside the brain and spinal cord). People with shingles need to seek immediate medical evaluation if they notice neurological symptoms outside the region of the primary shingles attack.

Can infection with VZV during pregnancy harm the baby?

Many mothers-to-be are concerned about any infection contracted during pregnancy, and rightly so because some infections can be transmitted across the mother's bloodstream to the fetus or can be acquired by the baby during the birth process. VZV infection during pregnancy poses some risk to the unborn child, depending upon the stage of pregnancy. During the first thirty weeks, maternal chickenpox may, in some cases, lead to congenital malformations. Such cases are rare and experts differ in their opinions on how great the risk is. Most experts agree that shingles in a pregnant woman, a rare event, is even less likely to cause harm to the unborn child.

If a pregnant woman gets chickenpox between twenty-one to five days before giving birth, her newborn can have chickenpox at birth or develop it within a few days. But the time lapse between the start of the mother's illness and the birth of the baby generally allows the mother's immune system to react and produce antibodies to fight the virus. These antibodies can be transmitted to the unborn child and thus help fight the infection. Still, a small percent of the babies exposed to chickenpox in the twenty-one to five days before birth develop shingles in the first five years of life because the newborn's immune system is not yet fully functional and capable of keeping the virus latent.

What if the mother contracts chickenpox at the time of birth?

In that case, the mother's immune system has not had a chance to mobilize its forces. And although some of the mother's antibodies will be transmitted to the newborn via the placenta, the newborn will have little ability to fight off the attack because its immune system is immature. If these babies develop chickenpox as a result, it can be fatal. They are given zoster immune globulin, a preparation made from the antibody-rich blood of adults who have recently recovered from chickenpox or shingles, to lessen the severity of their chickenpox.

How can a person catch chickenpox, but not catch shingles?

Chickenpox and shingles are caused by the same virus—varicella-zoster (VZV). When a person, usually a child, who has not received the chickenpox vaccine (which became available in the United States in 1995) is exposed to VZV, he or she usually develops chickenpox, a highly contagious disease that can be spread by breathing as well as by contact with the rash. The infection begins in the upper respiratory tract where the virus incubates for fifteen days or more. VZV then spreads to the bloodstream and migrates to the skin, giving rise to the familiar chickenpox rash.

In contrast, you cannot catch shingles from someone else. You must already have been exposed to chickenpox and harbor the virus in your nervous system to develop shingles. When reactivated, the virus travels down nerves to the skin, causing the painful shingles rash. In shingles, the virus does not normally spread to the bloodstream or lungs, so the virus is not shed in air. Because the shingles rash contains active virus particles, someone who has never had chickenpox can catch it from exposure to a shingles rash.

For More Information

VZV Research Foundation
Research on Varicella Zoster
1202 Lexington Ave., Suite 204
New York, NY 10028
Phone: 212-222-3390
Fax: 212-222-8627
Website: http://www.vzvfoundation.org
E-mail: vzv@vzvfoundation.org

Chapter 40

Shoulder Pain

The shoulder joint is made up of bones held in place by muscles, tendons, and ligaments. Tendons are tough cords of tissue that hold the shoulder muscles to bones. They help the muscles move the shoulder. Ligaments hold the three shoulder bones to each other and help make the shoulder joint stable.

Who gets shoulder problems?

Men, women, and children can have shoulder problems. They occur in people of all races and ethnic backgrounds. Shoulder problems occur most often in people more than sixty years old.

What causes shoulder problems?

Many shoulder problems are caused by the breakdown of soft tissues in the shoulder region. Using the shoulder too much can cause the soft tissue to break down faster as people get older. Doing manual labor and playing sports may cause shoulder problems.

Shoulder pain may be felt in one small spot, in a larger area, or down the arm. Pain that travels along nerves to the shoulder can be caused by diseases such as gall bladder, liver, or heart disease, or disease of the spine in the neck.

This chapter includes "Fast Facts about Shoulder Problems," National Institute of Arthritis and Musculoskeletal and Skin Diseases (NIAMS), November 2006; and, an illustration from "Questions and Answers about Shoulder Problems," NIAMS, NIH Publication No. 06–4865, March 2006.

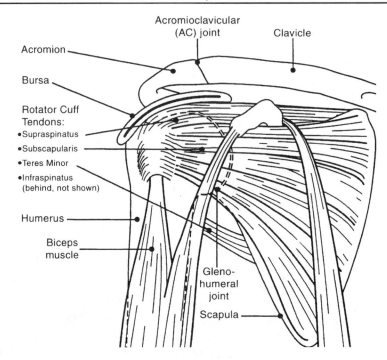

Acromioclavicular (AC) joint

Clavicle

Acromion

Bursa

Rotator Cuff Tendons:
- •Supraspinatus
- •Subscapularis
- •Teres Minor
- •Infraspinatus (behind, not shown)

Humerus

Biceps muscle

Gleno-humeral joint

Scapula

Figure 40.1. *Structure of the Shoulder*

How are shoulder problems diagnosed?

Doctors diagnose shoulder problems by using medical history, physical examination, and tests such as x-rays, ultrasound, and magnetic resonance imaging (MRI).

How are shoulder problems treated?

Shoulder problems are most often first treated with RICE (**R**est, **I**ce, **C**ompression, and **E**levation):

- **Rest:** Don't use the shoulder for 48 hours.

- **Ice:** Put an ice pack on the injured area for 20 minutes, four to eight times per day. Use a cold pack, ice bag, or a plastic bag filled with crushed ice wrapped in a towel.

- **Compression:** Put even pressure (compression) on the painful area to help reduce the swelling. A wrap or bandage will help hold the shoulder in place.

- **Elevation:** Keep the injured area above the level of the heart. Use a pillow to help keep the shoulder up.

If pain and stiffness persist, see a doctor to diagnose and treat the problem.

What are some common shoulder problems?

Dislocation: Dislocation occurs when the ball at the top of the bone in the upper arm pops out of the socket. It can happen if the shoulder is twisted or pulled very hard.

To treat a dislocation, a doctor performs a procedure to push the ball of the upper arm back into the socket. Further treatment may include the following:

- Wearing a sling or device to keep the shoulder in place
- Rest
- Ice three or four times a day
- Exercise to improve range of motion, strengthen muscles, and prevent injury

Once a shoulder is dislocated, it may happen again. This is common in young, active people. If the dislocation injures tissues or nerves around the shoulder, surgery may be needed.

Separation: A shoulder separation occurs when the ligaments between the collarbone and the shoulder blade are torn. The injury is most often caused by a blow to the shoulder or by falling on an outstretched hand.

Treatment for a shoulder separation includes the following:

- Rest
- A sling to keep the shoulder in place
- Ice to relieve pain and swelling
- Exercise, after a time of rest
- Surgery if tears are severe

Rotator cuff disease—tendonitis and bursitis: In tendonitis of the shoulder, tendons become inflamed (red, sore, and swollen) from being pinched by parts around the shoulder.

Bursitis occurs when the bursa—a small fluid-filled sac that helps protect the shoulder joint—is inflamed. Bursitis is sometimes caused by disease, such as rheumatoid arthritis. It is also caused by playing sports that overuse the shoulder or by jobs with frequent overhead reaching.

Tendonitis and bursitis may occur alone or at the same time. Treatment for tendonitis and bursitis includes the following:

- Rest

- Ice

- Medicines such as aspirin and ibuprofen that reduce pain and swelling

- Ultrasound (gentle sound-wave vibrations) to warm deep tissues and improve blood flow

- Gentle stretching and exercises to build strength

- Injection of corticosteroid drug if the shoulder does not get better in the first few weeks

- Surgery if the shoulder does not get better after 6–12 months

Rotator cuff tear: Rotator cuff tendons can become inflamed from frequent use or aging. Sometimes they are injured from a fall on an outstretched hand. Sports or jobs with repeated overhead motion can also damage the rotator cuff. Aging causes tendons to wear down which can lead to a tear. Some tears are not painful, but others can be very painful.

Treatment for a torn rotator cuff depends on age, health, how severe the injury is, and how long the person has had the torn rotator cuff. Treatment for torn rotator cuff includes the following:

- Rest

- Heat or cold to the sore area

- Medicines that reduce pain and swelling

- Electrical stimulation of muscles and nerves

- Ultrasound

- Cortisone injection

- Exercise to improve range-of-motion, strength, and function

- Surgery if the tear does not improve with other treatments

Frozen shoulder: Movement of the shoulder is very restricted in people with a frozen shoulder. Following are causes of frozen shoulder:

- Lack of use due to chronic pain
- Rheumatic disease that is getting worse
- Bands of tissue that grow in the joint and restrict motion
- Lack of the fluid that helps the shoulder joint move

Treatment for frozen shoulder includes the following:

- A doctor putting the bones into a position that will promote healing
- Medicines to reduce pain and swelling
- Heat
- Gentle stretching exercise
- Electrical stimulation of muscles and nerves
- Cortisone injection
- Surgery if the shoulder does not improve with other treatments

Fracture: A fracture is a crack through part or all of a bone. In the shoulder, a fracture usually involves the collarbone or upper arm bone. Fractures are often caused by a fall or blow to the shoulder.
Treatment for a fracture may include the following:

- A doctor putting the bones into a position that will promote healing
- A sling or other device to keep the bones in place
- Exercise to strengthen the shoulder and restore movement after the bone heals
- Surgery

Arthritis of the shoulder: Arthritis can be one of two types:

- Osteoarthritis: A disease caused by wear and tear of the cartilage
- Rheumatoid arthritis: An autoimmune disease causing one or more joints to become inflamed

Osteoarthritis of the shoulder is often treated with nonsteroidal anti-inflammatory drugs (NSAIDs) such as aspirin and ibuprofen. People with rheumatoid arthritis may need physical therapy and medicine such as corticosteroids. If these treatments for arthritis of the shoulder do not relieve pain or improve function, surgery may be needed.

Chapter 41

Sickle Cell Anemia
and Sickle Cell Crisis

Sickle cell anemia is a serious condition in which the red blood cells can become sickle-shaped (shaped like a C). Normal red blood cells are smooth and round like a doughnut without a hole. They move easily through blood vessels to carry oxygen to all parts of the body. Sickle-shaped cells do not move easily through blood. They are stiff and sticky and tend to form clumps and get stuck in blood vessels. The clumps of sickle cells block blood flow in the blood vessels that lead to the limbs and organs. Blocked blood vessels can cause pain, serious infections, and organ damage.

Sickle cell anemia is an inherited, lifelong condition. People who have sickle cell anemia are born with it. They inherit two copies of the sickle cell gene, one from each parent. People who inherit a sickle cell gene from one parent and a normal gene from the other parent have a condition called sickle cell trait.

Sickle cell trait is different from sickle cell anemia. People with sickle cell trait do not have the condition, but they have one of the genes that cause the condition. Like people with sickle cell anemia, people with sickle cell trait can pass the gene on when they have children.

Sickle cell anemia affects millions of people worldwide. There are excellent treatments for the symptoms and complications of the condition, but in most cases there is no cure. (Some researchers believe

Excerpted from "What Is Sickle Cell Anemia?" National Heart, Lung, and Blood Institute (NHLBI), May 2007. The full text is available at http://www.nhlbi.nih.gov/health/dci/Diseases/ScaSCA_WhatIs.html.

that bone marrow transplants may offer a cure in a small number of cases.)

Over the past 30 years, doctors have learned a great deal about the condition. They know what causes it, how it affects the body, and how to treat many of the complications. Today, with good health care, many people with the condition live close to normal lives and are in fairly good health much of the time. These people can live into their forties or fifties, or longer.

Anemia

Anemia is a condition in which a person's blood has a lower than normal number of red blood cells, or the red blood cells do not have enough hemoglobin. Hemoglobin is an iron-rich protein that gives blood its red color and carries oxygen from the lungs to the rest of the body.

Red blood cells are made in the spongy marrow inside the large bones of the body. Bone marrow constantly makes new red blood cells to replace old ones. Normal red blood cells last about 120 days in the bloodstream and then die. Their main role is to carry oxygen, but they also remove carbon dioxide (a waste product) from cells and carry it to the lungs to be exhaled.

In sickle cell anemia, a lower-than-normal number of red blood cells occurs because sickle cells do not last very long. Sickle cells die faster than normal red blood cells, usually after only about ten to twenty days. The bone marrow cannot make new red blood cells fast enough to replace the dying ones. The result is anemia.

Signs and Symptoms of Sickle Cell Anemia

The signs and symptoms of sickle cell anemia are different in each person. Some people have mild symptoms. Others have very severe symptoms and are often hospitalized for treatment. Although sickle cell anemia is present at birth, many infants do not show any signs until after four months of age. The most common signs and symptoms are linked to anemia and pain. Other signs and symptoms are linked to some of the complications of the condition.

Anemia

The general signs and symptoms of anemia are fatigue (tiredness), pale skin and nail beds, jaundice (yellowing of the skin and eyes), and shortness of breath.

Pain: Sickle Cell Crisis

Sudden episodes of pain throughout the body are a common symptom of sickle cell anemia and are often referred to as sickle cell crises. A sickle cell crisis occurs when the red blood cells sickle (become C shaped) and stick together in clumps. The clumps block the flow of blood through the small blood vessels (capillaries) in the limbs and organs.

Sickle crises can cause acute or chronic pain. Acute pain is the most common type. This is sudden pain that can range from mild to very severe. The pain usually lasts from hours to a few days. Chronic pain usually lasts for weeks to months. Chronic pain can be hard to bear and mentally draining. This pain may severely limit daily activities. Almost all people with sickle cell anemia have painful crises at some point in their lives. Some have a crisis less than once a year. Others may have 15 or more crises in a year.

Many factors can contribute to a sickle cell crisis. Often, more than one factor is involved and the exact cause cannot be identified. Factors that occur in your body and are not under your control can cause a sickle cell crisis, such as an infection. Factors that you can control also can affect whether you have a sickle cell crisis. For example, dehydration (when your body does not have enough fluid) can increase your chances of having a sickle cell crisis. Drinking plenty of fluids so your body is hydrated can often help decrease the chance of a crisis. The most common sites affected by sickle cell crises are the bones, lungs, abdomen, and joints. The blocked blood flow can cause pain and organ damage.

Complications of Sickle Cell Anemia

Complications of sickle cell anemia come from the effects of sickle cell crises on different parts of the body.

Hand-foot syndrome: When sickle cells block the small blood vessels in the hands or feet, pain and swelling along with fever can occur. One or both hands and/or feet may be affected at the same time. Pain may be felt in the many bones of the hands and feet. Swelling usually occurs on the back of the hands and feet and moves into the fingers and toes. This may be the first sign of sickle cell anemia in infants.

Splenic (sequestration) crisis: The spleen is an organ in the abdomen that filters out abnormal red blood cells and helps fight infection. Sometimes, the spleen traps many cells that should be in the bloodstream and it grows large. This causes anemia. Blood transfusions may be needed until the body can make more cells and recover. If the spleen becomes too clogged with sickle cells, it cannot work normally. It begins to shrink and stop working.

Infections: Both children and adults with sickle cell anemia have a hard time fighting infections. Sickle cell anemia can damage the spleen. Infants and young children with a damaged spleen are more likely to get infections that can kill them within hours or days. Pneumonia is the most common cause of death in young children who have sickle cell anemia. Meningitis, influenza, and hepatitis are other infections that are common in people with sickle cell anemia.

Acute chest syndrome: This is a life-threatening condition linked to sickle cell anemia. It is similar to pneumonia and is caused by an infection or by sickle cells trapped in the lungs. People with this condition usually have chest pain, fever, and an abnormal chest x-ray. Over time, lung damage may lead to pulmonary arterial hypertension.

Delayed growth and puberty in children: Children with sickle cell anemia often grow more slowly and reach puberty later than other children. A shortage of red blood cells (anemia) causes the slow growth rate. Adults with sickle cell anemia often are slender or small in size.

Stroke: Sickle-shaped red blood cells may stick to the walls of the tiny blood vessels in the brain. This can cause a stroke. This type of stroke occurs mainly in children. The stroke can cause learning disabilities or more severe problems.

Eye problems: The retina, a thin layer of tissue at the back of the eye, takes the images you see and sends them to your brain. When the retina does not get enough blood, it can weaken. A weak retina can cause serious problems, including blindness.

Priapism: Males with sickle cell anemia may have painful and unwanted erections called priapism. This happens because the sickle cells stop blood flow out of an erect penis. Over time, priapism can damage the penis and lead to impotence.

Gallstones: When red blood cells die, they release their hemoglobin, which the body breaks down into a compound called bilirubin. When there is too much bilirubin in the body, stones can form in the gallbladder. Gallstones can cause steady pain that lasts for 30 minutes or more in the upper right side of the belly, under the right shoulder, or between the shoulder blades. The pain may happen after eating fatty meals. People with gallstones may have nausea, vomiting, fever, sweating, chills, clay-colored stool, or jaundice (yellowish color of the skin or whites of the eyes).

Ulcers on the legs: Sickle cell ulcers (sores) usually begin as small, raised, crusted sores on the lower third of the leg. Leg sores occur more often in males than in females and usually appear between the ages of ten and fifty. The cause of leg ulcers is not clear. The number of ulcers can vary from one to many. Some heal rapidly, but others persist for years or come back after healing.

Pulmonary arterial hypertension (high blood pressure): Damage to the small blood vessels in the lungs makes it hard for the heart to pump blood through the lungs. This causes blood pressure in the lungs to increase. This condition is called pulmonary arterial hypertension. Excessive shortness of breath is an important symptom linked to this problem.

Multiple organ failure: Multiple organ failure is rare, but serious. It happens when a person has a sickle cell crisis that causes two out of three major organs (lungs, liver, or kidney) to fail. Symptoms linked to this complication are a fever and changes in mental status such as sudden tiredness and loss of interest in your surroundings.

Diagnosis of Sickle Cell Anemia

Early diagnosis of sickle cell anemia is very important so that children who have the condition can get proper treatment. In the United States, 44 States, the District of Columbia, Puerto Rico, and the U.S. Virgin Islands now test all newborns for sickle cell anemia. In the other six States, you can request a sickle cell test. Electrophoresis is usually used to diagnose older children and adults. It is also possible to identify sickle cell anemia before birth. This is done using a sample of amniotic fluid or tissue taken from the placenta. This test can be done as early as the first few months of pregnancy. It identifies the sickle gene, rather than the hemoglobin it makes.

Treatment of Sickle Cell Anemia

Effective treatments are available to help relieve the symptoms and complications of sickle cell anemia, but in most cases there is no cure.

Some researchers believe that bone marrow transplants may offer a cure in a small number of cases. Researchers are looking for new treatments for sickle cell anemia, including gene therapy and safer and more effective bone marrow transplants.

People who have sickle cell anemia need regular medical care. Some doctors and clinics specialize in treating people with the condition. Doctors specializing in sickle cell anemia are often hematologists (doctors who treat people with blood disorders)—or pediatric hematologists (if they also treat children).

Goals of Treatment

The goals of treating sickle cell anemia are to relieve pain; prevent infections, eye damage, and strokes; and control complications if they occur. The treatments include medicine, blood transfusions, and specific treatment for complications.

Treating Pain

Mild painful crises can be managed with treatments such as over-the-counter medicine and heating pads. However, severe pain may need to be treated in a hospital. Painful crises are the leading cause of emergency room visits and hospitalizations of people with sickle cell anemia.

The usual treatments for acute (short-term) pain crises are pain-killing medicines and fluids, given either by mouth or through a vein, to prevent dehydration (a condition in which your body does not have enough fluids). The pain-killing medicines most often used are acetaminophen, nonsteroidal anti-inflammatory drugs (NSAIDs), and narcotics such as meperidine, morphine, oxycodone, and others.

The treatment of patients who have mild-to-moderate pain usually begins with NSAIDs or acetaminophen. If pain continues, a narcotic may be added. Moderate-to-severe pain is often treated with narcotics. The narcotic may be used alone or together with NSAIDs or acetaminophen. Narcotic abuse and addiction are pain management issues that must be considered in any pain control plan.

A medicine called hydroxyurea may be given to adults and older adolescents with severe sickle cell anemia to reduce their number of painful crises. This medicine is used only to prevent these crises, not to treat them when they occur. Given daily, hydroxyurea can reduce the frequency of painful crises and of acute chest syndrome. People taking the medicine also may need fewer blood transfusions.

People taking hydroxyurea must be watched carefully because the medicine can cause serious side effects, including an increased risk of dangerous infections. Some evidence suggests that long-term use of hydroxyurea can cause tumors or leukemia. Because of these risks, the medicine is usually only used in adults and older teenagers with severe sickle cell anemia. Although hydroxyurea is being tested in infants and children at this time, it will not be approved for use in children until its long-term effects can be more closely studied.

Preventing Infections

Infection is a major complication of sickle cell anemia. In fact, pneumonia is the leading cause of death in children with the condition. Other infections common in people with sickle cell anemia include meningitis, influenza, and hepatitis. If a child with sickle cell anemia shows early signs of an infection, such as fever, seek treatment right away.

To prevent infections in babies and young children, treatments include the following:

- Daily doses of penicillin. Treatment may begin as early as two months of age and continue until the child is at least five years old.

- Vaccinations for pneumonia, meningitis, influenza, and hepatitis.

- A yearly flu shot.

Adults who have sickle cell anemia also should have flu shots every year and be vaccinated for pneumonia.

Preventing Eye Damage

Sickle cell anemia can damage the blood vessels in the eyes. Parents should ask their child's doctor about regular checkups with an eye doctor who specializes in diseases of the retina. Adults with sickle cell anemia also should have regular checkups with an eye doctor.

Preventing Strokes

Stroke prevention and treatment is now possible for children and adults who have sickle cell anemia. Starting at age two, children with sickle cell anemia often receive regular ultrasound scans of the head (this is called transcranial Doppler ultrasound). These scans are used to monitor blood flow in the brain.

The scans allow doctors to find out which children are at high risk for a stroke and treat them with regular blood transfusions. Routine blood transfusions have been found to greatly reduce the number of strokes in children.

Blood Transfusions

Blood transfusions are used to treat worsening anemia and sickle cell complications. A sudden worsening of anemia due to an infection or enlargement of the spleen is a common reason for a blood transfusion. Some, but not all, patients need transfusions to prevent life-threatening events such as stroke or pneumonia.

Regular blood transfusions do have side effects, and patients must be carefully watched. Side effects can include a dangerous buildup of iron in the blood (which must be treated) as well as an increased risk of infection from the transfused blood.

Treating Other Complications

Acute chest syndrome is a severe and life-threatening complication in children and adults who have sickle cell anemia. Treatment usually requires hospitalization and may include oxygen, blood transfusions, antibiotics, pain medicine, and monitoring the body's fluids.

Leg ulcers can be painful, and patients may be given strong pain medicines. Ulcers can be treated with cleansing solutions and medicated creams or ointments. Skin grafts may be needed if the condition continues. Bed rest and keeping the legs raised to reduce swelling are helpful, although not always possible.

Gallbladder surgery may be needed if the presence of gallstones leads to gallbladder disease. Priapism can be treated with fluids or surgery.

New Treatments

Today, research on sickle cell anemia is looking at bone marrow transplants, gene therapy, and new medicines. The hope is that these studies will provide better treatments for sickle cell anemia. Researchers also are looking for a way to predict the severity of the condition.

Coping with Pain

Pain is different for each person. Pain that one person can live with is too much for another person. Work with your doctor to make a pain management plan that works well for you. It may include both over-the-counter and prescription medicines. Talk with your doctor about how to safely use narcotic pain medicines.

Other ways to manage pain include using a heating pad, taking a hot bath, resting, or getting a massage. Physical therapy might help to relieve your pain if it can help you relax and strengthen your muscles and joints. Counseling and self-hypnosis may help. Also helpful are activities that keep your mind off the pain, such as watching television and talking on the phone.

Chapter 42

Somatization Disorder

Alternative name: Briquet syndrome

Definition

Somatization disorder is a chronic condition in which there are numerous physical complaints. These complaints can last for years, and result in substantial impairment. The physical symptoms are caused by psychological problems, and no underlying physical problem can be identified.

Causes

The disorder is marked by multiple physical complaints that persist for years, involving any body system. Most frequently, the complaints involve chronic pain and problems with the digestive system, the nervous system, and the reproductive system. The disorder usually begins before the age of 30 and occurs more often in women than in men. Recent research has shown higher percentages of this disorder in people with irritable bowel syndrome and chronic pain patients.

Somatization disorder is highly stigmatized, and patients are often dismissed by their physicians as having problems that are "all in your head." However, as researchers study the connections between the brain, the digestive system, and the immune system, somatization disorders are becoming better understood. They should not be seen as faked conditions that the patient could end if he or she chose to do so.

The symptoms are generally severe enough to interfere with work and relationships and lead the person to visit the doctor and even take medication. A lifelong history of "sickliness" is often present. However, despite thorough investigation, no specific underlying physical cause is ever identified to account for the symptoms. Stress often worsens the symptoms.

Symptoms

Some of the numerous symptoms that can occur with somatization disorder include:

- Vomiting
- Abdominal pain
- Nausea
- Bloating
- Diarrhea
- Pain in the legs or arms
- Back pain
- Joint pain
- Pain during urination
- Headaches
- Shortness of breath
- Palpitations
- Chest pain
- Dizziness
- Amnesia
- Difficulty swallowing
- Vision changes
- Paralysis or muscle weakness
- Sexual apathy
- Pain during intercourse
- Impotence
- Painful menstruation
- Irregular menstruation
- Excessive menstrual bleeding

It is important to note that many of these symptoms also occur in other medical and psychiatric disorders. If you experience any of these symptoms, be sure to work with your doctor to rule out possible causes before a diagnosis of somatization disorder is made.

Exams and Tests

- A thorough physical examination and diagnostic tests are performed to rule out physical causes. Which tests are done depends on the symptoms present.

- A psychological evaluation is performed to rule out related disorders.

Treatment

Once other causes have been ruled out and a diagnosis of somatization disorder is secured, the goal of treatment is to help the person learn to control the symptoms. There is often an underlying mood disorder which can respond to conventional treatment, such as antidepressant medications. Unfortunately, persons with this disorder rarely admit that it can be caused, at least in part, by mental health problems, and will usually refuse psychiatric treatment.

A supportive relationship with a sympathetic health care provider is the most important aspect of treatment. Regularly scheduled appointments should be maintained to review symptoms and the person's coping mechanisms. Test results should be explained.

You should not be told that your symptoms are imaginary. With the current understanding of the complex interactions between the brain and other body parts, scientists recognize that true physical symptoms can result from psychological stress.

Possible Complications

- Complications may result from invasive testing and from multiple evaluations that are performed while looking for the cause of the symptoms.

- A dependency on pain relievers or sedatives may develop.

- A poor relationship with the health care provider seems to worsen the condition, as does evaluation by many providers.

When to Contact a Medical Professional

A good relationship with a consistent primary health care provider is helpful. Call for an appointment if there is a significant change in symptoms.

Prevention

Counseling or other psychological interventions may help people who are prone to somatization learn other ways of dealing with stresses. This may help reduce the intensity of the symptoms.

Chapter 43

Sports Injuries: Acute and Chronic Pain

Sports injuries are injuries that happen when playing sports or exercising. Some are from accidents. Others can result from poor training practices or improper gear. Some people get injured when they are not in proper condition. Not warming up or stretching enough before you play or exercise can also lead to injuries. The most common sports injuries are:

- sprains and strains,
- knee injuries,
- swollen muscles,
- Achilles tendon injuries,
- pain along the shin bone,
- fractures, and
- dislocations.

Acute and Chronic Injury

There are two kinds of sports injuries: acute and chronic. Acute injuries occur suddenly when playing or exercising. Sprained ankles,

Excerpted from "Fast Facts about Sports Injuries," National Institute of Arthritis and Musculoskeletal and Skin Diseases (NIAMS), June 2005.

strained backs, and fractured hands are acute injuries. Following are signs of an acute injury:

- Sudden, severe pain
- Swelling
- Not being able to place weight on a leg, knee, ankle, or foot
- An arm, elbow, wrist, hand, or finger that is very tender
- Not being able to move a joint as normal
- Extreme leg or arm weakness
- A bone or joint that is visibly out of place

Chronic injuries happen after you play a sport or exercise for a long time. Signs of a chronic injury include the following:

- Pain when you play
- Pain when you exercise
- A dull ache when you rest
- Swelling

What should I do if I get injured?

Never try to work through the pain of a sports injury. Stop playing or exercising when you feel pain. Playing or exercising more only causes more harm. Some injuries should be seen by a doctor right away. Others you can treat yourself.

Call a doctor when:

- the injury causes severe pain, swelling, or numbness;
- you cannot put any weight on the area;
- an old injury hurts or aches;
- an old injury swells; or
- the joint doesn't feel normal or feels unstable.

If you do not have any of these signs, it may be safe to treat the injury at home. If the pain or other symptoms get worse, you should call your doctor. Use the RICE (**R**est, **I**ce, **C**ompression, and **E**levation) method to relieve pain, reduce swelling, and speed healing. Follow these four steps right after the injury occurs and do so for at least 48 hours:

- **Rest.** Reduce your regular activities. If you have injured your foot, ankle, or knee, take weight off of it. A crutch can help. If your right foot or ankle is injured, use the crutch on the left side. If your left foot or ankle is injured, use the crutch on the right side.

- **Ice.** Put an ice pack to the injured area for 20 minutes, four to eight times a day. You can use a cold pack or ice bag. You can also use a plastic bag filled with crushed ice and wrapped in a towel. Take the ice off after 20 minutes to avoid cold injury.

- **Compression.** Put even pressure (compression) on the injured area to help reduce swelling. You can use an elastic wrap, special boot, air cast, or splint. Ask your doctor which one is best for your injury.

- **Elevation.** Put the injured area on a pillow, at a level above your heart, to help reduce swelling.

Treatments for Sports Injuries

Treatment often begins with the RICE method. Here are some other things your doctor may do to treat your sports injury.

Nonsteroidal anti-inflammatory drugs (NSAIDs): Your doctor will suggest that you take a nonsteroidal anti-inflammatory drug (NSAID) such as aspirin, ibuprofen, ketoprofen, or naproxen sodium. These drugs reduce swelling and pain. You can buy them at a drug store. Another common drug is acetaminophen. It may relieve pain, but it will not reduce swelling.

Immobilization: Immobilization is a common treatment for sports injuries. It keeps the injured area from moving and prevents more damage. Slings, splints, casts, and leg immobilizers are used to immobilize sports injuries.

Surgery: In some cases, surgery is needed to fix sports injuries. Surgery can fix torn tendons and ligaments or put broken bones back in place. Most sports injuries do not need surgery.

Rehabilitation (exercise): Rehabilitation is a key part of treatment. It involves exercises that step by step get the injured area back to normal. Moving the injured area helps it to heal. The sooner this is done, the better. Exercises start by gently moving the injured body part through a range of motions. The next step is to stretch. After a while, weights may be used to strengthen the injured area.

As injury heals, scar tissue forms. After a while, the scar tissue shrinks. This shrinking brings the injured tissues back together. When this happens, the injured area becomes tight or stiff. This is when you are at greatest risk of injuring the area again. You should stretch the muscles every day. You should always stretch as a warmup before you play or exercise.

Do not play your sport until you are sure you can stretch the injured area without pain, swelling, or stiffness. When you start playing again, start slowly. Build up step by step to full speed.

Rest: Although it is good to start moving the injured area as soon as possible, you must also take time to rest after an injury. All injuries need time to heal; proper rest helps the process. Your doctor can guide you on the proper balance between rest and rehabilitation.

Other therapies: Other common therapies that help with the healing process include mild electrical currents (electrostimulation), cold packs (cryotherapy), heat packs (thermotherapy), sound waves (ultrasound), and massage.

Today, treating a sports injury is much better than in the past. Most people who get sports injuries play sports and exercise again. Doctors have many new ways to treat sports injuries. Some of these new ways include:

- arthroscopy (fiber optic scopes put through small cuts in the skin to see inside joints),

- tissue engineering (using a person's own tissues or cells to help heal injuries), and

- targeted pain relief (pain-reducing drug patches put directly on the injured area).

Chapter 44

Temporomandibular Muscle and Joint (TMJ) Disorders

Temporomandibular joint and muscle disorders (TMJ), are a group of conditions that cause pain and dysfunction in the jaw joint and the muscles that control jaw movement. We do not know for certain how many people have TMJ disorders, but some estimates suggest that over ten million Americans are affected. The condition appears to be more common in women than men.

For most people, pain in the area of the jaw joint or muscles does not signal a serious problem. Generally, discomfort from these conditions is occasional and temporary, often occurring in cycles. The pain eventually goes away with little or no treatment. Some people, however, develop significant, long-term symptoms.

What is the temporomandibular joint?

The temporomandibular joint connects the lower jaw, called the mandible, to the bone at the side of the head—the temporal bone. If you place your fingers just in front of your ears and open your mouth, you can feel the joints. Because these joints are flexible, the jaw can move smoothly up and down and side to side, enabling us to talk, chew, and yawn. Muscles attached to and surrounding the jaw joint control its position and movement.

Excerpted from "TMJ Disorders," National Institute of Dental and Craniofacial Research (NIDCR), NIH Publication No. 06–3487, September 2006.

319

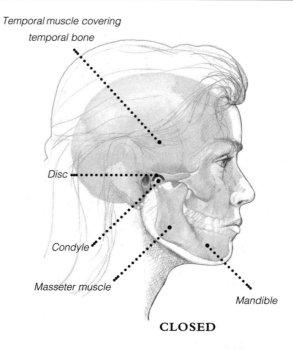

Temporal muscle covering temporal bone

Disc

Condyle

Masseter muscle

Mandible

CLOSED

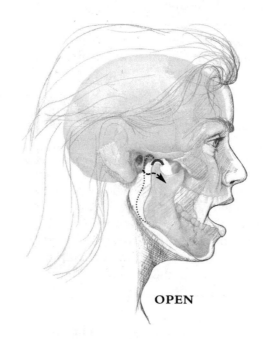

OPEN

Figure 44.1. Temporomandibular Joint

When we open our mouths, the rounded ends of the lower jaw, called condyles, glide along the joint socket of the temporal bone. The condyles slide back to their original position when we close our mouths. To keep this motion smooth, a soft disc lies between the condyle and the temporal bone. This disc absorbs shocks to the jaw joint from chewing and other movements.

What are TMJ disorders?

Disorders of the jaw joint and chewing muscles—and how people respond to them—vary widely. Researchers generally agree that the conditions fall into three main categories:

1. Myofascial pain, the most common temporomandibular disorder, involves discomfort or pain in the muscles that control jaw function.

2. Internal derangement of the joint involves a displaced disc, dislocated jaw, or injury to the condyle.

3. Arthritis refers to a group of degenerative and inflammatory joint disorders that can affect the temporomandibular joint.

A person may have one or more of these conditions at the same time. Some people have other health problems that co-exist with TMJ disorders, such as chronic fatigue syndrome, sleep disturbances, or fibromyalgia—a painful condition that affects muscles and other soft tissues throughout the body. It is not known whether these disorders share a common cause. People who have a rheumatic disease, such as rheumatoid arthritis, may develop TMJ disease as a secondary condition.

What are the signs and symptoms?

A variety of symptoms may be linked to TMJ disorders. Pain, particularly in the chewing muscles or jaw joint, is the most common symptom. Other likely symptoms include:

*   radiating pain in the face, jaw, or neck;

*   jaw muscle stiffness;

*   limited movement or locking of the jaw;

*   painful clicking, popping, or grating in the jaw joint when opening or closing the mouth; or

*   a change in the way the upper and lower teeth fit together.

How are TMJ disorders diagnosed?

There is no widely accepted, standard test now available to correctly diagnose TMJ disorders. Because the exact causes and symptoms are not clear, identifying these disorders can be difficult and confusing. Currently, health care providers note the patient's description of symptoms, take a detailed medical and dental history, and examine problem areas including the head, neck, face, and jaw. Imaging studies may also be recommended.

You may want to consult your doctor to rule out known causes of pain. Facial pain can be a symptom of many other conditions, such as sinus or ear infections, various types of headaches, and facial neuralgias (nerve-related facial pain). Ruling out these problems first helps in identifying TMJ disorders.

Treatments for TMJ Disorders

Because more studies are needed on the safety and effectiveness of most treatments for jaw joint and muscle disorders, experts strongly recommend using the most conservative, reversible treatments possible. Conservative treatments do not invade the tissues of the face, jaw, or joint, or involve surgery. Reversible treatments do not cause permanent changes in the structure or position of the jaw or teeth. Even when TMJ disorders have become persistent, most patients still do not need aggressive types of treatment.

Conservative Treatments

Because the most common jaw joint and muscle problems are temporary and do not get worse, simple treatment is all that is usually needed to relieve discomfort.

Self-care practices: There are steps you can take that may be helpful in easing symptoms, such as:

- eating soft foods,
- applying ice packs,
- avoiding extreme jaw movements (such as wide yawning, loud singing, and gum chewing),
- learning techniques for relaxing and reducing stress, and
- practicing gentle jaw stretching and relaxing exercises that may help increase jaw movement.

Your health care provider or a physical therapist can recommend exercises if appropriate for your particular condition.

Pain medications: For many people with TMJ disorders, short-term use of over-the-counter pain medicines or nonsteroidal anti-inflammatory drugs (NSAIDs), such as ibuprofen, may provide temporary relief from jaw discomfort. When necessary, your dentist or doctor can prescribe stronger pain or anti-inflammatory medications, muscle relaxants, or antidepressants to help ease symptoms.

Stabilization splints: Your doctor or dentist may recommend an oral appliance, also called a stabilization splint or bite guard, which is a plastic guard that fits over the upper or lower teeth. Stabilization splints are the most widely used treatments for TMJ disorders. Studies of their effectiveness in providing pain relief, however, have been inconclusive. If a stabilization splint is recommended, it should be used only for a short time and should not cause permanent changes in the bite. If a splint causes or increases pain, stop using it and see your health care provider.

The conservative, reversible treatments described are useful for temporary relief of pain—they are not cures for TMJ disorders. If symptoms continue over time, come back often, or worsen, tell your doctor.

Irreversible Treatments

Irreversible treatments that have not been proven to be effective—and may make the problem worse—include orthodontics to change the bite; crown and bridge work to balance the bite; grinding down teeth to bring the bite into balance, called occlusal adjustment; and repositioning splints, also called orthotics, which permanently alter the bite.

Surgery: Other types of treatments, such as surgical procedures, invade the tissues. Surgical treatments are controversial, often irreversible, and should be avoided where possible. There have been no long-term clinical trials to study the safety and effectiveness of surgical treatments for TMJ disorders. Nor are there standards to identify people who would most likely benefit from surgery. Failure to respond to conservative treatments, for example, does not automatically mean that surgery is necessary. If surgery is recommended, be sure to have the doctor explain to you, in words you can understand, the reason for the treatment, the risks involved, and other types of treatment that may be available.

Implants: Surgical replacement of jaw joints with artificial implants may cause severe pain and permanent jaw damage. Some of these devices may fail to function properly or may break apart in the jaw over time. If you have already had temporomandibular joint surgery, be very cautious about considering additional operations. Persons undergoing multiple surgeries on the jaw joint generally have a poor outlook for normal, pain-free joint function. Before undergoing any surgery on the jaw joint, it is extremely important to get other independent opinions and to fully understand the risks.

The U.S. Food and Drug Administration (FDA) monitors the safety and effectiveness of medical devices implanted in the body, including artificial jaw joint implants. Patients and their health care providers can report serious problems with TMJ implants to the FDA through MedWatch at http://www.fda.gov/medwatch, or telephone toll-free at 800-332-1088.

Prognosis

Remember that for most people, discomfort from TMJ disorders will eventually go away on its own. Simple self-care practices are often effective in easing symptoms. If treatment is needed, it should be based on a reasonable diagnosis, be conservative and reversible, and be customized to your special needs. Avoid treatments that can cause permanent changes in the bite or jaw. If irreversible treatments are recommended, be sure to get a reliable, independent second opinion.

Because there is no certified specialty for TMJ disorders in either dentistry or medicine, finding the right care can be difficult. Look for a health care provider who understands musculoskeletal disorders (affecting muscle, bone, and joints) and who is trained in treating pain conditions. Pain clinics in hospitals and universities are often a good source of advice, particularly when pain continues over time and interferes with daily life. Complex cases, often marked by prolonged, persistent, and severe pain; jaw dysfunction; co-existing conditions; and diminished quality of life, likely require a team of experts from various fields, such as neurology, rheumatology, pain management, and others, to diagnose and treat this condition.

Implant Registry

To learn more about TMJ implants and their medical effects on patients, the National Institute of Dental and Craniofacial Research (NIDCR) has launched a TMJ implant registry. The registry tracks the health of patients who receive implants, as well as those who already have the devices, or who have had them removed. Scientists also examine implants that have been removed to learn why problems developed in these patients. By increasing understanding of how temporomandibular joint implants perform and why they often fail, the study will help scientists design safer and more effective implants. To learn more about the TMJ implant registry, visit the registry online at http://tmjregistry.org.

Chapter 45

Tooth Pain

What is a toothache?

Toothache is pain typically around a tooth, teeth, or jaws. In most instances, toothaches are caused by a dental problem, such as a dental cavity, a cracked or fractured tooth, an exposed tooth root, or gum disease. Sometimes diseases of the jaw joint (temporomandibular joint), or spasms of the muscles used for chewing can cause toothache like symptoms.

The severity of a toothache can range from chronic and mild to sharp and excruciating. It can be a dull ache or intense. The pain may be aggravated by chewing or by thermal foods and liquids which are cold or hot. A thorough oral examination, proper tooth testing and evaluation, along with appropriate dental x-rays, can help determine the cause. What we want to know is whether the toothache is really coming from a tooth or somewhere else.

Aren't all toothaches caused by a tooth or several teeth?

No. Sometimes, a toothache may be caused by a problem not originating from a tooth or the jaw at all. Pain around the teeth and the jaws can be symptoms of diseases of the heart (angina, heart attack), ears (such as inner or external ear infections), and sinuses (air passages of the cheek bones) such as sinusitis (infection of the sinus cavities). For example, the pain of angina is usually located in the chest or the arm. However, in some patients with angina, a toothache or jaw pain is the only symptom of their heart problem. Infections and diseases of the ears and sinuses can also cause pain around the teeth and jaws. Therefore, evaluations by both dentists and doctors are sometimes necessary to diagnose medical illnesses causing a "toothache." Keep in mind, while rare, some chronic toothache-like pains are caused by neuralgias and other nerve ailments.

What are some dental causes of toothaches?

A dental cavity or decay which has inflamed the pulp. Left untreated this will progress to an abscessed tooth. Sometimes, in spite of the decay removal and restoration, the pulp has become so inflamed that it continues to degenerate.

Decay which has progressed to invade the pulp and cause the pulp tissue to become infected resulting in an abscessed tooth

Cracked, split, and fractured teeth can cause inflammation of the pulp and the tissues around the tooth.

Periodontal disease and receding gums can expose tooth roots making them more sensitive to hot and cold foods. Periodontal disease can cause pulpal inflammation via small canals that extend from the outside of the tooth to the inside called lateral or accessory canals.

Tooth and Oral Pain Symptoms Guide

Information provided in this guide is for educational purposes only. Your specific symptoms may require different actions than provided in this chapter. It should not be a substitute for professional medical and dental attention, diagnosis, and treatment.

Momentary Sensitivity to Hot or Cold Foods without Recent Dental Work

Potential Problem

If the discomfort lasts a fleeting moment to hot and cold foods it may not signal a problem. Unfortunately, it sometimes is a sign of another problem. The sensitivity may be caused by a loose filling, decay, crack or fracture in the tooth, or by minimal gum recession which exposes small areas of the root surface.

Action

1. Have the tooth area checked by your dentist or endodontist. It may be nothing important, but consider it could be an early indicator of a problem.

2. Treatment may be needed such as replacement of a loose filling, restoration, or some type of coverage over an exposed root.

3. In some cases, changing your brushing techniques or switching to a toothpaste for sensitive teeth may decrease the problem.

Lingering or Prolonged Sensitivity and Awareness to Hot or Cold Foods without Recent Dental Work

Potential Problem

This probably means the pulp has been irreversibly damaged by deep decay, crack or fracture, periodontal disease, or trauma.

Action

See your dentist or endodontist. You're probably going to need non-surgical endodontic therapy or root canal (RCT) to maintain your tooth. Waiting may cause the tooth to not be repairable or salvageable, so do it now.

Momentary Sensitivity to Hot or Cold Foods after Recent Dental Treatment.

Potential Problem

Dental work may inflame the pulp, inside the tooth, causing temporary sensitivity. This type of sensitivity lasts only a fleeting second and potentially may be quite intense. Fortunately, the pulp tissue usually recuperates from this trauma and the sensitivity diminishes within a few days to weeks.

Action

Wait four to six weeks. If the pain persists or worsens, see your dentist or endodontist.

Lingering or Prolonged Sensitivity to or Awareness of Hot or Cold Foods after Recent Dental Treatment

Potential Problem

Dental work inflamed the pulp such that the tissue inside the tooth is beginning to degenerate. Chances are your tooth is not going to repair the problem without intervention. Don't blame your dentist, most likely you had a cavity near the pulp tissue or were missing a substantial portion of the tooth prior to restoration.

Action

See your dentist or endodontist. There is a good chance nonsurgical endodontic therapy or root canal (RCT) is going to need to be performed to maintain your tooth.

Dull Ache Near a Tooth and/or Biting Sensitivity after Recent Dental Treatment

Potential Problem

Potentially an indicator that the pulp tissue is inflamed. Many of these require treatment, such as endodontic therapy to remove inflamed pulp. Occasionally, if just biting sensitive, it may be related to your bite.

Action

A trip to your dentist or endodontist for an endodontic evaluation is warranted. Many of these may require endodontic therapy to eliminate this problem.

Sometimes this can be bite related and may just require an adjustment. Repeated adjustments are a commonly a sign endodontic therapy may be needed.

Sharp Pain when Biting Down on Food

Potential Problem

There are a lot of problems which can cause this symptom. Here are a few:

- Loose filling
- Decay

- Cracked or split tooth
- Cuspal fracture
- Vertical root fracture
- Tooth that needs endodontic treatment
- A tooth that has already had endodontic therapy or root canal treatment which is not responding favorably (failing)

Action

You probably guessed the answer already. Go see your dentist or endodontist for an evaluation. Treatment will depend on the cause of the problem.

Constant and Severe Pain with Pressure, Swelling of the Gum, and Sensitivity to Touch

Potential Problem

A tooth may have become abscessed, causing the surrounding bone to become infected.

Action

See your dentist or endodontist for evaluation and treatment to relieve the pain and maintain the tooth. Many times you're going to require endodontic treatment of some type to maintain the tooth. If your tooth has already had endodontic therapy, retreatment or endodontic surgery may be needed to maintain your tooth.

A Tooth Hurts when I Tap on It with My Finger from the Side

Potential Problem

If this is your only symptom, there are a variety of reasons this might be occurring. I had a tooth treated once endodontically and it remained sensitive for 6 months like this. This is a marker that your periodontal ligament is probably inflamed.

Action

There are potentially several causes of this. See your dentist or endodontist for an evaluation of the tooth.

Gumboil That Sprouts and May Become Tender but Then Pops and Goes Away

Potential Problem

Either a periodontal (gum) abscess or an endodontic abscess.

Action

See your dentist, periodontist, or endodontist for diagnosis and treatment. If this is caused by an endodontic problem, endodontic therapy will be needed to maintain the tooth.

Dull Ache and Pressure in Upper Teeth and Jaw

Potential Problem

The pain of a sinus problem such as sinusitis or infection of the sinuses is often felt in the face and teeth. Grinding of teeth, a condition known as bruxism, can also cause this type of ache.

Action

If your sinuses seem to be the problem see your physician. If the muscles around your face or your TMJ (joint that connects your lower jaw to your skull) is sore, see your dentist.

Chronic Pain in Head, Neck, or Ear

Potential Problem

Sometimes pulp-damaged teeth cause pain in other parts of the head and neck, but other dental or medical problems may be responsible.

Action

See your endodontist for evaluation. If the problem is not related to the tooth, your endodontist will refer you to an appropriate dental specialist or a physician.

Specific Sharp, Jabbing Pain

Touching a specific spot in or near your mouth triggers a sharp, jabbing pain lasting a few seconds. Sometimes talking may also cause this to occur.

Potential Problem

Possibly a neurological condition known as trigeminal neuralgia.

Action

See your dentist or endodontist to rule out a possible dental cause. You will most likely be referred to a dentist that treats this type of pain or physician such as a neurologist. Neurologists specialize in treatment of nerve problems.

Clicking, Popping, or Pain when Opening or Closing Mouth

Clicking or pop is heard when opening your mouth. Opening or closing your mouth may be painful.

Potential Problem

Potentially your TMJ (temporomandibular joint) which connects your lower jaw to your skull has a problem. It's also known as TMD for temporomandibular dysfunction.

Action

See your dentist. Treatment will vary depending on the symptoms and severity of involvement.

How do you diagnose whether it's a tooth problem or something else?

Endodontic diagnosis requires a practitioner to be thorough and knowledgeable of anatomy of the region in addition to pain referral patterns. We will test your suspect tooth and other teeth in the area with many different tests. We always check if it is temperature sensitive to cold and possibly heat and/or electricity (sounds terrible but it's not so bad—I have had it done to myself). Other tests that we routinely complete include: tapping on your tooth to see if inflammation is present, rubbing the gum area near the end of the roots for sensitivity, and measuring your gums to check the periodontal health of the area including the "wiggliness" of your tooth. Sometimes we have you bite on a stick and/or use a fiber optic light to check for cracks or fractures which go through your tooth. Usually we will take x-rays at various angles. Not only are we looking for an abscess but also the anatomy of your tooth. Since you are three-dimensional and x-rays are two-dimensional, we lose information that we attempt to make up by taking specialized angles. X-rays alone are not sufficient for diagnosis. Just because there's nothing on the x-rays does not mean there is not a problem. Early stages of pulp degeneration and some small abscess are not visible on the x-rays. Hence, the reason we perform other tests.

Chapter 46

Trigeminal Neuralgia

Trigeminal neuralgia (TN), also called tic douloureux, is a chronic pain condition that affects the trigeminal, or fifth cranial nerve—one of the largest nerves in the head. The disorder causes extreme, sporadic, sudden burning or shock-like face pain that lasts anywhere from a few seconds to as long as two minutes per episode. The intensity of pain can be physically and mentally incapacitating.

The trigeminal nerve is one of twelve pairs of cranial nerves that originate at the base of the brain. The nerve has three branches that conduct sensations from the upper, middle, and lower portions of the face, as well as the oral cavity, to the brain. The ophthalmic, or upper, branch supplies sensation to most of the scalp, forehead, and front of the head. The maxillary, or middle, branch passes through the cheek, upper jaw, top lip, teeth and gums, and to the side of the nose. The nerve's mandibular, or lower, branch passes through the lower jaw, teeth, gums, and bottom lip. More than one nerve branch can be affected by the disorder.

The presumed cause of TN is a blood vessel pressing on the trigeminal nerve as it exits the brainstem. This compression causes the wearing away of the protective coating around the nerve (the myelin sheath). TN may be part of the normal aging process—as blood vessels lengthen they can come to rest and pulsate against a nerve. TN symptoms can also occur in people with multiple sclerosis, or may be

Excerpted from "Trigeminal Neuralgia Fact Sheet," National Institute of Neurological Disorders and Stroke (NINDS), NIH Publication No. 06–5116, updated January 10, 2008.

caused by damage to the myelin sheath by compression from a tumor. This deterioration causes the nerve to send abnormal signals to the brain. In some cases the cause is unknown.

What are TN symptoms?

TN is characterized by a sudden, severe, electric shock-like, stabbing pain that is typically felt on one side of the jaw or cheek. Pain may occur on both sides of the face, although not at the same time. The attacks of pain, which generally last several seconds and may repeat in quick succession, come and go throughout the day. These episodes can last for days, weeks, or months at a time and then disappear for months or years. In the days before an episode begins, some patients may experience a tingling or numbing sensation or a somewhat constant and aching pain.

The intense flashes of pain can be triggered by vibration or contact with the cheek (such as when shaving, washing the face, or applying makeup), brushing teeth, eating, drinking, talking, or being exposed to the wind. The pain may affect a small area of the face or may spread. The bouts of pain rarely occur at night, when the patient is sleeping.

Patients are considered to have Type 1 TN if more than 50 percent of the pain they experience is sudden, intermittent, sharp and stabbing, or shock-like. These patients may also have some burning sensation. Type 2 TN involves pain that is constant, aching, or burning more than 50 percent of the time.

TN is typified by attacks that stop for a period of time and then come back. The attacks often worsen over time, with fewer and shorter pain-free periods before they recur. The disorder is not fatal, but can be debilitating. Due to the intensity of the pain, some patients may avoid daily activities because they fear an impending attack.

Who is affected?

TN occurs most often in people over age 50, but it can occur at any age. The disorder is more common in women than in men. There is some evidence that the disorder runs in families, perhaps because of an inherited pattern of blood vessel formation.

How is TN diagnosed?

There is no single test to diagnose TN. Diagnosis is generally based on the patient's medical history and description of symptoms, a physical exam, and a thorough neurological examination by a physician. Other disorders, such as post-herpetic neuralgia, can cause similar facial pain, as do syndromes such as cluster headaches. Injury to the trigeminal nerve (perhaps the result of sinus surgery, oral surgery, stroke, or facial trauma) may produce neuropathic pain, which is characterized by dull, burning, and boring pain. Because of overlapping symptoms, and the large number of conditions that can cause facial pain, obtaining a correct diagnosis is difficult, but finding the cause of the pain is important as the treatments for different types of pain may differ.

Most TN patients undergo a standard magnetic resonance imaging (MRI) scan to rule out a tumor or multiple sclerosis as the cause of their pain. This scan may or may not clearly show a blood vessel on the nerve. Magnetic resonance angiography (MRA), which can trace a colored dye that is injected into the bloodstream prior to the scan, can more clearly show blood vessel problems and any compression of the trigeminal nerve close to the brainstem.

Treatment for TN

Treatment options include medicines, surgery, and complementary approaches.

Anticonvulsant medicines are used to block nerve firing and are generally effective in treating TN. These drugs include carbamazepine, oxcarbazepine, topiramate, clonazepam, phenytoin, lamotrigine, and valproic acid. Gabapentin or baclofen can be used as a second drug to treat TN and may be given in combination with other anticonvulsants.

Tricyclic antidepressants such as amitriptyline or nortriptyline are used to treat pain described as constant, burning, or aching. Typical analgesics and opioids are not usually helpful in treating the sharp, recurring pain caused by TN. If medication fails to relieve pain or produces intolerable side effects such as excess fatigue, surgical treatment may be recommended.

Neurosurgical Procedures

Several neurosurgical procedures are available to treat TN. The choice among the various types depends on the patient's preference, physical well-being, previous surgeries, presence of multiple sclerosis, and area of trigeminal nerve involvement (particularly when the upper or ophthalmic branch is involved). Some procedures are done on an outpatient basis, while others may involve a more complex operation that is performed under general anesthesia. Some degree of facial numbness is expected after most of these procedures, and TN might return despite the procedure's initial success. Depending on the procedure, other surgical risks include hearing loss, balance problems, infection, and stroke.

A rhizotomy is a procedure in which select nerve fibers are destroyed to block pain. A rhizotomy for TN causes some degree of permanent sensory loss and facial numbness. Several forms of rhizotomy are available to treat TN:

- *Balloon compression* works by injuring the insulation on nerves that are involved with the sensation of light touch on the face. The procedure is performed in an operating room under general anesthesia. A tube called a cannula is inserted through the cheek and guided to where one branch of the trigeminal nerve passes through the base of the skull. A soft catheter with a balloon tip is threaded through the cannula and the balloon is inflated to squeeze part of the nerve against the hard edge of the brain covering (the dura) and the skull. After one minute the balloon is deflated and removed, along with the catheter and cannula. Balloon compression is generally an outpatient procedure, although sometimes the patient may be kept in the hospital overnight.

- *Glycerol injection* is generally an outpatient procedure in which the patient is sedated intravenously. A thin needle is passed through the cheek, next to the mouth, and guided through the opening in the base of the skull to where all three branches of the trigeminal nerve come together. The glycerol injection bathes the ganglion (the central part of the nerve from which the nerve impulses are transmitted) and damages the insulation of trigeminal nerve fibers.

- *Radiofrequency thermal lesioning* is usually performed on an outpatient basis. The patient is anesthetized and a hollow needle is passed through the cheek to where the trigeminal nerve exits through a hole at the base of the skull. The patient is awakened and a small electrical current is passed through the needle, causing tingling. When the needle is positioned so that the tingling occurs in the area of TN pain, the patient is then sedated and that part of the nerve is gradually heated with an electrode, injuring the nerve fibers. The electrode and needle are then removed and the patient is awakened.

- *Stereotactic radiosurgery* uses computer imaging to direct highly focused beams of radiation at the site where the trigeminal nerve exits the brainstem. This causes the slow formation of a lesion on the nerve that disrupts the transmission of pain signals to the brain. Pain relief from this procedure may take several months. Patients usually leave the hospital the same day or the next day following treatment.

Microvascular decompression is the most invasive of all surgeries for TN, but it also offers the lowest probability that pain will return. This inpatient procedure, which is performed under general anesthesia, requires that a small opening be made behind the ear. While viewing the trigeminal nerve through a microscope, the surgeon moves away the vessels that are compressing the nerve and places a soft cushion between the nerve and the vessels. Unlike rhizotomies, there is usually no numbness in the face after this surgery. Patients generally recuperate for several days in the hospital following the procedure.

A *neurectomy*, which involves cutting part of the nerve, may be performed during microvascular decompression if no vessel is found to be pressing on the trigeminal nerve. Neurectomies may also be performed by cutting branches of the trigeminal nerve in the face. When done during microvascular decompression, a neurectomy will cause permanent numbness in the area of the face that is supplied by the nerve or nerve branch that is cut. However, when the operation is performed in the face, the nerve may grow back and in time sensation may return.

Complementary techniques are chosen by some patients to manage TN, usually in combination with drug treatment. These therapies offer varying degrees of success. Options include: acupuncture, biofeedback, vitamin therapy, nutritional therapy, and electrical stimulation of the nerves.

For More Information

Trigeminal Neuralgia Association
925 Northwest 56th Terrace, Suite C
Gainesville, FL 32605-6402
Toll-Free: 800-923-3608
Phone: 352-331-7009
Fax: 352-331-7078
Website: http://www.fpa-support.org
E-mail: patientinfo@tna-support.org

Part Three

Diagnosing and Treating Pain

Chapter 47

Talking with Your Doctor about Pain

What to Ask: Tips for Talking with Your Doctor

These tips are designed to help you understand the importance of regular check-ups and establishing open communication with your health care provider.

Some points you might want to think about:

- Establish a baseline (a time when you are well and feeling good) so that the health care provider will understand when you tell them how you are feeling at the time of a visit.

- You have the right to make another choice in health care providers if you do not like your treatment team.

- Your medical records belong to you and you have a right to take them if you change doctors.

- Find a new health care provider within the first three months if you move so that you can establish your baseline.

- New symptoms do not necessarily mean that your pain problems have progressed.

- Don't neglect your eyes and dental needs.

- "Flair ups" don't mean that you're failing at pain management.

Understand Your Medications

If you are given a prescription, it's important that you take it as directed. If you worry about remembering your doctor's or pharmacist's instructions, take along a copy of the American Chronic Pain Association (ACPA) Pharmacist's CARE (Compassionate, Accurate, Responsive, Educational) sheet and ask your provider to complete it with you. It's available online at http://www.theacpa.org/documents/PUP-CARE%20card%206-2.pdf.

Maintaining a Good Relationship with Your Doctor

Before you go to the doctor, write down exactly what you think is wrong. Also, include the following:

- list only the new symptoms
- include over-the-counter medicines taken
- methods of relief tried, for example, heat, message, exercise
- changes in your daily level of functioning
- changes in mood, appetite and sleep
- questions you have

The Doctor Visit Fact Sheet form can help to prepare for a visit to the doctor. It is available online at http://www.theacpa.org/nerve/pdf/Doctor_Visit_Fact_Sheet.pdf and is reprinted at the end of this chapter.

The ACPA Quality of Life Scale is available online at http://www.theacpa.org/documents/Quality_of_Life_Scale.pdf and is reprinted in chapter 48.

Here are a few things to keep in mind during a visit to your doctor:

- Restate instructions the doctor gave you to ensure that you understood.
- If you don't understand what he or she is saying, you have the right to ask for clarification.
- Don't discuss what others have told you or thought might be wrong with you. Your doctor is familiar with your case history; allow him or her to make the diagnosis.

- Before leaving the doctor's office, check your understanding by quickly summarizing what you've been told.

- If you are not sure about the recommendations of your doctor, get a second opinion, especially before having surgery.

It is important to understand that there won't always be an answer to your health care questions. Medicine is not an exact science. There are many things that doctors know. However, there are many things they still don't know. Health care research is ongoing. Just because current research may not explain the reason for your pain does not mean that your pain is not real. You feel the pain and, therefore, it is real to you and must be taken seriously. Following these guidelines will enable you to make the most of your visit with your doctor. You will have a clearer understanding of what you need to do to stay involved in your own recovery.

Having a Productive Conversation with Your Health Care Provider

1. Take charge of the conversation from the beginning.

2. Prepare a list of questions that you need to have answered.

3. State your concerns and the reason for the visit immediately.

4. If you need something from the doctor, tell him; don't wait for him to guess what you want.

5. State your main concern up front and briefly then if necessary, give the details.

6. Believe in yourself and what you are saying, don't stumble over words.

7. Don't be afraid to ask questions about what you do not understand. You are paying the doctor for her expertise.

Doctor Visit Fact Sheet

- Date: _____

- When did you first notice the pain?

- Reason for visit. List only the new symptoms and concerns you have.

- What were you doing when you realized you had increased pain?

- Compared to your "normal" level of pain, how severe is your pain now? 1 (not bad), 2 3 4 5 6 7 8 9 10 (very severe)

- What have you done to relieve your pain so far?

- Was it helpful? If yes, how did it help?

- Have you taken any over-the-counter medications to try to relieve your pain? (yes, no) If yes, what?

- Did you stop your exercise program because of the pain? (yes, no)

- On a scale from 1 to 10, 1 being no change and 10 being completely unable to participate in daily activity, what is your present level of functioning since the new symptoms occurred?

  - Unable to function 0 1 2 3 4 5 6 7 8 9 10 Full normal functioning

- What questions do you have for your doctor?

For More Information

American Chronic Pain Association
P.O. Box 850
Rocklin, CA 95677
Toll-Free: 800-533-3231
Phone: 916-632-0922
Fax: 916-632-3208
Website: http://www.theacpa.org
E-mail: acpa@pacbell.net

Chapter 48

Keeping a Pain Notebook

Target Chronic Pain Notebook

A pain notebook is created to help you record your pain experience (when it occurs, for how long, the level and type of pain, possible triggers), its impact on day-to-day life (what activities you can or cannot do), and how you respond to various treatments over time, including side effects and improvements in daily function and emotional wellness.

Use your pain notebook in a way that is most helpful to you. While you don't have to complete all of the sections, it's important to use your pain notebook every day—especially on the days you are most in pain. Your notebook will help you record important information about your physical and emotional comfort that will help your medical team find the most effective ways to treat your pain. It will also help you communicate with loved ones about what pain feels like and how it is interfering with certain activities and your enjoyment of life.

Editor's Note: To create your own pain notebook, you may print pages incorporating the following text and Figures 48.1 and 48.2 from the

American Pain Foundation's website at http://www.painfoundation
.org/publications/TargetNotebook.pdf.

Daily Pain Record

1. The first section, the "Daily Pain Chart" (Figure 48.1), helps
    you create a visual picture of your daily pain experience. Follow
    your pain level throughout the day choosing several times that
    fit your routine; for example, when you get in or out of bed, eat
    meals, take medicines, get the mail, or go for a walk. Make a
    mark that corresponds to your pain level at these times. For ex-
    ample, if you wake at 7 a.m. and your pain is a six, place an X
    where 7 a.m. and number six intersect on the pain scale.

2. The second section, the "Daily Pain Log," is where you can re-
    cord information about your pain—whether it's intermittent,
    persistent, or breakthrough—treatments, and side effects. Also,
    record days that you have no pain. In addition, use this section
    to look at how you are dealing and coping with pain. What has
    helped you most? What is not working? Make additional notes
    in this section to record pain producing activities, as well as
    times of pain relief. Also keep a record of things you did to re-
    lieve your pain. You can draw lines from the events on the chart
    to explanations in the log to show why pain levels went up or
    down.

3. Then, at the end of the day, use the "Daily Pain Summary"
    section to give an overview of your pain for the day. Using all
    of the sections will give your medical team the best descrip-
    tion of how your pain changes throughout the day. If it's easier
    for you to complete one part only, that's okay. The important
    thing is to track your pain each day. If you are unable to com-
    plete a page every day, find someone to help you with the task
    at least one week. This will still give your medical team an
    idea of changes in your pain over time. This information also
    may help your care team adjust your treatment.

Keeping a Pain Notebook

Daily Pain Log

Medicines: Record name(s) of medicine(s), dose(s), and time(s)
taken.

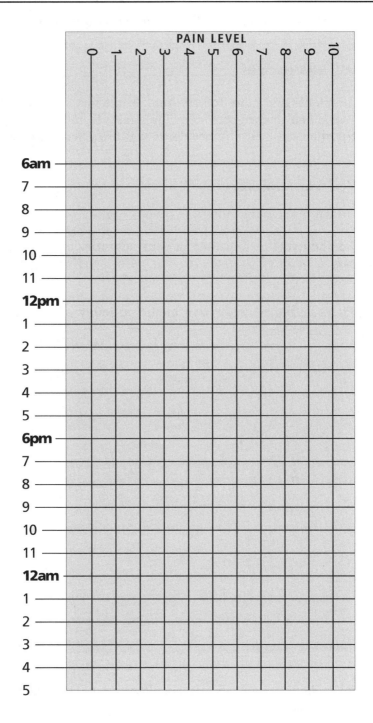

Figure 48.1. Daily Pain Chart (Connect the points on your Daily Pain Chart so your medical team can see when and why your pain level changed. Every day, start a new chart.)

Non-medicine therapy (other than prescription medicines):

_____

Activities/exercise:_____

Comments and more information: Make notes for and about visits with your health care provider, side effects from treatments you may be experiencing, and any problems you are having coping with your pain.

Daily Pain Summary

Did you have pain today? ____No ____Yes

Did you avoid or limit any of your activities or cancel plans today because of pain or changes in your pain? ____No ____Yes: What activities?

Did you take all your pain medicine today according to instructions? ____No ____Yes

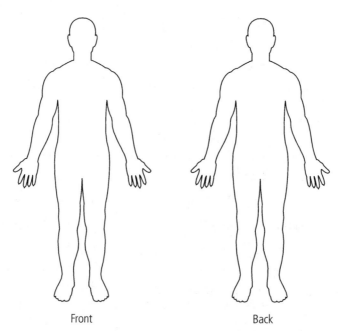

Front   Back

Figure 48.2. Put an X on the body diagram to show each place you've had pain today.

Even though you took your pain medicine for persistent pain on schedule , were there times during the day that you experienced un-relieved breakthrough pain? ____No ____Yes

- How many times did this happen today? 1, 2, 3, 4, 5, 6, 7, 8, 9, 10, more than 10

- Did any specific activity start your breakthrough pain? ____No ____Yes: What activities?

What was your average level of pain today? 0 (no pain), 1, 2, 3, 4, 5, 6, 7, 8, 9, 10 (severe pain)

Other than prescription medicine, did you do anything else today to relieve the pain? ____ No ____Yes (Check any of the following that you used.)

____ Non-prescription drugs (for example, acetaminophen, ibuprofen)
____ Herbal remedies
____ Hot or cold packs
____ Exercise
____ Changing position (such as lying down or elevating your legs)
____ Physical therapy
____ Massage
____ Acupuncture
____ Rest
____ Psychological counseling
____ Talk to trusted friend, family, clergy
____ Prayer, meditation, guided imagery
____ Relaxation technique (hypnosis, biofeedback)
____ Creative technique (art or music therapy)
____ Other (describe):_____

Check any of these common side effects that you've noticed after taking your pain medicine.

____ Drowsiness, sleepiness
____ Nausea, vomiting, upset stomach
____ Constipation
____ Lack of appetite
____ Other (describe):_____

Table 48.1. Quality of Life Scale: A Measure of Function for People with Pain

Scale Value	Activity Level
0 (Non-functioning)	Stay in bed all day Feel hopeless and helpless about life
1	Stay in bed at least half the day Have no contact with outside world
2	Get out of bed but don't get dressed Stay at home all day
3	Get dressed in the morning Minimal activities at home Contact with friends via phone, e-mail
4	Do simple chores around the house Minimal activities outside of home two days a week
5	Struggle but fulfill daily home responsi bilities No outside activity Not able to work/volunteer
6	Work/volunteer limited hours Take part in limitedsocial activities on weekends
7	Work/volunteer for a few hours daily Can be active atleast five hours a day Can make plans to do simple activities on weekends
8	Work/volunteer for at least six hours daily Have energy to make plans for one evening social activity during the week Active on weekends
9	Work/volunteer/be active eight hours daily Take part in family life Outside social activities limited
10 (Normal Quality of Life)	Go to work/volunteer each day Normal daily activities each day Have a social life outside of work Take an active part in family life

Did you skip any of your scheduled pain medicines today? ____No ____Yes: Why?

Did you call your doctor's office or clinic between visits because of pain? ____No ____Yes

Did you sleep through the night? ____No ____Yes

- If not, how many times was your sleep disrupted?_____
- How many hours did you sleep during the night? ___ hours

Overall, are you satisfied with your pain management? ____Yes ____No (Explain what makes you satisfied or not satisfied.)

What pain level overall would you find acceptable? 0 (no pain), 1, 2, 3, 4, 5, 6, 7, 8, 9, 10 (severe pain)

Pain is a highly personal experience. The degree to which pain interferes with the quality of a person's life is also highly personal.

The American Chronic Pain Association Quality of Life Scale looks at ability to function, rather than at pain alone. It can help people with pain and their health care team to evaluate and communicate the impact of pain on the basic activities of daily life. This information can provide a basis for more effective treatment and help to measure progress over time.

The scale is meant to help individuals measure activity levels. We recognize that homemakers, parents, and retirees often don't work outside the home, but activity can still be measured in the amount of time one is able to work at fulfilling daily responsibilities be that in a paid job, as a volunteer, or within the home.

With a combination of sound medical treatment, good coping skills, and peer support, people with pain can lead more productive, satisfying lives. The American Chronic Pain Association can help.

For More Information

American Chronic Pain Association
P.O. Box 850
Rocklin, CA 95677
Toll-Free: 800-533-3231
Phone: 916-632-0922
Fax: 916-632-3208

Website: http://www.theacpa.org
E-mail: acpa@pacbell.net

American Pain Foundation
201 N. Charles St., Suite 710
Baltimore, MD 21201-4111
Toll-Free: 888-615-7246
Website: http://www.painfoundation.org
E-mail: info@painfoundation.org

Chapter 49

Neurological Diagnostic Tests and Procedures

Diagnostic tests and procedures are vital tools that help physicians confirm or rule out the presence of a neurological disorder or other medical condition. A century ago, the only way to make a positive diagnosis for many neurological disorders was by performing an autopsy after a patient had died. But decades of basic research into the characteristics of disease, and the development of techniques that allow scientists to see inside the living brain and monitor nervous system activity as it occurs, have given doctors powerful and accurate tools to diagnose disease and to test how well a particular therapy may be working.

Perhaps the most significant changes in diagnostic imaging over the past 20 years are improvements in spatial resolution (size, intensity, and clarity) of anatomical images and reductions in the time needed to send signals to and receive data from the area being imaged. These advances allow physicians to simultaneously see the structure of the brain and the changes in brain activity as they occur. Scientists continue to improve methods that will provide sharper anatomical images and more detailed functional information.

Researchers and physicians use a variety of diagnostic imaging techniques and chemical and metabolic analyses to detect, manage, and treat neurological disease. Some procedures are performed in specialized settings, conducted to determine the presence of a particular

Excerpted from "Neurological Diagnostic Tests and Procedures," National Institute of Neurological Disorders and Stroke (NINDS), NIH Publication No. 05–5380, updated January 24, 2008.

disorder or abnormality. Many tests that were previously conducted in a hospital are now performed in a physician's office or at an outpatient testing facility, with little if any risk to the patient. Depending on the type of procedure, results are either immediate or may take several hours to process.

What are some of the more common screening tests?

Laboratory screening tests of blood, urine, or other substances are used to help diagnose disease, better understand the disease process, and monitor levels of therapeutic drugs. Certain tests, ordered by the physician as part of a regular check-up, provide general information, while others are used to identify specific health concerns. Blood tests are also used to monitor levels of therapeutic drugs used to treat epilepsy and other neurological disorders. Genetic testing of deoxyribonucleic acid (DNA) extracted from white cells in the blood can help diagnose Huntington disease and other congenital diseases. Analysis of the fluid that surrounds the brain and spinal cord can detect meningitis, acute and chronic inflammation, rare infections, and some cases of multiple sclerosis. Chemical and metabolic testing of the blood can indicate protein disorders, some forms of muscular dystrophy and other muscle disorders, and diabetes. Urinalysis can reveal abnormal substances in the urine or the presence or absence of certain proteins that cause diseases including the mucopolysaccharidoses.

What is a neurological examination?

A neurological examination assesses motor and sensory skills, the functioning of one or more cranial nerves, hearing and speech, vision, coordination and balance, mental status, and changes in mood or behavior, among other abilities. Items including a tuning fork, flashlight, reflex hammer, ophthalmoscope, and needles are used to help diagnose brain tumors, infections such as encephalitis and meningitis, and diseases such as Parkinson disease, Huntington disease, amyotrophic lateral sclerosis (ALS), and epilepsy. Some tests require the services of a specialist to perform and analyze results.

X-rays of the patient's chest and skull are often taken as part of a neurological work-up. X-rays can be used to view any part of the body, such as a joint or major organ system.

Fluoroscopy is a type of x-ray that uses a continuous or pulsed beam of low-dose radiation to produce continuous images of a body part in motion. The fluoroscope (x-ray tube) is focused on the area of interest and pictures are either videotaped or sent to a monitor for viewing. A contrast medium may be used to highlight the images. Fluoroscopy can be used to evaluate the flow of blood through arteries.

What are some diagnostic tests used to diagnose neurological disorders?

Based on the result of a neurological exam, physical exam, patient history, x-rays of the patient's chest and skull, and any previous screening or testing, physicians may order one or more of the following diagnostic tests to determine the specific nature of a suspected neurological disorder or injury. These diagnostics generally involve either nuclear medicine imaging, in which very small amounts of radioactive materials are used to study organ function and structure, or diagnostic imaging, which uses magnets and electrical charges to study human anatomy.

The following list of available procedures—in alphabetical rather than sequential order—includes some of the more common tests used to help diagnose a neurological condition.

Angiography is a test used to detect blockages of the arteries or veins. A cerebral angiogram can detect the degree of narrowing or obstruction of an artery or blood vessel in the brain, head, or neck. It is used to diagnose stroke and to determine the location and size of a brain tumor, aneurysm, or vascular malformation. This test is usually performed in a hospital outpatient setting and takes up to three hours, followed by a 6- to 8-hour resting period.

Biopsy involves the removal and examination of a small piece of tissue from the body. Muscle or nerve biopsies are used to diagnose neuromuscular disorders and may also reveal if a person is a carrier of a defective gene that could be passed on to children. A small sample of muscle or nerve is removed under local anesthetic and studied under a microscope. The sample may be removed either surgically, through a slit made in the skin, or by needle biopsy, in which a thin hollow needle is inserted through the skin and into the muscle.

Brain scans are imaging techniques used to diagnose tumors, blood vessel malformations, or hemorrhage in the brain. These scans are used to study organ function or injury, or disease to tissue or muscle. Types of brain scans include computed tomography, magnetic resonance imaging, and positron emission tomography.

357

Cerebrospinal fluid analysis involves the removal of a small amount of the fluid that protects the brain and spinal cord. The fluid is tested to detect any bleeding or brain hemorrhage, diagnose infection to the brain or spinal cord, identify some cases of multiple sclerosis and other neurological conditions, and measure intracranial pressure.

Computed tomography (CT), is a noninvasive, painless process used to produce rapid, clear two-dimensional images of organs, bones, and tissues. Neurological CT scans are used to view the brain and spine. They can detect bone and vascular irregularities, certain brain tumors and cysts, herniated discs, epilepsy, encephalitis, spinal stenosis (narrowing of the spinal canal), a blood clot or intracranial bleeding in patients with stroke, brain damage from head injury, and other disorders. Many neurological disorders share certain characteristics and a CT scan can aid in proper diagnosis by differentiating the area of the brain affected by the disorder.

Discography is often suggested for patients who are considering lumbar surgery or whose lower back pain has not responded to conventional treatments. This outpatient procedure is usually performed at a testing facility or a hospital. The physician numbs the skin with anesthetic and inserts a thin needle, using x-ray guidance, into the spinal disc. Once the needle is in place, a small amount of contrast dye is injected and CT scans are taken. The contrast dye outlines any damaged areas. More than one disc may be imaged at the same time.

An intrathecal contrast-enhanced CT scan (also called cisternography) is used to detect problems with the spine and spinal nerve roots. Following application of a topical anesthetic, the physician removes a small sample of the spinal fluid via lumbar puncture. The sample is mixed with a contrast dye and injected into the spinal sac located at the base of the lower back. The patient is then asked to move to a position that will allow the contrast fluid to travel to the area to be studied. The dye allows the spinal canal and nerve roots to be seen more clearly on a CT scan.

Electroencephalography (EEG), monitors brain activity through the skull. EEG is used to help diagnose certain seizure disorders, brain tumors, brain damage from head injuries, inflammation of the brain or spinal cord, alcoholism, certain psychiatric disorders, and metabolic and degenerative disorders that affect the brain. This painless, risk-free

358

test can be performed in a doctor's office or at a hospital or testing facility.

Electromyography (EMG), is used to diagnose nerve and muscle dysfunction and spinal cord disease. It records the electrical activity from the brain or spinal cord to a peripheral nerve root (found in the arms and legs) that controls muscles during contraction and at rest.

During an EMG, very fine wire electrodes are inserted into a muscle to assess changes in electrical voltage that occur during movement and when the muscle is at rest. The electrodes are attached through a series of wires to a recording instrument. Testing usually takes place at a testing facility and lasts about an hour but may take longer, depending on the number of muscles and nerves to be tested. Most patients find this test to be somewhat uncomfortable.

An EMG is usually done in conjunction with a nerve conduction velocity (NCV) test, which measures electrical energy by assessing the nerve's ability to send a signal. This two-part test is conducted most often in a hospital.

Electronystagmography (ENG) describes a group of tests used to diagnose involuntary eye movement, dizziness, and balance disorders, and to evaluate some brain functions.

Evoked potentials (also called evoked response) measure the electrical signals to the brain generated by hearing, touch, or sight. These tests are used to assess sensory nerve problems and confirm neurological conditions including multiple sclerosis, brain tumor, acoustic neuroma (small tumors of the inner ear), and spinal cord injury.

Auditory evoked potentials (also called brain stem auditory evoked response) are used to assess high-frequency hearing loss, diagnose any damage to the acoustic nerve and auditory pathways in the brainstem, and detect acoustic neuromas.

Visual evoked potentials detect loss of vision from optic nerve damage (in particular, damage caused by multiple sclerosis).

Somatosensory evoked potentials measure response from stimuli to the peripheral nerves and can detect nerve or spinal cord damage or nerve degeneration from multiple sclerosis and other degenerating diseases.

Magnetic resonance imaging (MRI) uses computer-generated radio waves and a powerful magnetic field to produce detailed images of body structures including tissues, organs, bones, and nerves. Neurological uses include the diagnosis of brain and spinal cord tumors, eye disease, inflammation, infection, and vascular irregularities that may lead to stroke. MRI can also detect and monitor degenerative disorders such as multiple sclerosis and can document brain injury from trauma.

Functional MRI (fMRI) uses the blood's magnetic properties to produce real-time images of blood flow to particular areas of the brain. An fMRI can pinpoint areas of the brain that become active and note how long they stay active. It can also tell if brain activity within a region occurs simultaneously or sequentially. This imaging process is used to assess brain damage from head injury or degenerative disorders such as Alzheimer disease and to identify and monitor other neurological disorders, including multiple sclerosis, stroke, and brain tumors.

Myelography involves the injection of a water- or oil-based contrast dye into the spinal canal to enhance x-ray imaging of the spine. Myelograms are used to diagnose spinal nerve injury, herniated discs, fractures, back or leg pain, and spinal tumors.

Positron emission tomography (PET) scans provide two- and three-dimensional pictures of brain activity by measuring radioactive isotopes that are injected into the bloodstream. PET scans of the brain are used to detect or highlight tumors and diseased tissue, measure cellular and tissue metabolism, show blood flow, evaluate patients who have seizure disorders that do not respond to medical therapy and patients with certain memory disorders, and determine brain changes following injury or drug abuse, among other uses. PET may be ordered as a follow-up to a CT or MRI scan to give the physician a greater understanding of specific areas of the brain that may be involved with certain problems.

Single photon emission computed tomography (SPECT), a nuclear imaging test involving blood flow to tissue, is used to evaluate certain brain functions. The test may be ordered as a follow-up to an MRI to diagnose tumors, infections, degenerative spinal disease, and stress fractures. As with a PET scan, a radioactive isotope, which binds to chemicals that flow to the brain, is injected intravenously into the body. Areas of increased blood flow will collect more of the isotope.

Thermography uses infrared sensing devices to measure small temperature changes between the two sides of the body or within a specific organ. Also known as digital infrared thermal imaging, thermography may be used to detect vascular disease of the head and neck, soft tissue injury, various neuromusculoskeletal disorders, and the presence or absence of nerve root compression.

Ultrasound imaging, also called ultrasound scanning or sonography, uses high-frequency sound waves to obtain images inside the body. Neurosonography (ultrasound of the brain and spinal column) analyzes blood flow in the brain and can diagnose stroke, brain tumors, hydrocephalus (build-up of cerebrospinal fluid in the brain), and vascular problems. It can also identify or rule out inflammatory processes causing pain. It is more effective than an x-ray in displaying soft tissue masses and can show tears in ligaments, muscles, tendons, and other soft tissue masses in the back. Transcranial Doppler ultrasound is used to view arteries and blood vessels in the neck and determine blood flow and risk of stroke.

Chapter 50

Over-the-Counter Medicines: What Is Right for You?

Advice for Americans about Self-Care

American medicine cabinets contain a growing choice of nonprescription, over-the-counter (OTC) medicines to treat an expanding range of ailments. OTC medicines often do more than relieve aches, pains, and itches. Some can prevent diseases like tooth decay, cure diseases like athlete's foot, and with a doctor's guidance, help manage recurring conditions like vaginal yeast infection, migraine, and minor pain in arthritis.

The U.S. Food and Drug Administration (FDA) determines whether medicines are prescription or nonprescription. The term prescription (Rx) refers to medicines that are safe and effective when used under a doctor's care. Nonprescription or OTC drugs are medicines the FDA decides are safe and effective for use without a doctor's prescription.

The FDA also has the authority to decide when a prescription drug is safe enough to be sold directly to consumers over the counter. This regulatory process allowing Americans to take a more active role in their health care is known as Rx-to-OTC switch. As a result of this process, more than 700 products sold over the counter today use ingredients or dosage strengths available only by prescription 30 years ago.

Text in this chapter is from "Over-the-Counter Medicines: What's Right for You?" U.S. Food and Drug Administration (FDA), March 7, 2006; and "The best way to take your over-the-counter pain reliever? Seriously," FDA, updated August 17, 2005.

Increased access to OTC medicines is especially important for our maturing population. Two out of three older Americans rate their health as excellent to good, but four out of five report at least one chronic condition. Fact is, today's OTC medicines offer greater opportunity to treat more of the aches and illnesses most likely to appear in our later years. As we live longer, work longer, and take a more active role in our own health care, the need grows to become better informed about self-care.

The best way to become better informed—for young and old alike— is to read and understand the information on OTC labels. Next to the medicine itself, label comprehension is the most important part of self-care with OTC medicines. With new opportunities in self-medication come new responsibilities and an increased need for knowledge. The FDA and the Consumer Healthcare Products Association (CHPA) have prepared the following information to help Americans take advantage of self-care opportunities.

OTC Know-How: It's on the Label

You would not ignore your doctor's instructions for using a prescription drug; so do not ignore the label when taking an OTC medicine. Here's what to look for:

- Product name

- Active ingredients: therapeutic substances in medicine

- Purpose: product category (such as antihistamine, antacid, or cough suppressant)

- Uses: symptoms or diseases the product will treat or prevent

- Warnings: when not to use the product, when to stop taking it, when to see a doctor, and possible side effects

- Directions: how much to take, how to take it, and how long to take it

- Other information: such as storage information

- Inactive ingredients: substances such as binders, colors, or flavoring

Other Tips

- You can help yourself read the label too. Always use enough light. It usually takes three times more light to read the same line at age 60 than at age 30. If necessary, use your glasses or contact lenses when reading labels.

- Always remember to look for the statement describing the tamper-evident feature(s) before you buy the product and when you use it.

- When it comes to medicines, more does not necessarily mean better. You should never misuse OTC medicines by taking them longer or in higher doses than the label recommends. Symptoms that persist are a clear signal that it is time to see a doctor.

- Be sure to read the label each time you purchase a product. Just because two or more products are from the same brand family does not mean they are meant to treat the same conditions or contain the same ingredients.

- Remember, if you read the label and still have questions, talk to a doctor, nurse, or pharmacist.

Drug Interactions: A Word to the Wise

Although mild and relatively uncommon, interactions involving OTC drugs can produce unwanted results or make medicines less effective. It is especially important to know about drug interactions if you are taking Rx and OTC drugs at the same time. Some drugs can also interact with foods and beverages, as well as with health conditions such as diabetes, kidney disease, and high blood pressure.

Here are a few drug interaction cautions for some common OTC ingredients:

- Avoid alcohol if you are taking antihistamines, cough or cold products with the ingredient dextromethorphan, or drugs that treat sleeplessness.

- Do not use drugs that treat sleeplessness if you are taking prescription sedatives or tranquilizers.

- Check with your doctor before taking products containing aspirin if you are taking a prescription blood thinner or if you have diabetes or gout.

- Do not use laxatives when you have stomach pain, nausea, or vomiting.

- Unless directed by a doctor, do not use a nasal decongestant if you are taking a prescription drug for high blood pressure or depression, or if you have heart or thyroid disease, diabetes, or prostate problems.

This is not a complete list. Read the label. Drug labels change as new information becomes available. That is why it is important to read the label each time you take medicine.

Time for a Medicine Cabinet Checkup

- Be sure to look through your medicine supply at least once a year.

- Always store medicines in a cool, dry place, or as stated on the label.

- Throw away any medicines that are past the expiration date.

- To make sure no one takes the wrong medicine, keep all medicines in their original containers.

Pregnancy and Breast-Feeding

Drugs can pass from a pregnant woman to her unborn baby. A safe amount of medicine for the mother may be too much for the unborn baby. If you are pregnant, always talk with your doctor before taking any drugs, Rx or OTC.

Although most drugs pass into breast milk in concentrations too low to have any unwanted effects on the baby, breast-feeding mothers still need to be careful. Always ask your doctor or pharmacist before taking any medicine while breast-feeding. A doctor or pharmacist can tell you how to adjust the timing and dosing of most medicines so the baby is exposed to the lowest amount possible, or whether the drugs should be avoided altogether.

Kids Are Not Just Small Adults

OTC drugs rarely come in one-size-fits-all. Here are some tips about giving OTC medicines to children:

- Children are not just small adults, so do not estimate the dose based on their size.

- Read the label. Follow all directions.

- Follow any age limits on the label.

- Be aware that some OTC products come in different strengths.

- Know the difference between abbreviations for tablespoon (T or tbs.) and teaspoon (tsp.)—they are very different doses.

- Be careful about converting dose instructions. If the label says two teaspoons, it's best to use a measuring spoon or a dosing cup marked in teaspoons, not a common kitchen spoon.

- Do not play doctor. Do not double the dose just because your child seems sicker than last time.

- Before you give your child two medicines at the same time, talk to your doctor or pharmacist.

- Never let children take medicine by themselves.

- Never call medicine candy to get your kids to take it. If they come across the medicine on their own, they're likely to remember that you called it candy.

Child-Resistant Packaging

Child-resistant closures are designed for repeated use to make it difficult for children to open. Remember, if you do not re-lock the closure after each use, the child-resistant device cannot do its job—keeping children out.

It is best to store all medicines and dietary supplements where children can neither see nor reach them. Containers of pills should not be left on the kitchen counter as a reminder. Purses and briefcases are among the worst places to hide medicines from curious kids.

If you find some packages too difficult to open—and do not have young children living with you or visiting—you should know the law allows one package size for each OTC medicine to be sold without child-resistant features. If you do not see it on the store shelf, ask.

Protect Yourself against Tampering

Makers of OTC medicines seal most products in tamper-evident packaging (TEP) to help protect against criminal tampering. TEP works by providing visible evidence if the package has been disturbed. But OTC packaging cannot be 100 percent tamper-proof. Here's how to help protect yourself:

- Be alert to the tamper-evident features on the package before you open it. These features are described on the label.

- Inspect the outer packaging before you buy it. When you get home, inspect the medicine inside.

- Do not buy an OTC product if the packaging is damaged.

- Do not use any medicine that looks discolored or different in any way.

- If anything looks suspicious, be suspicious. Contact the store where you bought the product. Take it back.

- Never take medicines in the dark.

The Best Way to Take Your Over-the-Counter Pain Reliever? Seriously

Over-the-counter (OTC) pain relievers and fever reducers (the kind you can buy without a prescription) are safe and effective when used as directed. However, they can cause serious problems when used by people with certain conditions or taking specific medicines. They can also cause problems in people who take too much, or use them for a longer period of time than the product's Drug Facts label recommends. That is why it is important to follow label directions carefully. If you have questions, talk to a pharmacist or health care professional.

What are pain relievers and fever reducers?

There are two categories of over-the-counter pain relievers and fever reducers: acetaminophen and nonsteroidal anti-inflammatory drugs (NSAIDs). Acetaminophen is used to relieve headaches, muscle aches, and fever. It is also found in many other medicines, such as cough syrup and cold and sinus medicines. OTC NSAIDs are used to help relieve pain and reduce fever. NSAIDs include aspirin, naproxen, ketoprofen, and ibuprofen, and are also found in many medicines taken for colds, sinus pressure, and allergies.

How do I use pain relievers and fever reducers safely?

These products, when used occasionally and taken as directed, are safe and effective. Read the labels of all your over-the-counter medicines so you are aware of the correct recommended dosage. If a measuring tool is provided with your medicine, use it as directed.

What can happen if I do not use pain relievers and fever reducers correctly?

Using too much acetaminophen can cause serious liver damage, which may not be noticed for several days. NSAIDs, for some people with certain medical problems, can lead to the development of stomach bleeding and kidney disease.

What if I need to take more than one medicine?

There are many OTC medicines that contain the same active ingredient. If you take several medicines that happen to contain the same active ingredient, for example a pain reliever along with a cough-cold-fever medicine, you might be taking two times the normal dose and not know it. So read the label, and avoid taking multiple medicines that contain the same active ingredient, or talk to your pharmacist or health care professional.

Chapter 51

Benefits and Risks of Non-Steroidal Anti-Inflammatory Drugs (NSAIDs)

Benefits and Risks of Pain Relievers

What are non-steroidal anti-inflammatory drugs (NSAIDs)?

NSAIDs are a group of drugs used to temporarily relieve pain and inflammation. They work by blocking the production of prostaglandins, or chemicals believed to be associated with pain and inflammation.

What conditions do NSAIDs treat?

Prescription NSAIDs are an important treatment for many debilitating conditions such as osteoarthritis and rheumatoid arthritis. Some prescription NSAIDs also are used to treat pain. Over-the-counter versions of some NSAIDs are used to treat fever and pain associated with dental problems, tendonitis, strains, sprains, and other injuries. NSAIDs are also commonly used to relieve pain associated with menstrual cramps.

This chapter includes text from "The Benefits and Risks of Pain Relievers," U.S. Food and Drug Administration (FDA), April 26, 2007; "Medication Guide for Non-Steroidal Anti-Inflammatory Drugs (NSAIDs)," FDA, updated April 19, 2007; and "NSAIDs and Peptic Ulcers," National Institute of Diabetes and Digestive and Kidney Diseases (NIDDK), NIH Publication No. 04–4644, September 2004.

What are non-selective NSAIDs and COX-2 selective NSAIDs?

Non-selective NSAIDs work by inhibiting two enzymes that are involved with inflammation—cyclooxygenase-1 and cyclooxygenase-2 (COX-1 and COX-2). There are several non-selective NSAIDs on the market, including diclofenac, ibuprofen, ketoprofen, meloxicam, naproxen, and oxaprozin. Ibuprofen, ketoprofen, and naproxen are available in both prescription and over-the-counter (OTC) versions. The doses in OTC NSAIDs are lower than the doses of prescription versions and should only be used for up to ten days without seeing a doctor. So, if you take OTC ibuprofen (Advil and Motrin) or naproxen (Aleve), the doses are about half the doses of prescription versions.

COX-2 selective inhibitors are a newer type of medicine that primarily blocks the COX-2 enzyme. The only COX-2 selective inhibitor currently on the market in the United States is the prescription drug Celebrex (celecoxib), which is marketed by Pfizer. It was believed that COX-2 inhibitors may be less likely to cause the stomach problems associated with the older NSAIDs, but all NSAIDs carry the risk of stomach problems.

What are the risks of taking NSAIDs?

Like all drugs, there is the potential for an allergic reaction to NSAIDs. Symptoms may include hives, facial swelling, wheezing, and skin rash.

There is the potential for gastrointestinal bleeding associated with all NSAIDs. The risk of bleeding is low for people who use NSAIDs intermittently. The risk of stomach problems goes up for people who take them every day or regularly, especially for people who are over 65, people with a history of stomach ulcers, and people who take blood thinners or corticosteroids (prednisone). Alcohol use can also increase the risk of stomach problems.

Long-term continuous use of all NSAIDs, except for aspirin, may increase the risk of heart attack or stroke. Aspirin is a non-selective NSAID, but it has been shown in clinical trials to reduce the risks of cardiovascular events. Aspirin is sold in generic forms and under brand names such as Bayer and St. Joseph's.

All NSAIDs also carry the risk of potential skin reactions. Patients should be alert for symptoms such as the skin reddening, rash, or blisters.

Which people are at highest risk for cardiovascular adverse events associated with NSAIDs?

People who have coronary artery disease (known angina or who have had a heart attack), people who have high blood pressure, and people who have had a stroke are at the greatest risk. Also, people who have just had cardiovascular bypass surgery are at risk for heart attacks with use of NSAIDs.

Which COX-2 selective inhibitors have been taken off the market?

Merck voluntarily withdrew Vioxx (rofecoxib) in 2004 after finding out the results of a study that showed patients who took Vioxx had a higher risk for heart attacks than patients who took a placebo. FDA asked Pfizer to withdraw Bextra (valdecoxib) from the market in 2005 because the overall risk to benefit profile was unfavorable. The request was based on many factors. Along with the other risks associated with NSAIDs, there was a higher than expected number of reports of serious and potentially life-threatening skin reactions, including death.

An increased risk of cardiovascular adverse events has been shown for all COX-2 inhibitors, including Celebrex, which is still on the market in the United States. Based on available data, FDA determined that the benefits of Celebrex outweigh the potential risks in properly selected and informed patients. FDA asked Pfizer to include a boxed warning on the Celebrex label, and asked manufacturers of all prescription NSAIDs to revise their labeling too. The boxed warning highlights the potential for increased risk of cardiovascular events as well as serious, potentially life-threatening, gastrointestinal bleeding. It is important to know that FDA also determined that the risk for cardiovascular events was most likely present for the non-selective NSAIDs as well, and all of the manufacturers of these drugs were asked to add important warnings to their labels.

What can consumers do to lower their risks with NSAIDs?

Tell your doctor about your complete medical history, including any history of cardiovascular disease or stomach ulcers. This will help you and your doctor weigh the risks and benefits. You can also ask your doctor what you can do to lessen the chance for stomach irritation such as taking medication with a meal. Also, ask what steps you can take to lower the risk of cardiovascular disease and report medication side effects to your doctor. Whether you're taking a prescription NSAID or an OTC NSAID, following directions is important. Available scientific data do not suggest an increased risk of serious cardiovascular events for short-term, low-dose use of OTC NSAIDs. But be aware that the OTC labeling states that if you take an NSAID for longer than ten days, you should see your doctor. The lowest effective dose should be used for the shortest time.

Medication Guide for NSAIDs

What is the most important information I should know about medicines called NSAIDs?

- NSAID medicines may increase the chance of a heart attack or stroke that can lead to death. This chance increases with longer use of NSAID medicines in people who have heart disease.

- NSAID medicines should never be used right before or after a heart surgery called a coronary artery bypass graft.

- NSAID medicines can cause ulcers and bleeding in the stomach and intestines at any time during treatment. Ulcers and bleeding can happen without warning symptoms and may cause death.

The following factors increase the chance of a person getting an ulcer or bleeding when taking a NSAID.

- taking medicines called corticosteroids and anticoagulants
- longer use
- smoking
- drinking alcohol
- older age
- having poor health

NSAID medicines should only be used:

- exactly as prescribed;
- at the lowest dose possible for your treatment; and
- for the shortest time needed.

What are the possible side effects of NSAIDs?

Serious Side Effects

- heart attack
- stroke
- high blood pressure
- heart failure from body swelling (fluid retention)
- kidney problems including kidney failure
- bleeding and ulcers in the stomach and intestine
- low red blood cells (anemia)
- life-threatening skin reactions
- life-threatening allergic reactions
- liver problems including liver failure
- asthma attacks in people who have asthma

Other Side Effects

- stomach pain
- constipation
- diarrhea
- gas
- heartburn
- nausea
- vomiting
- dizziness

Get Emergency Help Immediately for These Symptoms

- shortness of breath or trouble breathing
- chest pain
- weakness in one part or side of your body
- slurred speech
- swelling of the face or throat

Stop NSAID Medicine and Call Your Health Care Provider for These Symptoms

- nausea

- more tired or weaker than usual

- itching

- your skin or eyes look yellow

- stomach pain

- flu-like symptoms

- vomit blood

- there is blood in your bowel movement or it is black and sticky like tar

- unusual weight gain

- skin rash or blisters with fever

- swelling of the arms and legs, hands, and feet

These are not all the side effects with NSAID medicines. Talk to your health care provider or pharmacist for more information about NSAID medicines.

Other Information about NSAIDs

- Aspirin is an NSAID medicine but it does not increase the chance of a heart attack. Aspirin can cause bleeding in the brain, stomach, and intestines. Aspirin can also cause ulcers in the stomach and intestines.

- Some of these NSAID medicines are sold in lower doses without a prescription (over-the-counter). Talk to your health care provider before using over-the-counter NSAIDs for more than ten days.

NSAIDs and Peptic Ulcers

A peptic ulcer is a sore that forms in the lining of the stomach or the duodenum (the beginning of the small intestine). An ulcer can cause a gnawing, burning pain in the upper abdomen along with nausea, vomiting, loss of appetite, weight loss, and fatigue. Most peptic ulcers are caused by infection with the bacterium *Helicobacter pylori* (*H. pylori*). But some peptic ulcers are caused by prolonged use of nonsteroidal

Table 51.1. NSAID Medicines That Need a Prescription

Generic Name	Trade Name
Celecoxib	Celebrex
Diclofenac	Flector, Cataflam, Voltaren, Arthrotec (combined with misoprostol)
Diflunisal	Dolobid
Etodolac	Lodine, Lodine XL
Fenoprofen	Nalfon, Nalfon 200
Flurbiprofen	Ansaid
Ibuprofen	Motrin, Tab-Profen, Vicoprofen (combined with hydrocodone), Combunox (combined with oxycodone)
Indomethacin	Indocin, Indocin SR, Indo-Lemmon
Ketoprofen	Oruvail
Ketorolac	Toradol
Mefenamic Acid	Ponstel
Meloxicam	Mobic
Nabumetone	Relafen
Naproxen	Naprosyn, Anaprox, Anaprox DS, Naprelan, NapraPAC (copackaged with lansoprazole)
Oxaprozin	Daypro
Piroxicam	Feldene
Sulindac	Clinoril
Tolmetin	Tolectin, Tolectin DS, Tolectin 600

anti-inflammatory drugs (NSAIDs) such as aspirin, ibuprofen, and naproxen sodium.

Normally the stomach has three defenses against digestive juices: mucus that coats the stomach lining and shields it from stomach acid, the chemical bicarbonate that neutralizes stomach acid, and blood circulation to the stomach lining that aids in cell renewal and repair. NSAIDs hinder all of these protective mechanisms and with the stomach's defenses down, digestive juices can damage the sensitive stomach lining and cause ulcers.

NSAID-induced ulcers usually heal once the person stops taking the medication. To help the healing process and relieve symptoms in the meantime, the doctor may recommend taking antacids to neutralize the acid and drugs called H2-blockers or proton-pump inhibitors to decrease the amount of acid the stomach produces.

Medicines that protect the stomach lining also help with healing. Examples are bismuth subsalicylate which coats the entire stomach lining, and sucralfate which sticks to and covers the ulcer.

If a person with an NSAID ulcer also tests positive for *H. pylori*, he or she will be treated with antibiotics to kill the bacteria. Surgery may be necessary if an ulcer recurs or fails to heal, or if complications like severe bleeding, perforation, or obstruction develop.

Anyone taking NSAIDs who experiences symptoms of peptic ulcer should see a doctor for prompt treatment. Delaying diagnosis and treatment can lead to complications and the need for surgery.

Chapter 52

Opioid Analgesics Treat Pain

Pain Relief

Opioids are very effective for the relief of moderate to severe pain. Many patients with cancer pain, however, become tolerant to opioids during long-term therapy. Therefore, increasing doses may be needed to continue to relieve pain. A patient's tolerance of an opioid or physical dependence on it is not the same as addiction (psychological dependence). Mistaken concerns about addiction can result in under-treating pain.

Types of Opioids

There are several types of opioids. Morphine is the most commonly used opioid in cancer pain management. Other commonly used opioids include hydromorphone, oxycodone, methadone, and fentanyl. The availability of several different opioids allows the doctor flexibility in prescribing a medication regimen that will meet individual patient needs.

Text in this chapter titled "Pain Relief," is excerpted from PDQ® Cancer Information Summary. National Cancer Institute, Bethesda, MD. Pain (PDQ®): Supportive Care–Patient. Updated May 2007. Available at http://cancer.gov. Accessed February 26, 2008. The section titled "Abuse of Opioids," is from "NIDA InfoFacts: Prescription Pain and Other Medications," National Institute on Drug Abuse (NIDA), June 2006; and text titled, "FDA Warning about Methadone Use," is from "Methadone Hydrochloride Public Health Advisory," U.S. Food and Drug Administration (FDA), July 2007.

Guidelines for Giving Opioids

Most patients with cancer pain will need to receive pain medication on a fixed schedule to manage the pain and prevent it from getting worse. The doctor will prescribe a dose of the opioid medication that can be taken as needed along with the regular fixed-schedule opioid to control pain that occurs between the scheduled doses. The amount of time between doses depends on which opioid the doctor prescribes. The correct dose is the amount of opioid that controls pain with the fewest side effects. The goal is to achieve a good balance between pain relief and side effects by gradually adjusting the dose. If opioid tolerance does occur, it can be overcome by increasing the dose or changing to another opioid, especially if higher doses are needed.

Occasionally, doses may need to be decreased or stopped. This may occur when patients become pain free because of cancer treatments such as nerve blocks or radiation therapy. The doctor may also decrease the dose when the patient experiences opioid-related sedation along with good pain control.

Medications for pain may be given in several ways. When the patient has a working stomach and intestines, the preferred method is by mouth, since medications given orally are convenient and usually inexpensive. When patients cannot take medications by mouth, other less invasive methods may be used, such as rectally or through medication patches placed on the skin. Intravenous methods are used only when simpler, less demanding, and less costly methods are inappropriate, ineffective, or unacceptable to the patient. Patient-controlled analgesia (PCA) pumps may be used to determine the opioid dose when starting opioid therapy. Once the pain is controlled, the doctor may prescribe regular opioid doses based on the amount the patient required when using the PCA pump. Intraspinal administration of opioids combined with a local anesthetic may be helpful for some patients who have uncontrollable pain.

Side Effects of Opioids

Patients should be watched closely for side effects of opioids. The most common side effects of opioids include nausea, sleepiness, and constipation. The doctor should discuss the side effects with patients before starting opioid treatment. Sleepiness and nausea are usually experienced when opioid treatment is started and tend to improve within a few days. Other side effects of opioid treatment include vomiting, difficulty in thinking clearly, problems with breathing, gradual overdose, and problems with sexual function.

Opioids slow down the muscle contractions and movement in the stomach and intestines resulting in hard stools. The key to effective prevention of constipation is to be sure the patient receives plenty of fluids to keep the stool soft. The doctor should prescribe a regular stool softener at the beginning of opioid treatment. If the patient does not respond to the stool softener, the doctor may prescribe additional laxatives.

Patients should talk to their doctor about side effects that become too bothersome or severe. Because there are differences between individual patients in the degree to which opioids may cause side effects, severe or continuing problems should be reported to the doctor. The doctor may decrease the dose of the opioid, switch to a different opioid, or switch the way the opioid is given (for example, intravenous or injection rather than by mouth) to attempt to decrease the side effects.

Drugs Used with Pain Medications

Other drugs may be given at the same time as the pain medication. This is done to increase the effectiveness of the pain medication, treat symptoms, and relieve specific types of pain. These drugs include antidepressants, anticonvulsants, local anesthetics, corticosteroids, bisphosphonates, and stimulants. There are great differences in how patients respond to these drugs. Side effects are common and should be reported to the doctor. Certain bisphosphonates given for bone pain are linked to a risk of bone loss after dental work. Patients taking bisphosphonates should check with their doctor before having dental work done.

Abuse of Opioids

Opioids are commonly prescribed because of their effective analgesic, or pain relieving, properties. Studies have shown that properly managed medical use of opioid analgesic compounds is safe and rarely causes addiction. Taken exactly as prescribed, opioids can be used to manage pain effectively.

Among the compounds that fall within this class—sometimes referred to as narcotics—are morphine, codeine, and related medications. Morphine is often used before or after surgery to alleviate severe pain. Codeine is used for milder pain. Other examples of opioids that can be prescribed to alleviate pain include oxycodone (OxyContin—an oral, controlled release form of the drug); propoxyphene (Darvon); hydrocodone (Vicodin); hydromorphone (Dilaudid); and meperidine

(Demerol), which is used less often because of its side effects. In addition to their effective pain relieving properties, some of these medications can be used to relieve severe diarrhea (Lomotil, for example, which is diphenoxylate) or severe coughs (codeine).

Opioids act by attaching to specific proteins called opioid receptors, which are found in the brain, spinal cord, and gastrointestinal tract. When these compounds attach to certain opioid receptors in the brain and spinal cord, they can effectively change the way a person experiences pain. In addition, opioid medications can affect regions of the brain that mediate what we perceive as pleasure, resulting in the initial euphoria that many opioids produce. They can also produce drowsiness, cause constipation, and depress breathing. Taking a large single dose could cause severe respiratory depression or death.

Opioids may interact with other medications and are only safe to use with other medications under a physician's supervision. Typically, they should not be used with substances such as alcohol, antihistamines, barbiturates, or benzodiazepines. Since these substances slow breathing, their combined effects could lead to life-threatening respiratory depression.

Long-term use also can lead to physical dependence—the body adapts to the presence of the substance and withdrawal symptoms occur if use is reduced abruptly. This can also include tolerance, which means that higher doses of a medication must be taken to obtain the same initial effects. Note that physical dependence is not the same as addiction—physical dependence can occur even with appropriate long-term use of opioid and other medications. Addiction is defined as compulsive, often uncontrollable, drug use in spite of negative consequences.

Individuals taking prescribed opioid medications should not only be given these medications under appropriate medical supervision, but also should be medically supervised when stopping use in order to reduce or avoid withdrawal symptoms. Symptoms of withdrawal can include restlessness, muscle and bone pain, insomnia, diarrhea, vomiting, cold flashes with goose bumps (cold turkey), and involuntary leg movements.

Individuals who become addicted to prescription medications can be treated. Options for effectively treating addiction to prescription opioids are drawn from research on treating heroin addiction. Some pharmacological examples of available treatments follow:

- Methadone, a synthetic opioid that blocks the effects of heroin and other opioids, eliminates withdrawal symptoms and relieves craving. It has been used for over 30 years to successfully treat people addicted to opioids.

- Buprenorphine, another synthetic opioid, is a recent addition to the arsenal of medications for treating addiction to heroin and other opiates.

- Naltrexone is a long-acting opioid blocker often used with highly motivated individuals in treatment programs promoting complete abstinence. Naltrexone also is used to prevent relapse.

- Naloxone counteracts the effects of opioids and is used to treat overdoses.

FDA Warning about Methadone Use

The U.S. Food and Drug Administration (FDA) has received reports of death and life-threatening side effects in patients taking methadone. These deaths and life-threatening side effects have occurred in patients newly starting methadone for pain control and in patients who have switched to methadone after being treated for pain with other strong narcotic pain relievers. Methadone can cause slow or shallow breathing and dangerous changes in heart beat that may not be felt by the patient.

Prescribing methadone is complex. Methadone should only be prescribed for patients with moderate to severe pain when their pain is not improved with other nonnarcotic pain relievers. Pain relief from a dose of methadone lasts about 4–8 hours. However methadone stays in the body much longer—from 8–59 hours after it is taken. As a result, patients may feel the need for more pain relief before methadone is gone from the body. Methadone may build up in the body to a toxic level if it is taken too often, if the amount taken is too high, or if it is taken with certain other medicines or supplements.

To prevent serious complications from methadone, health care professionals who prescribe methadone should read and carefully follow the methadone (Dolophine) prescribing information.

FDA is issuing this public health advisory to alert patients and their caregivers and health care professionals to the following important safety information:

- Patients should take methadone exactly as prescribed. Taking more methadone than prescribed can cause breathing to slow or stop and can cause death. A patient who does not experience good pain relief with the prescribed dose of methadone, should talk to his or her doctor.

- Patients taking methadone should not start or stop taking other medicines or dietary supplements without talking to their health care provider. Taking other medicines or dietary supplements may cause less pain relief. They may also cause a toxic buildup of methadone in the body leading to dangerous changes in breathing or heart beat that may cause death.

- Health care professionals and patients should be aware of the signs of methadone overdose. Signs of methadone overdose include trouble breathing or shallow breathing; extreme tiredness or sleepiness; blurred vision; inability to think, talk, or walk normally; and feeling faint, dizzy, or confused. If these signs occur, patients should get medical attention right away.

FDA recently approved new prescribing information for methadone products approved for pain control. The information in the new prescribing information is based on a review of the scientific literature completed by FDA.

Chapter 53

Antidepressants, Anticonvulsants, and Adjuvant Medications Used to Treat Pain

Antidepressants

The analgesic benefits of tricyclic antidepressants have been well established and are generally considered first-line therapy for many neuropathic pain syndromes. Supporting evidence is strong for amitriptyline and desipramine, and there is endorsement of other newer antidepressants such as maprotiline and paroxetine. Patients with neuropathic pain characterized by continuous abnormal and disagreeable sensations from ordinary stimulation are generally believed to be the most likely to benefit from antidepressant management; however, a randomized placebo-controlled study of amitriptyline for neuropathic pain in cancer patients found only slight analgesic benefit with significantly worse adverse effects.

The most common side effects of tricyclic antidepressants are the following:

- Constipation
- Dry mouth
- Blurred vision
- Cognitive changes

Excerpted from PDQ® Cancer Information Summary. National Cancer Institute; Bethesda, MD. Pain (PDQ®) Supportive Care–Health Professional. Updated May 2007. Available at: http://cancer.gov. Accessed February 26, 2008.

- Tachycardia (rapid heart beat)
- Urinary retention

Caution has also been advised in treating patients with cardiac disease, and an electrocardiogram is sometimes recommended as a prudent measure. A slow upward titration is suggested as a good way to avoid side effects.

Anticonvulsants

The group of commonly used anticonvulsants as adjuvant analgesics for neuropathic pain includes carbamazepine, valproate, phenytoin, and clonazepam.

- Clinical experience with carbamazepine is extensive, but use of this drug is limited in the cancer population because of concern that it causes bone marrow suppression, in particular leukopenia. Other common adverse effects include nystagmus (involuntary eye movements), dizziness, double vision, cognitive impairment, and mood and sleep disturbance.

- Dosing guidelines for phenytoin are similar to those for the treatment for seizures. This drug can be administered using a loading dose, which may be particularly useful in patients with severe pain.

- Gabapentin is increasingly reported as useful for the management of neuropathic pain associated with cancer and its treatment. Commonly reported side effects include sleepiness, dizziness, incoordination, and fatigue.

- Clonazepam is an anticonvulsant from the benzodiazepine class and is commonly used for treating lancinating or paroxysmal neuropathic pain. The patient must be monitored carefully for drowsiness and cognitive impairment.

Local Anesthetics

The use of mexiletine has been described for chronic neuropathic pain. Side effects are reported as common and include gastrointestinal toxicity, in particular nausea, and central nervous system (CNS) side effects such as dizziness. Patients with a history of cardiac disease and those on higher doses are at increased risk of adverse effects, and it is recommended that they receive appropriate cardiac evaluation, including an electrocardiogram.

Corticosteroids

These drugs have achieved wide acceptance in the management of patients with cancer pain. They are indicated as adjuvant analgesics for cancer pain of bone, visceral, and neuropathic origin. Adverse effects include neuropsychiatric syndromes, gastrointestinal disturbances, proximal myopathy, hyperglycemia, aseptic necrosis, capillary fragility, and immunosuppression. The risk of adverse effects increases with the duration of use. As a result, use is often restricted to patients with a limited life expectancy; in addition, once effective pain control is obtained, it is commonly recommended that the dose be tapered as much as possible. Dosage recommendations vary from a trial of low-dose therapy such as dexamethasone 1–2 milligram (mg) or prednisone 5–10 mg once or twice daily, to a starting dose of dexamethasone 10 mg twice daily with subsequent tapering to the minimal effective dose.

Another suggested use of corticosteroids is in high doses for short periods in patients with severe pain. This empirical approach recommends a regime of a single large dose of dexamethasone 100 mg intravenous (IV) followed by a small amount given four times per day and then tapered over the next few weeks.

Although there is widespread acceptance of steroid therapy, mostly via the oral route but also subcutaneously and intravenously, data remain inadequate for definitive conclusions regarding efficacy and dosing guidelines.

Bisphosphonates

These drugs have been recommended for the management of bone pain as well as the prevention of skeletal complications in patients with metastatic bone disease. Their use in a study of breast cancer patients resulted in improved quality of life compared with that of patients not using bisphosphonates. The bisphosphonates most frequently used are clodronate, pamidronate, and zoledronic acid.

- Clodronate can be given orally or intravenously. Clodronate is not available in the United States.

- Pamidronate has been recommended in the dose range of 60–90 milligrams (mg) intravenous (IV) over two hours every 3–4 weeks;

however, pooled results from two multicenter, double-blind, randomized, placebo-controlled trials of 350 individuals using pamidronate (90 mg every three weeks) failed to demonstrate a benefit for bone pain.

- Zoledronic acid is a potent bisphosphonate that can be given as an IV dose over 15–30 minutes in the dose range of 4–8 mg; however, the 8 mg dose has been associated with deterioration of renal function. The few studies to date suggest administration at 3–4 week intervals.

- Ibandronate can be given orally or intravenously. Dosing recommendations are 50 mg orally daily or 6 mg intravenously every 3–4 weeks.

Despite the potential benefits, a caution was released by the U.S. Food and Drug Administration (FDA) regarding reports of osteonecrosis of the jaw in patients who received pamidronate disodium or zoledronic acid. Osteonecrosis occurred in patients who did not have malignancy in the head and neck region and who had not received radiation therapy to the jaw. Most of the cases were associated with dental procedures such as tooth extraction. While receiving these drugs, patients should avoid invasive dental procedures if possible.

Miscellaneous

Baclofen: This drug is generally used for spasticity but may also be used for the treatment of neuropathic pain. Side effects include drowsiness, dizziness, ataxia, confusion, nausea, and vomiting.

Calcitonin: Although the mechanism by which calcitonin produces analgesia is unknown; historically, it has been recommended for the treatment of both bone and neuropathic pain. However, a systematic review of randomized double-blind clinical trials assessing the efficacy of calcitonin for control of metastatic bone pain does not support its use. Because only two of these studies were evaluated as well designed, further research is necessary. The utility of calcitonin for bone pain is unclear.

Clonidine: This traditional antihypertensive can be given via the oral, epidural, or transdermal route and has been recommended as a trial for the management of neuropathic pain. Reported side effects include dry mouth, dizziness, low arterial blood pressure (hypotension), sedation, and constipation. The maximum recommended dose is 2.4 mg per day.

Psychostimulants: Psychostimulants such as dextroamphetamine, methylphenidate, and modafinil may enhance the analgesic effects of opioids. They may also be used to diminish opioid-induced sedation when reducing the dose is not possible.

N-methyl D-aspartate (NMDA) receptor antagonists: There is increasing evidence for the importance of NMDA receptors and the possibility that NMDA antagonists may have a role in refractory cancer pain management.

- *Ketamine* in subanesthetic doses has been used in this setting. The severe psychomimetic adverse effects associated with this treatment, including vivid hallucinations, limit widespread use of ketamine. Co-administration of a neuroleptic or benzodiazepine is recommended to limit the emergence of these effects.

- *Methadone,* particularly the racemic mixture, appears to have significant NMDA-antagonist properties. The d-isomer blocks the NMDA receptor and as a result may yield independent analgesic effects and perhaps reverse some analgesic tolerance to the opioid. This may explain the often-unanticipated high potency of methadone.

- *Dextromethorphan (DM)*, a commonly prescribed antitussive, may also have NMDA-blocking properties. The clinical significance of this effect, however, is unclear and studies have not been able to determine at what dose these effects may manifest.

Octreotide: Data from a case series of 16 patients with symptomatic liver metastases from a variety of nonneuroendocrine primary sites suggest that octreotide palliates pain and improves a variety of quality-of-life indices.

Chapter 54

Prescription Drugs: Abuse and Addiction

Although most people take prescription medications responsibly, there has been an increase in the nonmedical use or abuse of prescription drugs in the United States. Many prescription drugs can be abused, but there are several classifications of medications that are commonly abused. The three classes of prescription drugs that are most commonly abused are:

- opioids, which are most often prescribed to treat pain;

- central nervous system (CNS) depressants, which are used to treat anxiety and sleep disorders; and

- stimulants, which are prescribed to treat the sleep disorder narcolepsy and attention-deficit hyperactivity disorder (ADHD).

Opioids

Opioids are commonly prescribed because of their effective analgesic, or pain-relieving, properties. Medications that fall within this class—referred to as prescription narcotics—include morphine (Kadian, Avinza), codeine, oxycodone (OxyContin, Percodan, Percocet), and related drugs. Morphine, for example, is often used before and after surgical procedures to alleviate severe pain. Codeine, on the other hand,

Excerpted from "Prescription Drugs Abuse and Addiction," National Institute on Drug Abuse (NIDA), NIH Publication Number 05–4881, revised August 2005.

is often prescribed for mild pain. In addition to their pain-relieving properties, some of these drugs—codeine and diphenoxylate (Lomotil) for example—can be used to relieve coughs and diarrhea.

How do opioids affect the brain and body?

Opioids act on the brain and body by attaching to specific proteins called opioid receptors, which are found in the brain, spinal cord, and gastrointestinal tract. When these drugs attach to certain opioid receptors, they can block the perception of pain. Opioids can produce drowsiness, nausea, constipation, and, depending upon the amount of drug taken, depress respiration. Opioid drugs also can induce euphoria by affecting the brain regions that mediate what we perceive as pleasure. This feeling is often intensified for those who abuse opioids when administered by routes other than those recommended. For example, OxyContin often is snorted or injected to enhance its euphoric effects, while at the same time increasing the risk for serious medical consequences, such as opioid overdose.

What are the possible consequences of opioid use and abuse?

Taken as directed, opioids can be used to manage pain effectively. Many studies have shown that the properly managed, short-term medical use of opioid analgesic drugs is safe and rarely causes addiction—defined as the compulsive and uncontrollable use of drugs despite adverse consequences—or dependence, which occurs when the body adapts to the presence of a drug, and often results in withdrawal symptoms when that drug is reduced or stopped. Withdrawal symptoms include restlessness, muscle and bone pain, insomnia, diarrhea, vomiting, cold flashes with goose bumps (cold turkey), and involuntary leg movements. Long-term use of opioids can lead to physical dependence and addiction. Taking a large single dose of an opioid can cause severe respiratory depression that can lead to death.

Is it safe to use opioid drugs with other medications?

Only under a physician's supervision can opioids be used safely with other drugs. Typically, they should not be used with other substances that depress the CNS, such as alcohol, antihistamines, barbiturates, benzodiazepines, or general anesthetics, because these combinations increase the risk of life-threatening respiratory depression.

Central Nervous System (CNS) Depressants

CNS depressants, sometimes referred to as sedatives and tranquilizers, are substances that can slow normal brain function. Because of this property, some CNS depressants are useful in the treatment of anxiety and sleep disorders. Among the medications that are commonly prescribed for these purposes are the following:

- Barbiturates, such as mephobarbital (Mebaral) and pentobarbital sodium (Nembutal), are used to treat anxiety, tension, and sleep disorders.

- Benzodiazepines, such as diazepam (Valium), chlordiazepoxide HCl (Librium), and alprazolam (Xanax), are prescribed to treat anxiety, acute stress reactions, and panic attacks. The more sedating benzodiazepines, such as triazolam (Halcion) and estazolam (ProSom) are prescribed for short-term treatment of sleep disorders. Usually, benzodiazepines are not prescribed for long-term use.

How do CNS depressants affect the brain and body?

There are numerous CNS depressants; most act on the brain by affecting the neurotransmitter gamma-aminobutyric acid (GABA). Neurotransmitters are brain chemicals that facilitate communication between brain cells. GABA works by decreasing brain activity. Although the different classes of CNS depressants work in unique ways, it is through their ability to increase GABA activity that they produce a drowsy or calming effect that is beneficial to those suffering from anxiety or sleep disorders.

What are the possible consequences of CNS depressant use and abuse?

Despite their many beneficial effects, barbiturates and benzodiazepines have the potential for abuse and should be used only as prescribed. During the first few days of taking a prescribed CNS depressant, a person usually feels sleepy and uncoordinated, but as the body becomes accustomed to the effects of the drug, these feelings begin to disappear. If one uses these drugs long term, the body will develop tolerance for the drugs, and larger doses will be needed to achieve the same initial effects. Continued use can lead to physical dependence and—when use is reduced or stopped— withdrawal. Because all CNS depressants work by slowing the brain's activity, when an individual stops taking them, the brain's activity can rebound and race out of control, potentially leading to seizures and other harmful consequences. Although withdrawal from benzodiazepines can be problematic, it is rarely life threatening, whereas withdrawal from prolonged use of other CNS depressants can have life-threatening complications. Therefore, someone who is thinking about discontinuing CNS depressant therapy or who is suffering withdrawal from a CNS depressant should speak with a physician or seek medical treatment.

Is it safe to use CNS depressants with other medications?

CNS depressants should be used in combination with other medications only under a physician's close supervision. Typically, they should not be combined with any other medication or substance that causes CNS depression, including prescription pain medicines, some over-the-counter (OTC) cold and allergy medications, and alcohol. Using CNS depressants with these other substances—particularly alcohol—can slow both the heart and respiration and may lead to death.

Stimulants

As the name suggests, stimulants increase alertness, attention, and energy, as well as elevate blood pressure, and increase heart rate and respiration. Stimulants historically were used to treat asthma and other respiratory problems, obesity, neurological disorders, and a variety of other ailments. But as their potential for abuse and addiction became apparent, the medical use of stimulants began to wane. Now, stimulants are prescribed for the treatment of only a few health conditions, including narcolepsy, attention deficit hyperactivity disorder (ADHD), and depression that has not responded to other treatments.

How do stimulants affect the brain and body?

Stimulants, such as dextroamphetamine (Dexedrine and Adderall) and methylphenidate (Ritalin and Concerta), have chemical structures similar to a family of key brain neurotransmitters called monoamines which include norepinephrine and dopamine. Stimulants enhance the effects of these chemicals in the brain. Stimulants also increase blood pressure and heart rate, constrict blood vessels, increase blood glucose, and open up the pathways of the respiratory system. The increase in dopamine is associated with a sense of euphoria that can accompany the use of these drugs.

What are the possible consequences of stimulant use and abuse?

As with other drugs of abuse, it is possible for individuals to become dependent upon or addicted to many stimulants. Withdrawal symptoms associated with discontinuing stimulant use include fatigue, depression, and disturbance of sleep patterns. Repeated use of some stimulants over a short period can lead to feelings of hostility or paranoia. Further, taking high doses of a stimulant may result in dangerously high body temperature and an irregular heartbeat. There is also the potential for cardiovascular failure or lethal seizures.

Is it safe to use stimulants with other medications?

Stimulants should be used in combination with other medications only under a physician's supervision. Patients also should be aware of the dangers associated with mixing stimulants and OTC cold medicines that contain decongestants; combining these substances may cause blood pressure to become dangerously high or lead to irregular heart rhythms.

Trends in Prescription Drug Abuse

Although prescription drug abuse affects many Americans, some concerning trends can be seen among older adults, adolescents, and women. Several indicators suggest that prescription drug abuse is on the rise in the United States. According to the 2003 National Survey on Drug Use and Health (NSDUH), an estimated 4.7 million Americans used prescription drugs non-medically for the first time in 2002.

- 2.5 million used pain relievers

- 1.2 million used tranquilizers

- 761,000 used stimulants

- 225,000 used sedatives

Pain reliever incidence increased—from 573,000 initiates in 1990 to 2.5 million initiates in 2000—and remained stable through 2003. In 2002, more than half (55 percent) of the new users were females, and more than half (56 percent) were ages 18 or older.

The Drug Abuse Warning Network (DAWN), which monitors medications and illicit drugs reported in emergency departments (ED) across the United States., recently found that two of the most frequently reported prescription medications in drug abuse-related cases are benzodiazepines (diazepam, alprazolam, clonazepam, and lorazepam) and opioid pain relievers (oxycodone, hydrocodone, morphine, methadone, and combinations that include these drugs). In 2002, benzodiazepines accounted for 100,784 mentions that were classified as drug abuse cases, and opioid pain relievers accounted for more than 119,000 ED mentions. From 1994 to 2002, ED mentions of hydrocodone and oxycodone increased by 170 percent and 450 percent, respectively. While ED visits attributed to drug addiction and drug-taking for psychoactive effects have been increasing, intentional overdose visits have remained stable since 1995.

Older Adults

Persons 65 years of age and above comprise only 13 percent of the population, yet account for approximately one-third of all medications prescribed in the United States. Older patients are more likely to be prescribed long-term and multiple prescriptions, which could lead to unintentional misuse.

The elderly also are at risk for prescription drug abuse, in which they intentionally take medications that are not medically necessary. In addition to prescription medications, a large percentage of older adults also use OTC medicines and dietary supplements. Because of their high rates of comorbid illnesses, changes in drug metabolism with age, and the potential for drug interactions, prescription and OTC drug abuse and misuse can have more adverse health consequences among the elderly than are likely to be seen in a younger population.

Adolescents and Young Adults

Data from the 2003 NSDUH indicate that 4.0 percent of youth ages 12–17 reported nonmedical use of prescription medications in the past month. Rates of abuse were highest among the 18–25 age group (6.0 percent). Among the youngest group surveyed, ages 12–13, a higher percentage reported using psychotherapeutics (1.8 percent) than marijuana (1.0 percent).

The National Institute on Drug Abuse (NIDA) Monitoring the Future survey found that 5.0 percent of 12th-graders reported using OxyContin without a prescription in the past year, and 9.3 percent reported using Vicodin, making Vicodin one of the most commonly abused licit drugs in this population. Past year, nonmedical use of tranquilizers (Valium, Xanax) in 2004 was 2.5 percent for 8th-graders, 5.1

percent for 10th-graders, and 7.3 percent for 12th-graders. Also within the past year, 6.5 percent of 12th-graders used sedatives or barbiturates (Amytal, Nembutal) non-medically, and 10.0 percent used amphetamines (Ritalin, Benzedrine).

Youth who use other drugs are more likely to abuse prescription medications. According to the 2001 National Household Survey on Drug Abuse (now the NSDUH), 63 percent of youth who had used prescription drugs non-medically in the past year had also used marijuana in the past year, compared with 17 percent of youth who had not used prescription drugs non-medically in the past year.

Gender Differences

Studies suggest that women are more likely than men to be prescribed an abusable prescription drug, particularly narcotics and antianxiety drugs—in some cases, 55 percent more likely. Overall, men and women have roughly similar rates of nonmedical use of prescription drugs. An exception is found among 12- to 17-year-olds. In this age group, young women are more likely than young men to use psychotherapeutic drugs non-medically. In addition, research has shown that women are at increased risk for nonmedical use of narcotic analgesics and tranquilizers (benzodiazepines).

Preventing and Recognizing Prescription Drug Abuse

The risks for addiction to prescription drugs increase when the drugs are used in ways other than for those prescribed. Health care providers, primary care physicians, and pharmacists, as well as patients themselves, all can play a role in identifying and preventing prescription drug abuse.

Treating Prescription Drug Addiction

Years of research have shown that addiction to any drug (illicit or prescribed) is a brain disease that, like other chronic diseases, can be treated effectively. No single type of treatment is appropriate for all individuals addicted to prescription drugs. Treatment must take into account the type of drug used and the needs of the individual. Successful treatment may need to incorporate several components, including detoxification, counseling, and in some cases, the use of pharmacological therapies. Multiple courses of treatment may be needed for the patient to make a full recovery.

The two main categories of drug addiction treatment are behavioral and pharmacological. Behavioral treatments encourage patients to stop drug use and teach them how to: function without drugs, handle cravings, avoid drugs and situations that could lead to drug use, and handle a relapse should it occur. When delivered effectively, behavioral treatments—such as individual counseling, group or family counseling, contingency management, and cognitive-behavioral therapies—also can help patients improve their personal relationships and their ability to function at work and in the community.

Some addictions, such as opioid addiction, can be treated with medications. These pharmacological treatments counter the effects of the drug on the brain and behavior, and can be used to relieve withdrawal symptoms, treat an overdose, or help overcome drug cravings. Although a behavioral or pharmacological approach alone may be effective for treating drug addiction, research shows that, at least in the case of opioid addiction, a combination of both is most effective.

Patients addicted to barbiturates and benzodiazepines should not attempt to stop taking them on their own. Withdrawal symptoms from these drugs can be problematic, and—in the case of certain CNS depressants—potentially life threatening. Although no research regarding the treatment of barbiturate and benzodiazepine addiction exists, addicted patients should undergo medically supervised detoxification because the treatment dose must be gradually tapered.

Treatment of addiction to prescription stimulants, such as Ritalin, is often based on behavioral therapies that have proven effective in treating cocaine and methamphetamine addiction. At this time, there are no proven medications for the treatment of stimulant addiction.

Chapter 55

Fentanyl Pain Patches and Topical Compounded Pain Products

Proper Use of Fentanyl Pain Patches

Fentanyl skin patches provide convenient and effective relief for many people who experience chronic pain, and who have been taking pain medications for long periods of time. But health care providers and patients should be aware that deaths and other serious problems have resulted from accidental overdoses related to inappropriate use of the fentanyl patch, the U.S. Food and Drug Administration (FDA) says.

The patch is applied to the skin and delivers fentanyl—a potent, strong, opiate analgesic. The drug is slowly absorbed through the skin into the bloodstream and can relieve pain for up to three days from a single patch application. "After applying the first patch, it can take 12 to 18 hours to reach the peak of pain relief, with some early pain relief occurring at four to six hours after the first administration," says Donald R. Stanski, M.D., a professor of anesthesia at Stanford University who was involved with the clinical drug development of the first fentanyl patch in the 1980s.

The most frequent use of the fentanyl patch has been to treat pain in people with cancer, and it is only appropriate for patients who have

This chapter includes text from "Proper Use of Fentanyl Pain Patches," by Michelle Meadows, *FDA Consumer magazine*, March-April 2006, U.S. Food and Drug Administration (FDA); and "Warnings for Makers of Compounded Pain Products," by Michelle Meadows, *FDA Consumer magazine*, March-April 2007, FDA.

developed a degree of tolerance to the opiate analgesic effects because they have been previously using this type of drug, says Robert J. Meyer, M.D., director of the Office of Drug Evaluation II in the FDA's Center for Drug Evaluation and Research (CDER). "Because the patch provides slow, continuous drug delivery, people with constant pain are less likely to experience waxing and waning of pain control," as occurs when the traditional oral medication or injections of the opiate wear off, Meyer says. Some people can experience breakthrough pain, which may require additional analgesic medication. "With the patch, patients don't have to take multiple doses of oral medications to control the underlying chronic pain," Meyer says. "But in some reports of overdose, we have seen misunderstandings about the recommended use of the product." Proper use of the patch that follows the drug's label is crucial.

The FDA is investigating deaths and overdoses that have occurred with both brand-name and generic fentanyl patches. The brand Duragesic (fentanyl transdermal system), manufactured by Janssen L.P. of Titusville, New Jersey, was approved by the FDA in 1990. A generic version, manufactured by Mylan Laboratories Inc. of Canonsburg, Pennsylvania, was approved in 2005.

In July 2005, the FDA issued a public health advisory on the fentanyl patch. Meyer says the advisory focuses on improving education about the signs of an overdose, proper patch application, drug interactions, proper storage and disposal of the patch, and safeguards for children. The powerful pain-relieving properties of all opiates are countered by significant risks of depressed breathing that can cause unexpected death. Signs of an overdose include trouble breathing or shallow breathing, extreme sleepiness or sedation, an inability to walk or talk normally, and feeling faint, dizzy, and confused. People who experience these symptoms should seek emergency medical attention. Removing the patch will not reverse the problem; the drug is still absorbed into the body for more than 17 hours after the patch is removed.

Appropriate Use

The fentanyl patch should not be used for short-term acute pain, pain that is not constant, or pain after an operation. The patch is only for people who experience moderate-to-severe chronic pain that is expected to last for weeks or longer and that cannot be managed by acetaminophen-opioid combinations, nonsteroidal analgesics, or as-needed dosing with short-acting opioids.

The patch also should not be the first narcotic pain medicine that is prescribed. It should be used only in people who have been taking opiate analgesics for a period of time. It could be used if people have been taking at least 60 milligrams (mg) of oral morphine daily, at least 30 mg of oral oxycodone daily, at least 8 mg of oral hydromorphone daily, or an equally strong dose of another opioid for a week or longer. Stanski says, "This prior opiate dosing results in a degree of tolerance, or resistance to the opiate that is relevant when the patch is subsequently used." Children who are younger than two years should not use the fentanyl patch. It also shouldn't be used in children two years of age or older who are not already using other opioid narcotic pain medicines. Patches should always be prescribed at the lowest dose needed for pain relief.

"Understanding and following directions is so important because of the potential for respiratory depression associated with all opiate analgesic medications, and especially with the fentanyl patch," says Stanski. Some deaths have occurred because more than one patch was applied at the same time. Other problems associated with the patch include not removing one patch before applying another, and the failure of multiple caregivers to notice that someone else has applied a patch. The patches are clear, relatively transparent, and easily blend into the skin background.

Too much medication from a fentanyl patch also could be absorbed if a patch is damaged or broken. The effects may also be exaggerated if a person wearing a patch drinks alcohol, or takes other medicines that depress brain function. "As part of its pain-relieving effect, fentanyl also causes brain depression as seen by some sleepiness and sedation," Stanski says. "This can add to the effects of other drugs like sedatives and tranquilizers."

Fentanyl also should not be used with certain human immunodeficiency virus (HIV) drugs and antifungal medicines. "The HIV [human immunodeficiency virus] drugs slow the metabolism or breakdown of fentanyl in the body and can create an overdose situation," Stanski says. Patients should make sure their doctors know about all the medicines they are taking, including prescription and nonprescription medicines, vitamins, and herbal supplements.

Fentanyl patches should be stored in a secure place and kept out of reach of children. According to Duragesic's labeling, patches should be disposed of by folding the adhesive side of the patch together so that it sticks to itself. Flush it down the toilet right away.

Addiction and Abuse

Fentanyl is a Schedule II controlled substance, the highest level of control for drugs with a recognized medical use. It comes under the jurisdiction of the Drug Enforcement Administration (DEA). There have been reports of people extracting fentanyl from the patches and abusing the drug. Uncontrolled delivery of this potent drug is very dangerous and raises the risk of overdose.

In June 2005, researchers from the University of Florida at Gainesville presented results of a study that found that the number of sudden deaths from fentanyl overdoses has been climbing nationwide. The study cited Florida Department of Law Enforcement records showing that abuse of the fentanyl patch resulted in the deaths of 115 people in Florida in 2004. Researchers said that many people who overdosed removed the full three-day dose from the patch and took it through injection, ingestion, or smoking.

As with other opiate drugs, there is a risk of becoming either addicted to the substance in the fentanyl patch or tolerant to the drug. The risk goes up for people who have a history of mental problems, or who have been addicted to other medicines, street drugs, or alcohol.

Warnings for Makers of Compounded Pain Products

Shiri Berg was a 22-year-old college student who wanted to have hair removed from her legs without too much pain. According to FDA records, a spa gave her a topical anesthetic product and instructed her to spread it over her legs before coming in for a laser hair removal procedure. Berg also was advised to wrap her legs in cellophane to intensify the numbing effect. While driving to her appointment in December 2004, she felt ill and pulled over. She then had seizures in her car and went into a coma. Berg, who attended North Carolina State University, never regained consciousness. She died several days later in January 2005.

The product Berg used contained ten percent lidocaine and ten percent tetracaine, two drug ingredients that provide pain relief by blocking signals at nerve endings in the skin. It was a prescription product, and Berg received no written instructions or warnings, according to FDA records.

Berg received topical anesthetic products that were prepared by compounding pharmacies. "Some pharmacies promote these products to spas, cosmetic-service clinics, and doctors' offices," says Steve Silverman, assistant director of the Office of Compliance in the FDA's Center for Drug Evaluation and Research. In addition to being used for laser hair removal procedures, compounded topical anesthetic products have been used to lessen pain for tattoo applications and skin treatments.

"Compounded topical anesthetic products generally are not FDA-approved," Silverman says, "and these products may be dispensed to patients without appropriate precautions and explanations for use." The FDA is concerned about firms that behave like illegal manufacturers, not traditional compounding pharmacies, because they produce standardized varieties of topical anesthetic creams. To this end, the agency notes that the drugs made by these firms do not appear to be uniquely tailored to meet the specialized medical needs of individual patients.

Moreover, the FDA is especially concerned when compounded drugs are dangerous to health. Exposure to high concentrations of some local anesthetics can cause seizures, irregular heartbeats, and other serious reactions. "The risks are even greater when different anesthetics are combined into one product," according to Silverman. Small children and others with pre-existing heart disease or severe liver disease are especially susceptible, Silverman says. The potential harm may increase if the anesthetic is left on the body for long periods of time or applied to broad areas of the body, particularly if an area is then covered by a bandage, plastic, or other dressing.

Different from Traditional Compounding

Virtually all compounded drugs lack FDA approval, but the FDA has long recognized the important public health function served by traditional pharmacy compounding. In traditional compounding, pharmacists extemporaneously combine, mix, or alter drug ingredients to create a medication tailored to the specialized needs of a patient. For example, a compounding pharmacy might prepare a unique medicine for someone who is allergic to an ingredient in an FDA-approved drug.

This kind of compounding, which is done in accordance with a valid prescription from a licensed practitioner, follows a physician's decision that his or her patient has a special medical need that cannot be met by FDA-approved drugs. The FDA understands the benefits of traditional pharmacy compounding and is not targeting this practice. By contrast, the FDA is concerned that the five firms that received Warning Letters are producing standardized versions of topical anesthetic products for general distribution, which is opposite to the notion that patient-specific treatment underlies traditional compounding.

There are FDA-approved topical anesthetic products that are commercially available, properly labeled, and regularly used in health care settings. "The problem is when pharmacies create their own versions, without medical need, and those products reach consumers without appropriate warnings or directions for use," Silverman says.

Report Adverse Events

To report adverse events related to fentanyl patch products, compounded drugs, or compounded topical anesthetic products contact:

MedWatch
Office of the Center Director
Center for Drug Evaluation and Research
5515 Security Lane, Suite 5100
Rockville, MD 20852
Toll-Free: 800-332-1088
Fax: 800-332-0178
Website: http://www.fda.gov/medwatch

Chapter 56

Physical Rehabilitation for Pain Management

Physical methods have been used for pain relief for centuries. Reportedly, Hippocrates (420 BC)—considered the father of medicine—used a warm water bag to treat pain from sciatica. Today, there are a variety of skilled health care professionals with specialized training in the use of physical techniques that help reduce pain. Many work in the field of rehabilitative medicine, and include physiatrists (physicians who specialize in physical medicine), physical therapists, occupational therapists, and exercise physiologists.

Physiatry

Physiatry—also called Physical Medicine and Rehabilitation—is a branch of medicine focusing on the diagnosis, treatment, and management of disease primarily using physical methods of care, such as physical therapy and other methods. Physiatrists provide a wide variety of treatments for the musculoskeletal system (the muscles and bones) and do not perform surgery. Because the back is the core of the musculoskeletal system, many physiatrists are considered specialists in treating back pain. A number of physiatrists have additional training in special areas, like sports medicine, brain (for example, stroke) or spinal cord injury, pain management, or pediatric medicine.

Some physicians of rehabilitative medicine have had different training than others. They may be Doctors of Medicine (M.D.) or Doctors of Osteopathy (D.O.). D.O. have attended an independent medical school and received identical training in basic science and clinical medicine as M.D.; however, they are trained to use a holistic approach to health care that includes an additional 300–500 hours of training in osteopathic manipulative medicine (OMT). Most doctors of osteopathy practice no differently than doctors of medicine, and not all continue to use OMT. To find a D.O. who uses OMT in their practice, you must ask if they specialize or have additional interest in osteopathic manipulative medicine.

D.O. are different than chiropractors. Chiropractors are independent practitioners with limited licenses to practice spinal manipulation and may incorporate nutrition into their practices. Unlike D.O. or M.D., they cannot prescribe prescription medications, admit patients to hospitals or perform surgery.

Physical Therapy

Physical therapists provide services that help restore function, improve mobility, relieve pain, and prevent or limit permanent physical disabilities of those suffering from injuries or disease. They restore, maintain, and promote overall fitness and health. They work with accident victims, as well as individuals with disabling conditions, such as low-back pain, arthritis, heart disease, fractures, head injuries, and cerebral palsy.

Therapists first examine medical histories and then test and measure the individual's strength, range of motion, balance and coordination, posture, muscle performance, respiration, and motor function. They help determine one's ability to be independent and assist with the return to the community and workplace after an injury or illness. The overall goal is to improve and maximize how an individual performs in their work setting and at home.

Physical therapists use a variety of treatment methods to relieve pain and reduce swelling including electrical stimulation, hot packs, cold compresses, traction, deep-tissue massage, and ultrasound. They also teach patients to use assistive or adaptive devices, such as crutches, prostheses, and wheelchairs. Exercise training is often provided, which can be performed at home to help advance recovery by reducing immobility and improving flexibility, strength, and endurance. As treatment continues, physical therapists document the individual's progress, conduct periodic examinations, and modify therapies when necessary. Besides tracking progress, they help identify areas that may require more or less attention.

Physical therapists consult and practice with a variety of other professionals, such as physicians, dentists, nurses, educators, social workers, occupational therapists, speech-language pathologists, and audiologists. Some treat a wide range of conditions; others specialize in areas such as pediatrics, geriatrics, orthopedics, sports medicine, neurology, pain management, and cardiopulmonary physical therapy.

Occupational Therapy

Occupational therapists help people perform tasks required for daily living and in the work setting. They work with those who have mentally, physically, developmentally, or emotionally disabling conditions. Occupational therapists help to improve their basic movement and thinking skills, as well as adaptive behaviors when there is a permanent loss of function. Their overall goal is to help individuals have independent, productive, and satisfying lives.

Occupational therapists assist in performing activities of all types ranging from using a computer to mastering everyday needs such as dressing, cooking, and eating. Physical exercises may be used to increase strength and skillfulness. Therapists instruct those with disabilities in the use of adaptive equipment, including wheelchairs, splints, and aids for eating and dressing. They can design or make special equipment needed at home or at work.

Some occupational therapists treat individuals whose ability to perform in a work environment has been impaired. Occupational therapists can help arrange for work re-training or new employment, and may team up with the individual and the employer to evaluate the work environment, plan work activities, and provide a progress report on work performance. If needed, they help modify the work environment so that work can be successfully completed.

Exercise Physiology

Exercise physiologists are commonly seen working in wellness or fitness centers. Their duties include developing exercise routines and educating people about the benefits of exercise. Exercise physiologists may also work in clinical settings prescribing exercise for individuals with special risks, such as cardiac and pulmonary disease. Services they may provide include:

- Assessment of functional abilities, including monitoring cardio-vascular and metabolic state

- Risk profile for various exercise modes and intensities

- Health-behavior change counseling and management

- Specific physical activity prescription (to accommodate current health status)

- Exercise supervision or delivery for individual or group settings

They provide the pain management team regular reports on individual progress.

Rehabilitative Techniques

The most common physical methods for pain management offered by rehab services are:

Exercise

Exercise and physical activity are beneficial not only for the body, but also the mind, spirit, and soul. Making a commitment to carve out a little time for exercise everyday is challenging for those who do not live with pain. It is much more difficult when simple movements like walking and changing positions cause pain.

Exercise not only keeps you healthy, it also helps reduce pain over time. Weight-bearing and cardiovascular exercise strengthens your heart, lungs, bones, and muscles. This becomes even more important as we age. Physical activity protects against falls and bone fractures in older adults. Research also suggests that exercise may help control joint swelling and pain caused by arthritis. If we don't "use it, we lose it." Exercise helps preserve strength, agility, and independence as we age.

The benefits of exercise are not only physically tangible; exercise has a profound effect on your mental state as well. Regular physical activity helps you cope with stress, improve your self-image, and ease anxiety and depression by releasing pleasure chemicals in our brains called endorphins. Research even suggests that physical fitness can make you more mentally alert. By incorporating group exercise with friends or family into your routine, you can also use exercise to strengthen your bonds with others. Connecting with friends and family is a key aspect of good emotional health. Too often, living with pain, leads to isolation.

Here are a few tips:

- Find something that you enjoy.

- Remember your routine need not start out at a vigorous pace. Try walking. Look into yoga classes to help you stretch and become more flexible. Tai Chi offers a low impact workout that promotes physical and mental well-being.

- Ask your instructors if they have experience working with those who live with chronic pain.

- Consult your health care professional before beginning any exercise program.

Hydrotherapy, Heat and Cold

Hydrotherapy is the use of water to maintain health or promote healing. Water has been part of health care since the beginning of civilization. Today, aspects of hydrotherapy are taught as part of health care training. Also known as aquatic or pool therapy, the use of therapeutically warm water and exercise may help ease painful muscles and joints. Gentle movement may help build strength, relax stiff joints and sore muscles. Water buoyancy greatly reduces the pressure on joints, making it easier to perform range of motion exercises.

The use of ice packs, hot water bottles, heating pads, and counter-irritant preparations, like Tiger Balm, Icy Hot, or Ben Gay, are familiar in popular culture. For example, many use the application of ice to a sprained ankle or soaking in a hot tub to soothe sore muscles. Steam can open clogged sinuses; ice packs can relieve swelling. Cold-based hydrotherapies, such as ice packs and cold compresses, decrease swelling and pain by constricting blood vessels and numbing nerve endings. On the other hand, heat-based hydrotherapies, such as whirlpools and hot compresses, have the opposite effect. As the body attempts to throw off the excess heat and keep body temperature from rising, dilation of blood vessels occurs, providing increased circulation to the area being treated. This helps relax muscle spasms and relieve pain.

Today hydrotherapy is a part of the physical therapy department of virtually every hospital and medical center. Various techniques using water are considered standard strategies for rehabilitation and pain relief. Many forms of hydrotherapy are also available at health spas and resorts. Be sure to check with your health care provider and verify the credentials of the spa before going.

Myofascial Therapy

A gentle blend of stretching and massage, myofascial release therapy uses hands-on manipulation of muscle and skin to relieve pain and promote healing. According to practitioners of myofascial release, scarring or injury to this network of connective tissue and muscle is a major cause of pain and restricted motion. The easy stretch is aimed to alleviate these problems by breaking up, or releasing, constrictions or snags in the fascia. People with longstanding back pain, fibromyalgia, recurring headaches, sports injuries, and other chronic pain disorders may benefit from this technique.

Myofascial release is part of a larger philosophy of healing that emphasizes the importance of mind-body interactions and preventive care. It is based on the idea that poor posture, physical injury, illness, and emotional stress can throw the body out of alignment which causes the fascia and muscle to become tight and constricted. Scarring or adhesions form. The gentle and sustained stretching of myofascial release is believed to free adhesions and soften and lengthen the fascia. The stretch may be held for one to two minutes, and sometimes for up to five minutes, before a softening, or release, is felt. The release indicates that the muscle is relaxing, fascial adhesions are slowly breaking down, or the fascia has realigned to its normal position. The process is then repeated until the tissues are fully elongated.

Sessions typically last 30 minutes to an hour and may be given one to three times a week depending on your condition. Some people immediately feel better—even free of pain—and are able to move their joints more freely as soon as the session is over. Others feel some discomfort that night or the next day. Any soreness should subside within a day or two, and you should feel less pain and be able to move more easily than you did before.

Exercises are tailored to your individual needs, and you should be given exercises to do at home. Unlike stretching routines for specific sports, these exercises will be designed to lengthen the muscles and connective tissues in various directions. To relieve tightness in the pelvic region, for instance, you may lie with your hip resting on a small foam ball for several minutes.

Osteopathic Manipulation Treatment (OMT)

Osteopathic medicine is a form of conventional medicine that highlights diseases arising in the musculoskeletal system. This practice follows an underlying belief that all of the body's systems work together,

410

and disturbances in one system may affect function elsewhere in the body. The use of a hands-on technique called osteopathic manipulation treatment (OMT) may be considered to help reduce pain, restore function, and promote health and well-being.

OMT covers a wide range of services including spinal manipulation, connective tissue release, soft-tissue techniques, muscle energy, and cranial osteopathy. It is considered more comprehensive than a chiropractic spinal adjustment. OMT works to release blockages in a person's body to promote health. By removing restrictions in the muscles, nerves, blood vessels, and ligaments, the patient's body is able to move more freely allowing it to heal itself more effectively. As previously stated, some doctors of osteopathy practice osteopathic manipulation, particularly those who specialize in physical medicine.

Splints

Casts, splints, and braces are more commonly known as tools to support and protect injured bones and tissue following an injury. By shielding the injury, they allow for more rapid healing and help prevent further injury. They can also help reduce pain, swelling, and muscles spasms.

At times, pain from inflammation, like in arthritis, causes swelling, which, in turn, increases pain. Your provider may suggest a splint to help you rest the affected area. Periodic rest with support and elevation may help to reduce the swelling and pain that has already occurred.

Wearing splints or braces during certain activities may also be recommended to help prevent pain, particularly when repetitive motion is a primary cause. Whether you are advised to wear a splint all day or only at night, this technique may help decrease additional irritation and lessen the degree of swelling and pain that might occur without one.

Protective devices such as light compression gloves or socks, or splints, may be recommended if you have neuropathic pain that affects your hands and/or feet. These may help reduce swelling and decrease pain from light touch or light pressure.

Transcutaneous Electrical Nerve Stimulation (TENS)

TENS is a method commonly managed by physical therapy as a means to decrease pain without needles or surgery. The TENS unit is designed to block or prevent pain by providing opposing stimulation to compete with the unpleasant signals that cause pain. The TENS sensation(s) interrupt pain signals in the body. The mechanisms by which TENS can relieve pain are not understood.

TENS can be used in the treatment of acute and chronic pain, including pain of the lower back, neck, pelvis, nerves (complex regional pain syndrome/reflex sympathetic dystrophy syndrome [CRPS/RSD], neuritis), and muscles (fibromyalgia, myofascial).

Used properly, TENS units are very safe and do not hurt to apply or wear. The best time to wear TENS is during activities or times of the day when your pain is generally the most severe. The sensation should feel comfortable or pleasurable when the unit is turned on. They are battery-operated (9-volt). A TENS unit will not electrocute you. To prevent an unintentional shock, they should not be worn in the shower or bath tub, or be turned up too high. It is not recommended to be used with a demand-type cardiac pacemaker. Also, there are specific areas of the body that should be avoided, like over the larger blood vessels (arteries) in the neck.

Additional Physical Methods

There are other physical methods that may be offered to aid in pain reduction and improvement of movement. Depending on the practice, size, location, and experience of the providers may determine the scope of services. These methods may be performed by a physical therapist with special training or a complementary practitioner.

Chiropractic

Note: Information about chiropractic care is available in the "Complementary and Alternative Medicine," section of *Treatment Options: A Guide for People Living with Pain*, available online at http://www.painfoundation.org/Publications/TreatmentOptions2006.pdf, or through the American Pain Foundation, 201 N. Charles Street, Suite 710, Baltimore, MD 21201-4111.

Craniosacral Therapy

A gentle form of manipulation, craniosacral therapy is a hands-on healing technique typically practiced by physical therapists, massage therapists, and chiropractors. Craniosacral therapists believe the movement of spinal fluid within and around the central nervous system creates a vital body rhythm, no less important to health and well-being than the heartbeat or breath. Health problems develop, they contend, when blockages occur. Practitioners assert that craniosacral therapy reestablishes the normal flow of fluids and thus restores health. By law, craniosacral therapists are not allowed to make a medical diagnosis. For this reason, the technique should not be confused with cranial osteopathy, a diagnostic and therapeutic method of treatment that is practiced by highly trained osteopathic physicians. A session usually lasts from 20 minutes to an hour.

Feldenkrais (Functional Integration)

The Feldenkrais Method is a form of somatic education that uses gentle movement and directed attention to improve movement and enhance human functioning. Through this method, you learn to improve your ease of motion, increase your range of motion, expand your flexibility and coordination, and rediscover your ability to move gracefully and effectively. These improvements may enhance functioning in other aspects of your life, such as pain reduction. The Feldenkrais Method is based on principles of physics, biomechanics, and an understanding of learning and human development. By expanding the self-image through movement sequences that bring attention to the parts of the self that are out of awareness, the method enables you to include more of yourself in your everyday activities.

Rolfing (Structural Integration)

Rolfing emerged from the concept that humans function most efficiently and comfortably when key parts of the body, such as the head, torso, pelvis, and legs, are properly aligned. There are different versions of Rolfing. Rolfing is a form of myofascial massage guided by the contours of the body. Rolfers use their fingers, hands, elbows, and knees to place deep pressure and shift bones into proper alignment. Their goal is to increase range of motion and make movement easier by correcting posture misalignments. Rolfing can sometimes be painful.

Trager Approach

The Trager Approach is a form of movement consisting of a series of gentle, passive movements, along with rotation and traction of arms and legs to relieve muscular tightness without pain. This was technique was developed in the early 1900s to help polio victims. Some with chronic pain due to muscle spasm have reported noticeable pain relief beginning with the first session. The practitioner moves select parts of the body in a light rhythmical fashion so that you can experience the

413

feeling of this light, effortless movement. The goal of each session is to help reduce stress and to find more effective ways to deal with stressful situations. Added benefits are enhanced conscious awareness, greater flexibility, improved self image, greater energy, and reduced constriction and rigidity.

The following are commonly recommended techniques, which can be done at home as part of a self-care program:

Icing: Ideal for pain related to recent injury, re-injury, or inflammation like with strains, sprains, and bruises. It can easily be done anywhere. Cold has a numbing effect. However, placing ice directly on your skin can cause nerve damage. Be sure to place a thin towel or pillow case between your skin and the cold source, whether using ice cubes in a plastic bag, a frozen pack of peas (or corn), or a gel pack. Ice for 20 minutes, and then remove it until the surrounding skin returns to normal temperature before re-applying. This can be repeated on a regular basis every two hours throughout the day.

Compresses: To make a wet compress, soak a cloth in hot or cold water and squeeze out the excess until the desired amount of moisture remains. Single or double compresses may be used. Grain pillows, gel-packing, and certain heating pads (follow the manufacturer directions) can be used. A single compress involves the use of the wet cloth over the affected area. A double compress includes placing a dry material such as wool or flannel over the wet compress.

A cold compress can be used to decrease swelling, reduce blood flow to an area, or inhibit inflammation. Cold should not be used in the presence of circulation disorders, like peripheral vascular disease, certain heart conditions, and diabetes, unless pre-approved by your health care professional.

A hot compress can have an analgesic effect, thereby decreasing pain. When using hot water, the double compress serves to retain the heat. Hot compresses can also be used to lessen the discomfort from muscle cramping or spasm and improve blood flow to a particular part of the body. Separate, alternating, or simultaneous use of hot or cold compresses can be applied for pain relief depending on the individual preference. When using a microwave to heat a gel pack or grain pillow, please follow the directions to avoid extreme heat that could cause skin burn.

Baths: Either immersing the entire body or simply the affected part of the body can be helpful. Hot, full-immersion baths can help with arthritic discomfort and conditions where muscles are in painful spasm, such as fibromyalgia. For a neutral (or tepid) bath, the temperature should be neither too hot, nor too cold. These are mainly used for relaxation purposes and to treat stress-related ailments such as insomnia, anxiety, and nervous exhaustion. Cool baths can relieve swelling or inflammation.

Sitz baths: Taking sitz baths involves partially immersing the pelvic region. A hot sitz bath can help reduce pain from hemorrhoids, abdominal cramping, or sciatica. A special sitz bath seat can be purchased at most pharmacies.

Cold friction rubs: A friction rub involves massaging a particular area of the body with a rough washcloth, terry towel, or loofah that has first been place in ice water. Friction rubs have a toning effect that helps to increase circulation and tighten muscles.

Counter-irritants: Better known as heating or cooling creams, lotions, or salves applied to the skin over the painful area. They are either gently rubbed around the skin surface or used with massage or myofascial release treatments. They can be used as a single agent for either the preferred heat or cooling effects, alternating between the two sensations, or in combination with a therapy that provides the opposite effect.

Alternating: Use one preparation that heats, wait for effect to wear off, and skin returns to normal temperature; wash off remaining product before applying opposite preparation that cools.

Combination: Apply product that heats. Be sure to protect the skin by placing plastic wrap over area, then place ice pack on top. Remove ice pack within 15–20 minutes and wait 30 minutes before reapplication of ice pack.

Whenever these preparations are used, it is important to avoid using two therapies that enhance the same temperature effect to avoid heat or cold burns to the skin. For example, if you plan to take a hot shower or apply a heating pad to an area previously treated, wait for the product effect to wear away, and wash off any remaining product.

Chapter 57

Injection and Infusion Therapies for Pain

Injection and infusion therapies may be used for the management of both acute and chronic pain. Acute pain, which you might experience after surgery or a major trauma, may be controlled optimally with pain medications delivered directly into your vein (intravenous) or your spine (intraspinal, which includes epidural or intrathecal), or with local anesthetics injected prior to your procedure (regional anesthesia). Persistent or chronic pain, which is defined as pain lasting longer than three months, may require injection (nerve block) or infusion therapies if other therapies (for example; oral medications, physical therapy) do not provide adequate pain relief.

Injection Therapies

Injection therapies may be used to treat painful conditions in many areas of the body. The term nerve block was originally used for an injection that targeted specific nerves. It is now associated with any procedure involving placing a needle into a muscle, joint, spine, or around a specific group of nerves, followed by the injection of medication(s) or delivery of some other treatment such as electricity, heat, or cold.

Nerve blocks can be used to:

- **Diagnose pain (diagnostic nerve blocks):** This can help determine if your pain is coming from a nerve, muscle, or joint. It may also help identify nerve pathways causing your pain.

- **Predict the effects of permanent nerve blocks (prognostic nerve blocks):** Certain nerve blocks are first done with a numbing (local anesthetic medication). If you have relief from this type of block, a more permanent type of block, which will provide longer lasting pain relief may be recommended. The local anesthetic block may predict what kind of result you will have with the permanent block.

- **Prevent development of chronic pain syndromes (prophylactic nerve blocks):** Development and spread of certain types of sympathetic nerve pain conditions may be slowed or stopped by using prophylactic nerve blocks.

- **Provide pain relief (therapeutic nerve blocks):** When the cause of your pain is known, a therapeutic nerve block may provide a reduction in pain that serves as a complement to other pain treatment options.

Prior to any procedure, your pain specialist may perform a complete pain assessment in order to select the most appropriate injection therapy. This usually includes a complete physical exam and a review of your full medical history, including any testing you may have had (x-rays, computed tomography [CT] scans, magnetic resonance imaging [MRI], or others), as well as your personal preferences. This will allow your provider to develop a treatment plan tailored to your specific condition and needs. Your pain specialist should go over the type of block, benefits and risks, and potential side effects in detail before getting your consent to perform the procedure.

The most common medications injected include local anesthetics, corticosteroids, and neurolytic drugs.

- **Local anesthetics** can numb a painful area by blocking sensory and pain pathways. Commonly used local anesthetics are lidocaine and bupivacaine.

- **Corticosteroids** reduce inflammation around the nerves to decrease pain. Commonly used corticosteroids are methylprednisolone acetate and triamcinolone.

- **Neurolytic drugs** destroy nerve pathways to produce a more permanent effect. These drugs include absolute alcohol and phenol which are otherwise not commonly used in chronic pain management.

In all cases, the area to be injected will be cleaned with an antiseptic solution before any medication or solution is injected into the affected area, which will be numbed with a local anesthetic. Fluoroscopy (a special x-ray) is used for some nerve blocks in order to guide the placement of the needle.

What to Expect Prior to the Procedure (Preparation)

What you may need to do to prepare for each injection therapy will depend on the type of injection and the setting in which the pain specialist will perform the procedure (private office, ambulatory surgery center, hospital center). Particularly for nerve blocks or minimally invasive surgery, you might need to consider:

- **Food and liquids:** You may be asked to refrain from eating or drinking for a certain period of time prior to your procedure.

- **Transportation:** You may be asked to have someone drive you home after the procedure.

- **Medications:** You may be asked to stop certain medications (blood thinners) prior to your procedure.

- **Intravenous (IV):** You may have an IV placed prior to your procedure with or without IV fluids running.

- **Conscious sedation:** You may be given medications either before or during your procedure to calm you, make you sleepy while remaining aware and able to follow directions, or to relieve your pain. You should be given specific instructions prior to receiving any type of sedation. These medications may interfere with your memory and functioning, which is why you need to bring a friend or family member with you to listen to your discharge instructions and drive you home.

- **Positioning:** You may be asked to get onto an exam or x-ray table and lie still for a period of time. Be sure to let the pain specialist know if you will require any special assistance.

- **Allergies:** It is very important that you report if you are allergic to any medications, especially any reactions you may have had to local anesthetics, corticosteroids, iodine, IV dye, or shellfish.

- **Risk of exposure to radiation (if x-ray or fluoroscopy is used):** This is a particular concern in pregnancy.

General Risks

As with any procedure, there are risks of serious complications. While these are uncommon, your pain specialist will be prepared to treat them immediately. Admission to the hospital for at least an overnight observation could be recommended for any of the following:

- Uncontrolled bleeding

- Unplanned perforation of a vital organ located close to the treatment area

- Unplanned nerve damage causing weakness or numbness to the surrounding area of treatment

- Allergic reaction from the local anesthetic causing difficulty breathing

Types of Injection-Based Therapies (Such as Nerve Blocks) and How They Are Used

Diagnostic Injection

Discogram: A discogram is a procedure used to determine which disc(s) in your lower back is causing your back or leg pain. Fluoroscopy is used and x-ray pictures of the discs are taken. This procedure may be performed by a pain specialist or a specialty trained radiologist. You may be asked to take copies of your x-rays back to the physician who ordered the discogram for their review if that is preferred over a written report of findings by the performing physician.

Conscious sedation is commonly used for this procedure. You will be placed in the prone (face down) position on an x-ray table. A thin needle will be placed into each disc being tested and solution will be injected to increase pressure in the disc in an attempt to recreate your pain. You will be asked if the injection of the solution reproduces your pain or not. If it does, then this may be the disc that is causing your pain and further treatment options may be available.

Injections

Botulinum toxin injection: An injection of botulinum toxin into the muscle or muscle group causing you pain. This toxin causes temporary paralysis of these muscles. This injection may be done if you have dystonia—a disorder characterized by cramping muscles, certain headaches, or other conditions where muscles are in chronic spasm causing pain.

The dosage of botulinum toxin is very small. The relief effect takes time to notice. It may take 2–3 days before muscle relaxation is achieved. This effect generally lasts months, but requires follow-up before a repeat injection is recommended. If a poor response, or no response, occurs with a previous injection, the value of proceeding with further injections should be reviewed first.

Sacroiliac (SI) joint injections : An SI joint injection is the injection of medication into the sacroiliac joint in your buttock region. This may be done if you have a certain type of low back or buttock pain.

Fluoroscopy may be used to guide placement of a needle into the SI joint, and inject a local anesthetic or local anesthetic and steroid solution.

Trigger point injections (TPI): TPI are the injection of medications into your muscles. These muscle trigger points are usually painful when you press directly on them.

TPI may be done to treat trigger point pain from chronic spasm, myofascial syndrome, or fibromyalgia. A needle will be inserted into the painful trigger points and a local anesthetic with or without steroid will be injected.

Nerve Blocks

The nerve blocks described are a representation of the most common nerve blocks done for pain conditions. Ask your health care provider about these and nerve blocks not discussed in this section.

Axillary block: An axillary block is an injection of a local anesthetic around a group of nerves located in your underarm area. This type of block may be done if you have complex regional pain syndrome (CRPS), nerve pain in your arm, or for diagnostic purposes.

You will lie flat with the affected arm stretched out with your palm up. A needle will be inserted into your underarm and a local anesthetic is injected. You may feel a sharp tingling sensation at the time of injection. Don't worry, this is normal. This confirms that the needle is in the proper place.

Celiac plexus/hypogastric plexus block: These blocks involve the injection of a local anesthetic into the area of a group of nerves which supply the abdominal organs, called celiac plexus nerves. These blocks are performed most commonly for the treatment of upper abdominal pain due to chronic pancreatitis, cancer, and pelvic pain. Fluoroscopy is used to guide the placement of needle to the area. After the needle is in the proper area, local anesthetic will be injected in the area of the celiac plexus nerves.

Epidural steroid injection (ESI): An ESI is the injection of a small amount of steroid into the epidural space that surrounds the spinal cord and spinal nerves. This can be done in the neck (cervical), mid back (thoracic) or low back (lumbar or caudal).

An ESI may be performed if you have back, leg, neck, or arm pain. The pain may be due to a herniated spinal disc, spinal stenosis (narrowing of the spinal canal space), degeneration of your spinal bones (vertebrae), or compression fractures. All of these conditions may cause irritation and inflammation, which may be the root cause your pain.

Fluoroscopy is commonly used as a guide for needle placement, so typically, you will be lying face down on an x-ray table. If x-ray is not used, you may be sitting or lying on your side during the procedure. Conscious sedation may be optional and would require IV placement prior to the procedure. Sometimes, IV placement is required for the first procedure, or if you have a history of fainting or sudden drops in your blood pressure during medical procedures (better known as a vagal response).

The needle may not be placed in exactly the same site as your pain; the medication injected will float to coat the nearby nerves. You may feel some pressure in the area of the injection or some re-creation of your pain symptoms as the medication (steroid or steroid and local anesthetic) is injected. This feeling is normal and will go away in a short period of time.

Facet nerve blocks: A facet nerve block is performed if it is suspected that your back or neck pain may be caused by irritation or inflammation of the small nerves near the facet joints of the spine. Pain from facet nerves can occur from injuries that involve twisting and straining while lifting heavy objects or falling. Facet joints are on the back of your spine, one on each side, near the boney spine, but not near the spinal cord.

Fluoroscopy is used to guide the placement of needles to the area. After correct needle placement is confirmed, a small amount of local anesthetic will be injected near the facet nerve.

Intercostal nerve blocks: An intercostal nerve block is the injection of a local anesthetic or a neurolytic agent in the area between two ribs. This may be performed for pain due to nerve injury around the rib area. A needle will be inserted into the intercostal space and a local anesthetic, local anesthetic and steroid, or neurolytic solution is injected.

Because the pain specialist is working close to your lung, you should be made aware that a pneumothorax (collapsed lung) is a possible complication. A highly, skilled practitioner, a calm, quiet environment, along with very small and short needles are used to avoid this complication. It is very important that you do not move during the injection phase of this procedure.

Lumbar sympathetic block: A lumbar sympathetic block is the injection of local anesthetic around a group of nerves (lumbar sympathetic nerve chain or plexus) in your low back (lumbar) region. This is typically recommended if you have complex regional pain syndrome/reflex sympathetic dystrophy (CRPS/RSD) syndrome, severe peripheral vascular disease, or neuropathic pain (pain coming from the nerves). Fluoroscopy is used to guide the placement of the needle to the area. After the needle is in the proper area, local anesthetic will be injected in the area of the lumbar plexus nerves.

Stellate ganglion block: A stellate ganglion block is the injection of local anesthetic around a group of nerves (cervical sympathetic nerve chain or plexus) in the base of the front of your neck. This type of block may be done if you have CRPS/RSD or severe peripheral vascular disease.

You may experience a temporary drooping of your eyelid, blurred vision on the side that was injected, or minor swallowing difficulties. You should be monitored closely by skilled health care professionals until these go away and you are able to swallow liquids without difficulty.

Occipital nerve block: An occipital nerve block is the injection of local anesthetic around the occipital nerves, which are located in the back of your neck near the base of the skull. This may be useful in the diagnosis and treatment of headache and jaw pain. A needle is inserted around your occipital nerve and a local anesthetic or local anesthetic and steroid solution is injected.

Selective nerve root block: A nerve root block is the injection of a local anesthetic and steroid solution around a nerve root after it leaves the spine, also called the paraspinal region. This may be performed to diagnose a particular pain problem (to determine if your pain is coming from a nerve, muscle, or joint) or as an alternative treatment approach to an epidural steroid injection (for a herniated spinal disc or spinal stenosis, which is the narrowing of the spinal space).

Fluoroscopy is used to guide the placement of a needle to the area of the involved nerve root. You may experience a small electric shock-like sensation (similar to when you hit your funny bone). This will confirm if the needle is in the right place. A small amount of local anesthetic and steroid or steroid solution will be injected.

Other Information

Epidural Blood Patch

An epidural blood patch is done when a person has a spinal headache, usually from a myelogram or lumbar puncture. This type of headache can occur when there is a hole or tear in the dura (the covering of the spinal cord), which causes spinal fluid to leak through. A severe headache results. This headache is usually different from a typical headache; it usually is not present when you lie down and is painful when you stand up. Nausea and vomiting commonly occur when the pain is severe.

The blood patch is the injection of your own blood, which is first taken from your arm, into the epidural space in your spine. An IV (intravenous) will be started in your arm prior to the procedure.

The pain specialist will insert a needle into the epidural space in your spine. An assistant will then draw blood from your arm through the IV. This is done in sterile conditions. Your blood is then injected through the needle in your back. That needle is removed. The blood remains in your epidural space where it will clot or patch the hole or tear.

What to Expect after a Procedure

Different injection procedures will have all, some, or none of the following considerations. The antiseptic solution will usually be washed off of the area that was injected, and a small dressing (Band-Aid®) will be placed over the injection site. Your provider may monitor your vital signs (blood pressure, pulse, respirations) for a period of time. If you had an IV, it will be removed. You will be given instructions of what to expect when you go home, which might include:

- **Numbness:** Common if a local anesthetic was used. Use caution with any area that is numb. Do not walk or drive with a numb leg, or apply heat or ice to the area until all feeling has returned.

- **Soreness:** Common at the injection site after any type of injection. You may put ice on the area.

- **Low blood pressure:** May be common for a short period of time if you have had a sympathetic block. You will be monitored until your blood pressure is within your normal limits.

- **Mild to moderate headache:** May be from steroids if they were used. An over-the-counter medication of your choice may be used. If you have a severe headache, with or without nausea and vomiting, please call your pain specialist as soon as possible.

- **Increase in pain level or change in pain location:** Common for the first 24 hours after the injection or block.

- **Hot flashes, facial redness, mood changes, increased appetite, and menstrual irregularities:** Common for the first few days to weeks post injection or block. This is due to the effects of the steroid that was injected. These will go away with time.

- **Increased blood sugar:** If you are a diabetic, your blood sugar may be higher than normal for the first 3–5 days after an injection or block. Please contact the health care provider who treats your diabetes for any advice before the procedure is scheduled to make plans on what to do when/if this happens after the procedure.

- **Activity after a blood patch:** Your activity should be minimal for the first 24 hours. Rest is necessary so as not to dislodge the patch. All other injections or blocks often do not restrict activity. Use your judgment and be careful not to overdo it just because you may be feeling better; this can prevent re-injury.

Please call your pain specialist if you experience any of the following:

- Redness, swelling, or drainage around or from the injection or block site

- Persistent bleeding from injection or block site

- Severe headache (may or may not be accompanied by nausea and vomiting)

- Fever

- Stiff neck

- Weakness not present prior to the injection

Neuroablative Therapies

Neuroablative therapies usually produce a longer lasting effect than nerve blocks. These therapies use thermal (heat or cold) or chemical agents (alcohol or phenol) to destroy certain nerves or nerve chain pain pathways, thereby providing you with prolonged pain relief. Your pain specialist might choose one of the following therapies if your pain is severe, expected to persist, and cannot be lessened by other therapies. However, in some cases, special cautions must be given about potential nerve damage and return of pain that can be the same, or even worse, than before.

Thermal Therapies

Radiofrequency facet rhizotomy: A facet rhizotomy destroys facet nerve(s) either in the lower back (lumbar) or the neck (cervical) region using radiofrequency (heat) waves. This procedure is done if you have pain due to disease in the facet joints of your spine, and you have had pain relief from your facet nerve blocks.

You will be placed in the prone position. Your back or neck will be cleaned with an antiseptic solution, and the skin area will be numbed with a local anesthetic. Fluoroscopy is used to guide the placement of the needle probe to the area of the facet nerve. Radiofrequency waves are transmitted to lesion (destroy with heat) the involved nerve(s). This temporarily stops sensation from that area, which may last for an average of six months or more.

Intra discal electro thermal therapy (IDET): IDET may be considered if you have cracks or fissures in the wall of one of your spinal discs, or if the inner disc tissue has herniated into the fissure. Since these fissures are filled with small nerve endings, this may be a source of chronic back pain.

IDET is the application of thermal energy (heat) to a section of a spinal disc wall. This may result in the contraction or closure of that crack in the spinal disc wall or a reduction in the bulge of the inner disc material.

An IV will be placed in your arm and you will be given sedation. You will be placed in the prone position on an x-ray table. Fluoroscopy is used to guide a needle into place. An electrothermal treatment catheter is inserted through the needle, and the heating element is started. Once the heating is done, the catheter and needle are removed.

You should be given special instructions after this procedure with regard to activity, physical rehabilitation, and other considerations.

Cryoanalgesia: Cryoanalgesia is the application of thermal energy (cold) to a nerve or nerve chain to freeze it with nitrous oxide or carbon dioxide gas. Cryoanalgesia may still be available in some pain specialty practices, but it is limited due to the unavailability of equipment from old or new manufacturers.

Cryoanalgesia may be done if you have rib pain, pain after lung or chest surgery, facial pain, or pain from a neuroma.

Your positioning will depend on the area being treated. The cryoanalgesia probe will be placed around the nerve to be frozen when the gas is activated. This process forms an ice ball around the nerve to freeze it. This temporarily stops sensation from that area, which may last for an average of 3–6 months and sometimes more.

Chemical Therapies

Celiac plexus (destructive) block: A celiac plexus destructive block is the injection of an alcohol or phenol in the area of a group of nerves which innervate (supply) the abdominal organs. It is performed most commonly for the treatment of upper abdominal pain due to chronic pancreatitis or cancer, and usually after you have had pain relief from a diagnostic celiac plexus block.

After the needle is in the proper area, alcohol or phenol will be injected in the area of the celiac plexus or hypogastric plexus nerves.

Lumbar sympathetic (destructive) block: A lumbar sympathetic block is the injection of alcohol or phenol around a group of nerves (lumbar sympathetic nerve chain) in your low back (lumbar) region. This may be done if you have CRPS/RSD, severe peripheral vascular disease, or neuropathic pain (pain coming from the nerves), and you have had pain relief from a diagnostic lumbar sympathetic block.

Fluoroscopy is used to guide placement of a needle to the grouping of nerves in your low back. After correct needle placement, alcohol or phenol will be injected.

Minimally Invasive Surgery

Vertebroplasty (therapeutic): Percutaneous vertebroplasty is a procedure that allows health professionals to stabilize vertebrae damaged by compression fractures by injecting bone cement into the collapsed vertebrae. The aim of a vertebroplasty is to improve the strength and stability of the injured vertebrae and to eliminate pain.

When conservative treatment fails to alleviate pain associated with vertebral compression fractures, this method may be suggested. The most common complication following vertebroplasty is a transient increase in pain at the injected level. This is readily treated with non-steroid anti-inflammatory drugs (NSAID) and typically resolves within 48 hours.

Your care after any of these procedures will be similar to that after having an injection or nerve block. Your pain specialist may provide you with additional instructions depending on the type of procedure performed.

Kyphoplasty: Like vertebroplasty, kyphoplasty is used to treat bone fractures due to osteoporosis—the loss of calcium from bones resulting in weakened bone structure that increases the risk of fracture. Kyphoplasty includes an additional step when compared to vertebroplasty. Prior to injecting the cement-like material, a special balloon is inserted and gently inflated inside the fractured vertebrae. The goal of this step is to restore height to the bone, thus reducing deformity of the spine. Pain is reduced which allows you to return to normal daily activities after either procedure.

Infusion Therapies

Infusion therapies, especially intravenous (IV) drug delivery, are a convenient and effective way to control your pain. Giving pain medications through a catheter placed in your vein or spine means you may get faster and more effective pain relief, especially after surgery, injury, or trauma. The following are common infusion therapies.

Subcutaneous (SC): The SC route is usually used for chronic pain, not acute pain, because pain medication given this way will take longer to work. A small needle is placed under your skin into your subcutaneous or fatty tissue. The needle is connected to a hollow tubing and infusion pump which will deliver the pain medication into the SC tissue. The medication is then absorbed by your body and distributed to relieve your pain. SC infusion can successfully be used in the home setting, but requires visits from home health personnel.

IV bolus: Small amounts of pain medication are given through an IV catheter by a doctor or nurse. IV boluses are good for fast control of severe or acute pain on a short-term basis. IV boluses can provide immediate pain relief, but this might only last for 45–60 minutes, so additional boluses will have to be given. IV boluses are usually only used in a hospital setting.

IV continuous infusion: When moderate to severe pain over a long period of time (for example, a few days after surgery) is expected, a continuous infusion may be used. A continuous dose of pain medication is delivered through an IV by an infusion pump, which means you will have a constant level of pain relief. This is usually started after your pain has been controlled with IV boluses. IV continuous infusions are usually only used in a hospital setting, where a health care provider can monitor you.

IV patient-controlled analgesia (PCA): IV PCA is a method of pain relief to help you feel comfortable. It is routinely used after surgery or during a painful illness. By pushing the patient control button for the PCA infusion pump, you can give yourself small amounts of pain medication. Your doctor will order the amount of pain medication and indicate how often you can have it. The benefits of PCA are rapid pain relief when you need it, the possibility of using less pain medicine, having fewer side effects, and a sense of control over your pain. You will be given specific instructions on using PCA by your provider. IV PCA is usually used in a hospital setting, but may be used at home for severe, chronic pain.

Intraspinal drug delivery: Infusing pain medications and/or local anesthetics directly into the epidural—in front of the spinal fluid space (epidural analgesia) or spinal fluid space (intrathecal analgesia)—is a method of pain relief used after surgery, painful injury, or illness. This can help you get better pain relief and help you move better after surgery. It is also possible to use less pain medicine and have fewer side effects, which should help your recovery. With epidural analgesia, a small hollow tube (catheter) is placed in the space between the covering around the spinal cord and the bones of the spine; with intrathecal analgesia, the catheter is placed in the spinal fluid. The catheter may be inserted in the operating room before surgery, on a hospital floor/ intensive care unit, or as an outpatient in a pain center or outpatient surgical center. A dressing will be put over the area where the catheter goes into your skin, and the catheter will be taped along your back up to your shoulder. An anesthesiologist (doctor specializing in giving anesthesia), or pain management specialist will order the amount of pain medicine to be given by a specialized infusion pump. Special training is required for nurses who assist in the monitoring and care of this infusion system.

Epidural/intrathecal analgesia is usually used in a hospital setting, but may be used at home for cancer pain.

IV regional blocks: IV regional blockade, also known as a Bier block, is a method of producing pain relief (analgesia) in an arm or leg by injecting medications intravenously while the blood supply (circulation) in the arm or leg is cut off (occluded). This may cause temporary numbing (anesthesia) of the extremity, if a local anesthetic drug is used. Many patients are sent for physical therapy after the block, so their arm or leg can be exercised without pain. Your doctor may recommend this type of block if you have severe pain from CRPS or nerve injury.

Anesthetic infusions: IV anesthetic infusion is the infusion of a local anesthetic such as lidocaine through an IV catheter. This method can be used to treat chronic neuropathic pain (pain coming from nerves). The local anesthetic is given over a 30–60 minute period of time; you will be monitored for a period of time after that determined by your pain specialist. This may be done in an outpatient or ambulatory care setting.

Disposable anesthetic systems: PainBuster and ON~Q are two of the systems available that provide a continuous infusion of local anesthetic directly into the surgical wound. Your health care provider might recommend this method of pain control if you are having knee, hip, shoulder, or abdominal surgery. The advantage to this system is it can be used on an outpatient basis. A small catheter is placed directly into the surgical site, and your skin closed around the catheter. A small device will deliver local anesthetic to the wound site for 24–48 hours. You will be instructed on care and removal of the catheter.

Chapter 58

Painless Drug Delivery

Transdermal patches—medicated adhesive pads placed on the skin that release drugs gradually for up to a week—have been available in the United States for more than 20 years. The first transdermal patch, approved by the U.S. Food and Drug Administration (FDA) in 1979, delivered scopolamine to treat motion sickness. Since then, more than 35 transdermal patch products have been approved. Examples include the nicotine patch that helps people quit smoking, the lidocaine patch for relieving pain, and a patch containing hormone derivatives for preventing pregnancy.

Transdermal patches have several advantages compared with other methods of drug delivery: they are painless, the drugs are not degraded in the gastrointestinal tract, and they provide a constant dosage without the need for patients to remember to take their medications. In addition, delivering drugs by way of patches can reduce the side effects of some drugs. For example, estrogen patches, unlike estrogen pills, do not cause adverse effects on the liver when used to treat menopausal symptoms. However, due to permeability constraints of the outer skin layer, the number of drugs that can be administered via transdermal patches is limited.

"Painless Drug Delivery," National Institute of Biomedical Imaging and Bioengineering (NIBIB), January 11, 2008.

Microneedle Arrays Expand Transdermal Applications

To expand the number of compounds that can be delivered via the skin, researchers are developing novel transdermal technologies, including microneedle arrays that consist of tiny needles with diameters smaller than a strand of hair. The microneedles create micrometer-scale holes in the outer skin layer, thereby allowing passage of large molecules and other compounds that ordinarily could not traverse the skin. The microneedles are painless because they are too small to touch the nerves located deeper in the skin.

Although microneedles were first proposed in the 1970s, the technology needed to make microneedles did not become widely available until the 1990s. Using techniques developed in the microelectronics industry, National Institutes of Health (NIH)-supported researchers devised methods for inexpensively mass-producing microneedles from materials such as silicon, metals, and glass. The researchers also showed that microneedles can be made from polymers that will harmlessly degrade in the body, thereby preventing problems should a microneedle break off in the skin. The investigators further demonstrated that microneedles can be constructed to be solid or hollow, and both types can be made with different geometries to allow the administration of different-sized compounds, including drugs, proteins, and vaccines.

One drug-delivery technique uses solid microneedles to create micropores in the skin, and then the drug is applied over this area. NIH-funded scientists recently used this technique to administer insulin to diabetic rats. An array of solid metal microneedles was pressed into the skin, and then a glass chamber filled with insulin solution was placed over the microneedle array. Over a four-hour time period, blood glucose levels steadily dropped by as much as 80 percent. Another drug-delivery method involves coating solid microneedles with a drug which is then released from the needles when they are embedded in the skin.

Still another method employs hollow microneedles which allow drug solutions to be infused through the needles using a microprocessor-controlled pump. NIH-supported scientists recently inserted hollow glass microneedles into the skin of diabetic rats to deliver insulin for 30 minutes. Over a five-hour period after the insulin was administered, the blood glucose level dropped by as much as 70 percent. Because people would require minimal training to apply microneedles, these devices may prove useful for immunization programs in developing countries, or for mass vaccination or antidote administration in bioterrorism incidents.

Increasing Skin Permeability with Low-Frequency Ultrasound

Another transdermal technology being developed is low-frequency sonophoresis (LFS), which uses low-frequency ultrasound to create pores in the skin that stay open for several hours. In studies with animals, LFS has delivered insulin to diabetic rabbits and the anticoagulant heparin to rats. Recently, scientists used LFS to administer local anesthetics through the skin to human volunteers. To improve the design of LFS systems, NIH-funded researchers have been studying the mechanisms by which LFS increases skin permeability. Scientists found that an ultrasound frequency of 20 kilohertz induces the formation of low-pressure air bubbles on the skin surface. These bubbles grow rapidly and then collapse violently, producing microjets and shock waves that create temporary micropores in the skin. With this understanding of the mechanism of pore formation, investigators can design LFS systems to focus the ultrasound waves so that they maximize bubble formation on the skin surface.

Researchers have also experimented with viscous substances known as porous resins to increase skin permeability during sonophoresis. When dissolved in a solution of water and alcohol, these resins release air bubbles that trigger the formation of larger bubbles when LFS is applied. Investigators discovered that adding a porous resin to the solution surrounding pig skin increased permeability to the drug mannitol during sonophoresis. Mannitol promotes urine excretion, which is useful for treating brain swelling and other conditions that involve excess fluid. The results of this study suggest that adding a porous resin to the fluid that bathes the skin might enhance drug administration by sonophoresis.

Transporting Drugs Using Electroporation

Still another transdermal technology under development is electroporation, the application of short, high-voltage, electrical pulses to create temporary micropores in the skin. Electroporation has been used to transport several drugs through the skin in humans, including insulin, heparin, and the local anesthetic lidocaine. Studies also suggest that electroporation could be used to deliver compounds that would ameliorate skin aging, such as particular genes or vitamin C. NIH-supported scientists have found that transdermal drug delivery via electroporation can be enhanced through the use of mild heat, alkaline solutions, and sodium dodecyl sulfate (a detergent used in various household products, including toothpaste, shampoo, and cosmetics).

Because the drug reservoir remains outside the body, transdermal drug delivery devices provide the opportunity to easily adjust the quantity and delivery rate of medications. Transdermal systems could be controlled by a miniature computer, which would allow for accurate dosing as needed by the patient. These systems might also include sensors that monitor blood levels of compounds, such as glucose in diabetics, and then adjust the release of a drug, such as insulin. These and other developments in transdermal drug delivery technologies hold promise for improving patient compliance by making drug administration effortless and painless.

Chapter 59

Joint Replacement Surgery May Help Relieve Pain

What is joint replacement surgery?

Joint replacement surgery is removing a damaged joint and putting in a new one. A joint is where two or more bones come together, like the knee, hip, and shoulder. The surgery is usually done by a doctor called an orthopaedic surgeon. Sometimes, the surgeon will not remove the whole joint, but will only replace or fix the damaged parts.

The doctor may suggest a joint replacement to improve how you live. Replacing a joint can help you relieve pain and move and feel better. Joints that can be replaced include the shoulders, fingers, ankles, and elbows. Hips and knees are replaced most often.

What can happen to my joints?

Joints can be damaged by arthritis and other diseases, injuries, or other causes. Arthritis or simply years of use may cause the joint to wear away. This can cause pain, stiffness, and swelling. Bones are alive, and need blood to be healthy, grow, and repair. Diseases and damage inside a joint can limit blood flow, causing problems.

Excerpted from "Joint Replacement Surgery and You," National Institute of Arthritis and Musculoskeletal and Skin Diseases (NIAMS), NIH Publication No. 06–5149, October 2005.

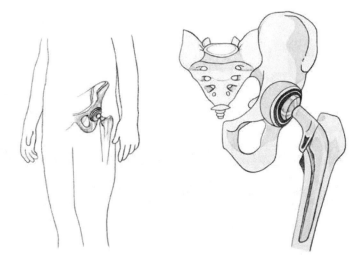

Figure 59.1. New Hip Joint

What is a new joint like?

A new joint, called a prosthesis, can be made of plastic, metal, or both. It may be cemented into place or not cemented, so that your bone will grow into it. Both methods may be combined to keep the new joint in place.

A cemented joint is used more often in older people who do not move around as much and in people with weak bones. The cement holds the new joint to the bone. An uncemented joint is often recommended for younger, more active people and those with good bone quality. It may take longer to heal, because it takes longer for bone to grow and attach to it. New joints generally last at least 10–15 years. Therefore, younger patients may need to have the same damaged joint replaced more than once.

Do many people have joints replaced?

Joint replacement is becoming more common. About 435,000 Americans have a hip or knee replaced each year. Research has shown that even if you are older, joint replacement can help you move around and feel better.

Any surgery has risks. Risks of joint surgery will depend on your health before surgery, how severe your arthritis is, and the type of surgery done. More hospitals and doctors have been replacing joints for several decades, and this experience results in better patient outcomes.

For answers to their questions, some people talk with their doctors, or someone who has had the surgery. A doctor specializing in joints will probably work with you before, during, and after surgery to make sure you heal quickly and recover successfully.

Do I need to have my joint replaced?

Only a doctor can tell if you need a joint replaced. He or she will look at your joint with an x-ray machine or other machines. The doctor may put a small, lighted tube (arthroscope) into your joint to look for damage. A small sample of your tissue could also be tested.

After looking at your joint, the doctor may say that you should consider exercise, walking aids like braces or canes, physical therapy, or medicines and supplements. Medicines for arthritis include drugs that reduce inflammation. Depending on the type of arthritis, the doctor may prescribe corticosteroids or other drugs. However, all drugs may cause side effects, including bone loss.

If these treatments do not work, the doctor may suggest an operation called an osteotomy, where the surgeon aligns the joint. Here, the surgeon cuts the bone or bones around the joint to improve alignment. This may be simpler than replacing a joint, but it may take longer to recover. However, it is not commonly done today.

Joint replacement is often the answer if you have constant pain and cannot move the joint well; for example, if you have trouble with things like walking, climbing stairs, and taking a bath.

What happens during surgery?

First, the surgical team will give you medicine so you will not feel pain (anesthesia). The medicine may block the pain only in one part of the body (regional), or it may put your whole body to sleep (general). The team will then replace the damaged joint with a prosthesis.

Each surgery is different. How long it takes depends on how badly the joint is damaged and how the surgery is done. To replace a knee or a hip takes about two hours or less, unless there are complicating factors. After surgery, you will be moved to a recovery room for 1–2 hours until you are fully awake or the numbness goes away.

What happens after surgery?

With knee or hip surgery, you may be able to go home in 3–5 days. If you are elderly or have additional handicaps, you may then need to spend several weeks in an intermediate care facility before going home. How long you stay in the hospital will be determined by you and your team of doctors.

After hip or knee replacement, you will often stand and begin walking sometimes even the day of surgery. At first, you will walk with a walker or crutches. You may have some temporary pain in the new joint because your muscles are weak from not being used. Also, your body is healing. The pain can be helped with medicines and should end in a few weeks or months.

Physical therapy can begin the day after surgery to help strengthen the muscles around the new joint and help you regain motion in the joint. If you have your shoulder joint replaced, you can usually begin exercising the same day of your surgery. A physical therapist will help you with gentle, range-of-motion exercises. Before you leave the hospital (usually two or three days after surgery), your therapist will show you how to use a pulley device to help bend and extend your arm.

Will the surgery be successful?

The success of your surgery depends a lot on what you do when you come home. Follow your doctor's advice about what you eat, what medicines to take, and how to exercise. Talk with your doctor about any pain or trouble moving.

Joint replacement is usually a success in more than 90 percent of people who have it. When problems do occur, most are treatable. Possible problems include the following:

- **Infection:** Areas in the wound or around the new joint may get infected. It may happen while in the hospital or after you go home. It may even occur years later. Minor infections in the wound are usually treated with drugs. Deep infections may need a second operation to treat the infection or replace the joint.

- **Blood clots:** If your blood moves too slowly, it may begin to form lumps of blood parts called clots. If pain and swelling develop in your legs after hip or knee surgery, blood clots may be the cause. The doctor may suggest drugs to make your blood thin, or special stockings, exercises, or boots to help your blood move faster. If swelling, redness, or pain occurs in your leg after you leave the hospital, contact your doctor right away.

- **Loosening:** The new joint may loosen, causing pain. If the loosening is bad, you may need another operation. New ways to attach the joint to the bone should help.

- **Dislocation:** Sometimes after hip or other joint replacement, the ball of the prosthesis can come out of its socket. In most cases, the hip can be corrected without surgery. A brace may be worn for a while if a dislocation occurs.

- **Wear:** Some wear can be found in all joint replacements. Too much wear may cause loosening. The doctor may need to operate again if the prosthesis comes loose. Sometimes, the plastic can wear thin, and the doctor may just replace the plastic and not the whole joint.

- **Nerve and blood vessel injury:** Nerves near the replaced joint may be damaged during surgery, but this does not happen often. Over time, the damage often improves and may disappear. Blood vessels may also be injured.

As you move your new joint and let your muscles grow strong again, pain will lessen, flexibility will increase, and movement will improve.

Chapter 60

Pain Control after Surgery

Pain control following surgery is a major priority for both you and your doctors. While you should expect to have some pain after your surgery, your doctor will make every effort to safely minimize your pain.

We provide the following information to help you understand your options for pain treatment, to describe how you can help your doctors and nurses control your pain, and to empower you to take an active role in making choices about pain treatment.

Be sure to inform your doctor if you are taking pain medication at home on a regular basis and if you are allergic to or cannot tolerate certain pain medications.

Why is pain control so important?

In addition to keeping you comfortable, pain control can help you recover faster and may reduce your risk of developing certain complications after surgery, such as pneumonia and blood clots. If your pain is well controlled, you will be better able to complete important tasks such as walking and deep breathing exercises.

"What You Need to Know about Pain Control After Surgery," © 2007 The Cleveland Clinic Foundation, 9500 Euclid Avenue, Cleveland, OH 44195, www.clevelandclinic.org. Additional information is available from the Cleveland Clinic Health Information Center, 216-444-3771, toll-free 800-223-2273 extension 43771, or at http://www.clevelandclinic.org/health. Reprinted with permission.

What kinds of pain will I feel after surgery?

You may be surprised at where you experience pain after surgery. Often times the incision is not the only area of discomfort. You may or may not feel the following:

- **Muscle pain:** You may feel muscle pain in the neck, shoulders, back, or chest from lying on the operating table.

- **Throat pain:** Your throat may feel sore or scratchy.

- **Movement pain:** Sitting up, walking, and coughing are all important activities after surgery, but they may cause increased pain at or around the incision site.

What can I do to help keep my pain under control?

Important: Your doctors and nurses want and need to know about pain that is not adequately controlled. If you are having pain, please tell someone. Don't worry about being a bother.

You can help the doctors and nurses "measure" your pain. While you are recovering, your doctors and nurses will frequently ask you to rate your pain on a scale of 0 to 10, with "0" being "no pain" and "10" being "the worst pain you can imagine." Reporting your pain as a number helps the doctors and nurses know how well your treatment is working and whether to make any changes. Keep in mind that your comfort level (for example, ability to breathe deeply or cough) is more important than absolute numbers (for example, a pain score).

Who is going to help manage my pain?

You and your surgeon will decide what type of pain control would be most acceptable for you after surgery. Your surgeon may choose to consult the Acute Pain Management Service to help manage your pain following surgery. Doctors on this service are specifically trained in the types of pain control options described on the next several pages.

You are the one who ultimately decides which pain control option is most acceptable. The manager of your post-surgical pain—your surgeon or the Acute Pain Management Service doctor—will review your medical and surgical history, check the results from your laboratory tests and physical exam, then advise you about which pain management option may be best suited to safely minimize your discomfort.

After surgery, you will be assessed frequently to ensure that you are comfortable and safe. When necessary, adjustments or changes to your pain management regimen will be made.

Types of Pain-Control Treatments

You may receive more than one type of pain treatment, depending on your needs and the type of surgery you are having. All of these treatments are relatively safe, but like any therapy, they are not completely free of risk. Dangerous side effects are rare. Nausea, vomiting, itching, and drowsiness can occur. These side effects are usually easily treated in most cases.

Intravenous Patient-Controlled Analgesia (PCA)

Patient-controlled analgesia (PCA) is a computerized pump that safely permits you to push a button and deliver small amounts of pain medicine into your intravenous (IV) line, usually in your arm. There is no injection of needles into your muscle. PCA provides stable pain relief in most situations. Many patients like the sense of control they have over their pain management.

The PCA pump is programmed to give a certain amount of medication when you press the button. It will only allow you to have so much medication, no matter how often you press the button, so there is little worry that you will give yourself too much.

One way that you may get too much medication from the PCA pump is if a family member presses the PCA button for you. This removes the patient control aspect of the therapy, which is a major safety feature. Do not allow family members or friends to push your PCA pump button for you. You need to be awake enough to know that you need pain medication.

Patient-Controlled Epidural Analgesia

Many people are familiar with epidural anesthesia because it is frequently used to control pain during childbirth. Patient-controlled epidural analgesia uses a PCA pump to deliver pain-control medicine into an epidural catheter (a very thin plastic tube) that is placed into your back.

Placing the epidural catheter (to which the PCA pump is attached) usually causes no more discomfort than having an IV started. A sedating medication, given through your IV, will help you relax. The skin of your back will be cleaned with a sterile solution and numbed with a local anesthetic. Next, a thin needle will be carefully inserted into an area called the epidural space. A thin catheter will be inserted through this needle into the epidural space, and the needle will then be removed. During and after your surgery, pain medications will be

443

infused through this epidural catheter with the goal of providing you with excellent pain control when you awaken. If additional pain medication is required, you can press the PCA button.

Epidural analgesia is usually more effective in relieving pain than intravenous medication. Patients who receive epidural analgesia typically have less pain when they take deep breaths, cough, and walk, and they may recover more quickly. For patients with medical problems such as heart or lung disease, epidural analgesia may reduce the risk of serious complications such as heart attack and pneumonia.

Epidural analgesia is safe, but like any procedure or therapy, not risk free. Sometimes the epidural does not adequately control pain. In this situation, you will be given alternative treatments or be offered replacement of the epidural. Nausea, vomiting, itching, and drowsiness can occur. Occasionally, numbness and weakness of the legs can occur, which disappears after the medication is reduced or stopped. Headache can occur, but this is rare. Severe complications such as nerve damage and infection are extremely rare.

Nerve Blocks

You may be offered a nerve block to control your pain after surgery. Whereas an epidural controls pain over a broad area of your body, a nerve block is used when pain from surgery affects a smaller region of your body, such as an arm or leg. Sometimes a catheter similar to an epidural catheter is placed for prolonged pain control. There are several potential advantages of a nerve block. It may allow for a significant reduction in the amount of opioid (narcotic) medication, which may result in fewer side effects such as nausea, vomiting, itching, and drowsiness.

In some cases, a nerve block can be used as the main anesthetic for your surgery. In this case, you will be given medications during your surgery to keep you sleepy, relaxed, and comfortable. This type of anesthesia provides the added benefit of pain relief both during and after your surgery. It may reduce your risk of nausea and vomiting after surgery. You, your anesthesiologist, and your surgeon will decide before surgery if a nerve block is a suitable pain management or anesthetic option for you.

Pain Medications Taken by Mouth

At some point during your recovery from surgery, your doctor will order pain medications to be taken by mouth (oral pain medications). These may be ordered to come at a specified time, or you may need to ask your nurse to bring them to you. Make sure you know whether or not you need to ask for the medication. Most oral pain medications can be taken every four hours.

Important: Do not wait until your pain is severe before you ask for pain medications. Also, if the pain medication has not significantly helped within 30 minutes, notify your nurse. Extra pain medication is available for you to take. You do not have to wait four hours to receive more medication.

What Are Some of the Risks and Benefits Associated with Pain Medication?

Opioids (Narcotics) after Surgery: Medications such as Morphine, Fentanyl, Hydromorphone

Benefits: Strong pain relievers. Many options are available if one is causing significant side effects.

Risks: May cause nausea, vomiting, itching, drowsiness, and constipation. The risk of becoming addicted is extremely rare.

Opioids (Narcotics) at Home: Percocet®, Vicodin®, Darvocet®, Tylenol #3®

Benefits: Effective for moderate to severe pain. Many options are available.

Risks: Nausea, vomiting, itching, drowsiness, constipation. Stomach upset can be lessened if the drug is taken with food. Should not drive or operate machinery while taking these medications. Note: These medications often contain acetaminophen (Tylenol®). Make sure that other medications that you are taking do not contain acetaminophen, as too much of it may damage your liver.

Be sure to tell your doctor about all medications (prescribed and over-the-counter), vitamins, and herbal supplements you are taking. This may affect which drugs are prescribed for your pain control.

Non-Opioid (Non-Narcotic) Analgesics: Tylenol®, FeverAll®

Benefits: Effective for mild to moderate pain. They have very few side effects and are safe for most patients. They often decrease the requirement for stronger medications, which may reduce the incidence of side effects.

Risks: Liver damage may result if more than the recommended daily dose is used. Patients with pre-existing liver disease or those who drink significant quantities of alcohol may be at increased risk.

Nonsteroidal Anti-inflammatory Drugs (NSAIDs): Ibuprofen (Advil®), Naproxen Sodium (Aleve®), Celecoxib (Celebrex®)

Benefits: These drugs reduce swelling and inflammation and relieve mild to moderate pain. Ibuprofen and naproxen sodium are available without a prescription, but you should ask your doctor about taking them. They may reduce the amount of opioid analgesic you need, possibly reducing side effects such as nausea, vomiting, and drowsiness. If taken alone, there are no restrictions on driving or operating machinery.

Risks: The most common side effects of nonsteroidal anti-inflammatory medication (NSAIDs) are stomach upset and dizziness. You should not take these drugs without your doctor's approval if you have kidney problems, a history of stomach ulcers, heart failure or are on blood thinner medications such as Coumadin® (warfarin), Lovenox® injections, or Plavix®.

Are there ways I can relieve pain without medication?

Yes, there are other ways to relieve pain, and it is important to keep an open mind about these techniques. When used along with medication, these techniques can dramatically reduce pain.

Relaxation tapes, or guided imagery, is a proven form of focused relaxation that coaches you in creating calm, peaceful images in your mind—a mental escape. For the best results, practice using the tape or compact disk (CD) before your surgery and then use it twice daily during your recovery. You can get relaxation tapes at a bookstore, or rent them from your library. Finally, you can bring a battery-operated tape recorder or CD player to the hospital to play prior to surgery and during your hospital stay.

Listening to soft music or changing your position in bed are additional methods to relieve or lessen pain.

At home, heat or cold therapy may be an option that your surgeon may choose to help reduce swelling and control your pain. Specific instructions for the use of these therapies will be discussed with you by your surgical team.

If you have an abdominal or chest incision, you will want to splint the area with a pillow when you are coughing or deep breathing to decrease motion near your incision. You will be given a pillow in the hospital. Continue to use it at home as well.

Lastly, make sure you are comfortable with your treatment plan. Talk to your doctor and nurses about your concerns and needs. This will help avoid miscommunication, stress, anxiety, and disappointment, which may make pain worse. Keep asking questions until you have satisfactory answers. You are the one who will benefit.

How can I control pain at home?

You may be given prescriptions for pain medication to take at home. These may or may not be the same pain medications you took in the hospital. Talk with your doctor about which pain medications will be prescribed at discharge.

Note: Make sure your doctor knows about pain medications that have caused you problems in the past. This will prevent possible delays in your discharge from the hospital.

Preparation for Your Discharge

Your doctors may have already given you your prescription for pain medication prior to your surgery date. If this is the case, it is best to be prepared and have your medication filled and ready for you when you come home from the hospital. You may want to have your pain pills with you on your ride home if traveling a long distance. Check with your insurance company regarding your prescription plan and coverage for your medication. Occasionally, a pain medication prescribed by your doctor is not covered by your insurance company.

If you haven't received your prescription for pain medication until after the surgery, make sure a family member takes your prescription and either gets it filled at the hospital pharmacy or soon after your discharge from the hospital. It is important that you are prepared in case you have pain.

Make sure you wear comfortable clothes and keep your coughing and deep breathing pillow with you.

You may want to have your relaxation tapes and player available for your travels.

If you are traveling by plane, make sure you have your pain pills in your carry-on luggage in case the airline misplaces your checked luggage.

While at Home

Remember to take your pain medication before activity and at bedtime. Your doctor may advise you to take your pain medication at regular intervals (such as every four to six hours).

Be sure to get enough rest. If you are having trouble sleeping, talk to your doctor.

Use pillows to support you when you sleep and when you do your coughing and deep breathing exercises.

Try using the alternative methods discussed earlier. Heating pads or cold therapy, guided imagery tapes, listening to soft music, changing your position in bed, and massage can help relieve your pain.

Note: If you need to have stitches or staples removed and you are still taking pain medications, be sure to have a friend or family member drive you to your clinic appointment. Commonly, you should not drive or operate equipment if you are taking opioid (narcotic)-containing pain medications. Check the label of your prescription for any warnings or ask your doctor, nurse, or pharmacist.

Frequently Asked Questions

I am nervous about getting hooked on pain pills. How do I avoid this?

The risk of becoming addicted to pain medication after surgery is very small. The bigger risk is a possible prolonged recovery if you avoid your pain medications, and cannot effectively do your required activities. If you are concerned about addiction, or have a history of substance abuse (alcohol or any drug), talk with your doctors. They will monitor you closely during your recovery. If issues arise following surgery, they will consult the appropriate specialists.

I am a small person who is easily affected by medicine. I am nervous that a normal dose of pain medication will be too much for me. What should I do?

During recovery, your health care team will observe how you respond to pain medication and make changes as needed. Be sure to communicate with your doctors any concerns you have prior to surgery. The relatively small doses of pain medication given after surgery are highly unlikely to have an exaggerated effect based on your body size.

I don't have a high tolerance for pain. I am afraid that the pain will be too much for me to handle. What can I do?

Concern about pain from surgery is very normal. The most important thing you can do is to talk with your surgeon and anesthesiologist about your particular situation. Setting pain control goals with your doctors before surgery will help them better tailor your pain treatment plan. Treating pain early is easier than treating it after it has set in. If you have had prior experiences with surgery and pain control, let your doctor know what worked or what did not. As listed earlier in this document, there are usually many options available to you for pain control after surgery.

I normally take Tylenol® if I get a headache. Can I still take Tylenol® for a headache if I am on other pain medication?

As discussed earlier, before taking any other medication, be sure to talk to your doctor. Some of the medications prescribed for use at home contain acetaminophen (Tylenol®) and if too much is taken, you may become ill. In order to avoid getting too much of any medication, discuss this issue with your doctor before you leave the hospital.

Play an Active Role in Your Pain Control

Ask your doctors and nurses about:

- Pain and pain control treatments and what you can expect from them. You have a right to the best level of pain relief that can be safely provided.
- Your schedule for pain medicines in the hospital.
- How you can participate in a pain-control plan.

Inform your doctors and nurses about:

- Any surgical pain you have had in the past.
- How you relieved your pain before you came to the hospital.
- Pain you have had recently or currently.

- Pain medications you have taken in the past and cannot tolerate.

- Pain medications you have been taking prior to surgery.

- Any pain that is not controlled with your current pain medications.

You should:

- Help the doctors and nurses measure your pain and expect staff to ask about pain relief often and to respond quickly when you do report pain.

- Ask for pain medicines as soon as pain begins.

- Tell us how well your pain is relieved and your pain relief expectations.

- Use other comfort measures for pain control—listening to relaxation tapes or soft music, repositioning in bed.

Your doctors are committed to providing you with the safest and most effective pain management strategy that is most acceptable to you.

Pain Facts

- Pain is different for everyone.

- Treating pain early usually brings quicker and better results.

- Healing occurs faster when pain is under control.

- Pain affects blood pressure, heart rate, appetite, and general mood.

- Pain may be sharp, dull, stabbing, cramping, throbbing, constant, on and off, and so forth.

Chapter 61

Psychosocial Interventions Can Alleviate Pain

Psychosocial Interventions

Pain is complex and unique to each individual. As with other aspects of life, each of us brings pre-existing thoughts, feelings, beliefs, expectations, and behavior patterns to any health experience. Understanding the impact of pain requires that we expand our view to consider the whole person—the mind, body, and spirit.

Research shows that pain can affect your emotions and behavior and interfere with your ability to concentrate, manage everyday tasks, and cope with stress. Likewise, stress and emotional pressures can make pain worse, provoking flare ups and contributing to alterations in the immune system response. These relationships are not always easily recognized or readily fixed by medical procedures or medications alone.

As the science of pain moves forward, there is growing evidence that interventions (drug and non-drug) used to influence emotions, thinking, and behavior can aid in the reduction of pain and associated distress. For example, studies are uncovering a biological link between the brain systems involved in depression and pain regulation. Some antidepressant medications may have analgesic properties, which may be because these systems have shared properties.

Some people experience depression due to chronic pain. Others may begin to realize that depression was present before their pain began. Depression can make the experience of living with persistent pain more difficult and should be diagnosed and treated.

Others may falsely believe that referral for psychological pain treatment means that their pain is not physical, or feel they are being labeled as having a mental illness rather than a physical problem. You may feel hesitant to try psychosocial therapies due to the associated stigma, or the fear that your provider will no longer treat the physical symptoms of your pain or try new treatment options. Don't let these fears interfere with your willingness to try a broad class of potentially safe and effective treatments. Consider these a gift to yourself—an investment in your peace of mind and quality of life.

Psychological Consultation and Counseling

Consultation

Many people believe knowledge is power. In fact, you may be reading this book to increase your pain knowledge and put it to good use. While reading, ask yourself:

1. How does your pain affect the way you think and act?

2. How does your pain affect your loved ones and co-workers?

3. How do they react to you?

4. Does this help or hinder your recovery and healing?

5. Are there ongoing stressors in your life?

For example, you may find that previous relationship patterns are no longer working for you. Stress and emotions, such as fear and anger, increase pain, which can then heighten stress levels. These kinds of cycles are important to recognize and modify. This action may decrease your pain and, at the same time, boost your sense of control over your life. Change is difficult. Working with a skilled therapist who understands chronic pain may help you recognize the unhealthy stressors in your life and guide you through making necessary life changes.

Your health care providers may recommend that you consult a behavioral health professional. This could be a social worker, psychologist, or psychiatrist, or a therapist with special training in chronic pain. No, they do not think that you are crazy or that your pain is only in your head. This evaluation may include testing and interviews to help assess how you cope with pain. It is important to:

- Identify how your pain interferes with your daily life and relationships

- Understand the stressors that worsen your pain and distress

- Determine which coping skills are helpful and which are harmful

When people have had pain for a long time, they develop ways to deal with pain, which are called coping strategies. Some of these strategies may help, while other may not. As a result, you may need to learn new ways to cope. There are a range of strategies that can help in this process. The following therapies may be recommended:

- Relaxation therapy (relaxation, mindfulness, imagery)

- Biofeedback training

- Behavioral modification

- Stress management training

- Hypnotherapy

- Counseling (individual, family, or group)

Cognitive Techniques

Some techniques used in stress management include relaxation training, meditation, hypnosis, biofeedback, and behavior modification. Common to these approaches is the belief that people have the ability to self-manage some aspects of pain, such as changing attitudes, thoughts, feelings, or behaviors.

Relaxation therapies teach people how to relax tense muscles, reduce anxiety, and alter their mental state. Both physical and mental tension can make pain worse. Headaches or back pain, muscle tension or spasms can be part of the problem. Meditation, which aims to produce a state of conscious relaxation, is sometimes combined with therapies that assist you in thinking of pain as a distant part of you. This skill of detachment helps to regain a sense of control. This approach may be particularly helpful when fear or anxiety accompanies pain.

Mindfulness meditation is a concentration practice during which people focus their attention on a specific object, most commonly on breathing patterns. For example, the focus might be on the experience of the breath entering the nostrils when inhaling and again when exhaling. When our minds wander off the breath (which is natural to do), we acknowledge that it has wandered and bring it back to the breath. Conscious awareness can bring about a sense of calm, patience, reduced muscle tension and pain, and a clear sense of reality. When beginning this practice, you may experience anxiety or increased pain. This is because you may not have spent time being quiet with yourself. It is best to start a meditation practice with the help of a meditation teacher who can give you suggestions on how to proceed when these feelings arise.

Once mastered, meditation can be used in many situations, such as reducing the intensity of pain during flare ups, decreasing anxiety while sitting in the dentist chair, and reducing the urge to scream during a traffic jam.

Guided imagery is a conscious meditation technique. Advocates of imagery believe our imagination is a potent healer which has been overlooked by practitioners of Western medicine. Imagery may help relieve pain, promote healing from injury or illness, and ease depression, anxiety, and sleeplessness. Thoughts have a direct influence on feelings and behavior. Negative thoughts may promote sadness and hopelessness, while positive thoughts breed pleasure and drive.

Imagery has been found to be very effective for the treatment of stress. Imagery relaxes the body by aiding the release of brain chemicals that serve as the body's natural tranquilizers. These chemicals lower blood pressure, heart rate, and anxiety levels. Practitioners who specialize in imagery may recommend it for a variety of different conditions such as headaches, chronic pain in the neck and back, high blood pressure, spastic colon, and cramping due to premenstrual syndrome. Several studies suggest that imagery can also boost the immune system and, therefore, promote healing.

Most guided imagery techniques begin with relaxation followed by the visualization of a mental image. For example, imagine a color for pain and then gradually replace that color with one that is more pleasing. Another is visualizing a peaceful scene, such as the ocean surf, wooded forest, fishing at a quiet pond, or watching the sunset. Practicing guided imagery with music or aromatherapy may enhance the overall experience. This eventually may stimulate the ability to relax and create a mental image when those favorite sounds or scents are present.

Biofeedback training teaches people how to recognize their physical reaction to stress and tension by using a variety of monitoring procedures and equipment. Physical responses that might be monitored include brain activity, blood pressure, muscle tension, and heart rate. These involuntary responses generally increase with stress (known as the stress response), which can accompany pain. By measuring these physical reactions, you can learn relaxation and breathing techniques to help return these responses to normal levels of activity. Often, when the stress response is lowered, so is the intensity of pain.

Behavioral modification (sometimes called operant conditioning) is aimed at changing habits, behaviors, and attitudes that can develop from living with chronic pain. Some people are overwhelmed by pain and may become dependent, anxious, homebound, or perhaps even bedridden. Living with pain is influenced and sometimes complicated by social, family, legal, insurance, and political factors. For example, some people are told they will lose financial benefits or other types of critical support if they improve. Those involved in lengthy lawsuits may hesitate to get better or gain function due to the fear that they will lose any chance of financial compensation, which they believe they deserve. In some instances, pain has spurred an unhappy employee to leave a job in which they never felt valued. At times, having pain becomes a way of saying no to situations or people we have never been able to refuse. In some families, pain becomes a way to express anger, get care, or be excused from responsibilities. These situations are damaging far beyond what is happening in your body. It is very important to understand how pain fits into the larger context of your life so you can identify ways to diminish harmful influences.

When appropriate, vocational counseling and rehabilitation can help to create a gradual path to more productive, fulfilling employment so that worries about the loss of compensation are replaced with possibilities. Behavioral modification can help people separate the multitude of issues surrounding pain and devise a step-by-step approach to confronting challenges through behavior change and shifting attitudes.

Chapter 62

Complementary Therapy for Pain Relief

Chapter Contents

457

Section 62.1

Complementary Therapy Overview

Excerpted from "What Is CAM?" National Center for Complementary and Alternative Medicine (NCCAM), NCCAM Publication No. D347, updated February 2007.

There are many terms used to describe approaches to health care that are outside the realm of conventional medicine as practiced in the United States. This section explains how the National Center for Complementary and Alternative Medicine (NCCAM), a component of the National Institutes of Health, defines some of the key terms used in the field of complementary and alternative medicine (CAM).

What is CAM?

CAM is a group of diverse medical and health care systems, practices, and products that are not presently considered to be part of conventional medicine. Conventional medicine is medicine as practiced by holders of M.D. (medical doctor) or D.O. (doctor of osteopathy) degrees and by their allied health professionals, such as physical therapists, psychologists, and registered nurses. Some health care providers practice both CAM and conventional medicine. While some scientific evidence exists regarding some CAM therapies, for most there are key questions that are yet to be answered through well-designed scientific studies—questions such as whether these therapies are safe and whether they work for the diseases or medical conditions for which they are used.

The list of what is considered to be CAM changes continually, as those therapies that are proven to be safe and effective become adopted into conventional health care and as new approaches to health care emerge.

Are complementary medicine and alternative medicine different from each other?

Yes, they are different.

- **Complementary medicine is used together with conventional medicine.** An example of a complementary therapy is using aromatherapy to help lessen a patient's discomfort following surgery.

- **Alternative medicine is used in place of conventional medicine.** An example of an alternative therapy is using a special diet to treat cancer instead of undergoing surgery, radiation, or chemotherapy that has been recommended by a conventional doctor.

What is integrative medicine?

Integrative medicine combines treatments from conventional medicine and CAM for which there is some high-quality evidence of safety and effectiveness. It is also called integrated medicine.

Major Types of Complementary and Alternative Medicine

NCCAM groups CAM practices into four domains, recognizing there can be some overlap. In addition, NCCAM studies CAM whole medical systems which cut across all domains.

Whole Medical Systems

Whole medical systems are built upon complete systems of theory and practice. Often, these systems have evolved apart from and earlier than the conventional medical approach used in the United States. Examples of whole medical systems that have developed in Western cultures include homeopathic medicine and naturopathic medicine. Examples of systems that have developed in non-Western cultures include traditional Chinese medicine and Ayurveda.

Mind-Body Medicine

Mind-body medicine uses a variety of techniques designed to enhance the mind's capacity to affect bodily function and symptoms. Some techniques that were considered CAM in the past have become mainstreamed (for example, patient support groups and cognitive-behavioral therapy). Other mind-body techniques are still considered CAM, including meditation, prayer, mental healing, and therapies that use creative outlets such as art, music, or dance.

Biologically-Based Practices

Biologically-based practices in CAM use substances found in nature, such as herbs, foods, and vitamins. Some examples include dietary supplements, herbal products, and the use of other so-called natural, but as yet scientifically unproven, therapies (for example, using shark cartilage to treat cancer).

Manipulative and Body-Based Practices

Manipulative and body-based practices in CAM are based on manipulation and/or movement of one or more parts of the body. Some examples include chiropractic or osteopathic manipulation and massage.

Energy Medicine

Energy therapies involve the use of energy fields. They are of two types:

Biofield therapies are intended to affect energy fields that purportedly surround and penetrate the human body. The existence of such fields has not yet been scientifically proven. Some forms of energy therapy manipulate the biofield by applying pressure and/or manipulating the body by placing the hands in, or through, these fields. Examples include qi gong, Reiki, and Therapeutic Touch.

Bio-electromagnetic-based therapies involve the unconventional use of electromagnetic fields, such as pulsed fields, magnetic fields, or alternating-current or direct-current fields.

Section 62.2

Acupuncture

Excerpted from "Acupuncture," National Center for Complementary and Alternative Medicine (NCCAM), NCCAM Publication Number D404, December 2007.

The term acupuncture describes a family of procedures involving the stimulation of anatomical points on the body using a variety of techniques. The acupuncture technique that has been most often studied scientifically involves penetrating the skin with thin, solid, metallic needles that are manipulated by the hands or by electrical stimulation.

Practiced in China and other Asian countries for thousands of years, acupuncture is one of the key components of traditional Chinese medicine (TCM). In TCM, the body is seen as a delicate balance of two opposing and inseparable forces: yin represents the cold, slow, or passive principle, while yang represents the hot, excited, or active principle. According to TCM, health is achieved by maintaining the body in a balanced state; disease is due to an internal imbalance of yin and yang. This imbalance leads to blockage in the flow of qi (vital energy) along pathways known as meridians. Qi can be unblocked, according to TCM, by using acupuncture at certain points on the body that connect with these meridians. Sources vary on the number of meridians, with numbers ranging from 14 to 20. One commonly cited source describes meridians as 14 main channels "connecting the body in a weblike interconnecting matrix" of at least 2,000 acupuncture points.

Acupuncture became better known in the United States in 1971, when *New York Times* reporter James Reston wrote about how doctors in China used needles to ease his pain after surgery. American practices of acupuncture incorporate medical traditions from China, Japan, Korea, and other countries.

Acupuncture Use in the United States

The report from a Consensus Development Conference on Acupuncture held at the National Institutes of Health (NIH) in 1997 stated that

461

acupuncture is being widely practiced—by thousands of physicians, dentists, acupuncturists, and other practitioners—for relief or prevention of pain and for various other health conditions. According to the *2002 National Health Interview Survey*—the largest and most comprehensive survey of CAM use by American adults to date—an estimated 8.2 million U.S. adults had ever used acupuncture, and an estimated 2.1 million U.S. adults had used acupuncture in the previous year.

Acupuncture Side Effects and Risks

The U.S. Food and Drug Administration (FDA) regulates acupuncture needles for use by licensed practitioners, requiring that needles be manufactured and labeled according to certain standards. For example, the FDA requires that needles be sterile, nontoxic, and labeled for single use by qualified practitioners only.

Relatively few complications from the use of acupuncture have been reported to the FDA, in light of the millions of people treated each year and the number of acupuncture needles used. Still, complications have resulted from inadequate sterilization of needles and from improper delivery of treatments. Practitioners should use a new set of disposable needles taken from a sealed package for each patient and should swab treatment sites with alcohol or another disinfectant before inserting needles. When not delivered properly, acupuncture can cause serious adverse effects, including infections and punctured organs.

Status of Acupuncture Research

There have been many studies on acupuncture's potential health benefits for a wide range of conditions. Summarizing earlier research, the 1997 NIH Consensus Statement on Acupuncture found that, overall, results were hard to interpret because of problems with the size and design of the studies.

In the years since the Consensus Statement was issued, the National Center for Complementary and Alternative Medicine (NCCAM) has funded extensive research to advance scientific understanding of acupuncture. Some recent NCCAM-supported studies have looked at the following:

- Whether acupuncture works for specific health conditions such as chronic low-back pain, headache, and osteoarthritis of the knee

- How acupuncture might work, such as what happens in the brain during acupuncture treatment

- Ways to better identify and understand the potential neurological properties of meridians and acupuncture points

- Methods and instruments for improving the quality of acupuncture research

Finding a Qualified Practitioner

Health care providers can be a resource for referral to acupuncturists, and some conventional medical practitioners—including physicians and dentists—practice acupuncture. In addition, national acupuncture organizations (which can be found through libraries or online search engines) may provide referrals to acupuncturists.

- Check a practitioner's credentials. Most states require a license to practice acupuncture; however, education and training standards and requirements for obtaining a license to practice vary from state to state. Although a license does not ensure quality of care, it does indicate that the practitioner meets certain standards regarding the knowledge and use of acupuncture.

- Do not rely on a diagnosis of disease by an acupuncture practitioner who does not have substantial conventional medical training. If you have received a diagnosis from a doctor, you may wish to ask your doctor whether acupuncture might help.

What to Expect from Acupuncture Visits

During your first office visit, the practitioner may ask you at length about your health condition, lifestyle, and behavior. The practitioner will want to obtain a complete picture of your treatment needs and behaviors that may contribute to your condition. Inform the acupuncturist about all treatments or medications you are taking and all medical conditions you have.

Acupuncture needles are metallic, solid, and hair-thin. People experience acupuncture differently, but most feel no, or minimal, pain as the needles are inserted. Some people feel energized by treatment, while others feel relaxed. Improper needle placement, movement of the patient, or a defect in the needle can cause soreness and pain during treatment. This is why it is important to seek treatment from a qualified acupuncture practitioner.

Treatment may take place over a period of several weeks or more.

Treatment Costs

Ask the practitioner about the estimated number of treatments needed and how much each treatment will cost. Some insurance companies may cover the costs of acupuncture. It is important to check with your insurer before you start treatment to see whether acupuncture is covered for your condition and, if so, to what extent.

References

1. Acupuncture. Natural Standard Database website. Accessed at http://www.naturalstandard.com on June 28, 2007.

2. Barnes PM, Powell-Griner E, McFann K, Nahin RL. Complementary and alternative medicine use among adults: United States, 2002. *CDC Advance Data Report #343*. 2004.

3. Berman BM, Lao L, Langenberg P, et al. Effectiveness of acupuncture as adjunctive therapy in osteoarthritis of the knee: a randomized, controlled trial. *Annals of Internal Medicine*. 2004;141(12):901–910.

4. Eisenberg DM, Cohen MH, Hrbek A, et al. Credentialing complementary and alternative medical providers. *Annals of Internal Medicine*. 2002;137(12):965–973.

5. Ernst E. Acupuncture—a critical analysis. *Journal of Internal Medicine*. 2006;259(2):125–137.

6. Kaptchuk, TJ. Acupuncture: theory, efficacy, and practice. *Annals of Internal Medicine*. 2002;136(5):374–383.

7. Lao L. Safety issues in acupuncture. *Journal of Alternative and Complementary Medicine*. 1996;2(1):27–31.

8. MacPherson H, Thomas K. Short-term reactions to acupuncture—a cross-sectional survey of patient reports. *Acupuncture in Medicine*. 2005;23(3):112–120.

9. National Cancer Institute. *Acupuncture (PDQ)*. National Cancer Institute website. Accessed at http://www.cancer.gov/cancertopics/pdq/cam/acupuncture on August 16, 2007.

10. National Institutes of Health Consensus Panel. *Acupuncture: National Institutes of Health Consensus Development Conference Statement*. National Institutes of Health website. Accessed at http://consensus.nih.gov/1997/1997acupuncture107html.htm on June 22, 2007.

11. Reston J. Now, about my operation in Peking; Now, let me tell you about my appendectomy in Peking.... *New York Times.* July 26, 1971:1.

12. U.S. Food and Drug Administration. Acupuncture needles no longer investigational. *FDA Consumer.* 1996;30(5). Also available at http://www.fda.gov/fdac/departs/596_upd.html.

Section 62.3

Mind-Body Medicine

National Center for Complementary and Alternative Medicine (NCCAM), NCCAM Publication No. D239, updated May 2007.

Mind-body medicine focuses on the interactions among the brain, mind, body, and behavior, and on the powerful ways in which emotional, mental, social, spiritual, and behavioral factors can directly affect health. It regards as fundamental an approach that respects and enhances each person's capacity for self-knowledge and self-care, and it emphasizes techniques that are grounded in this approach.

Mind-body medicine typically focuses on intervention strategies that are thought to promote health, such as relaxation, hypnosis, visual imagery, yoga, biofeedback, tai chi, qi, cognitive-behavioral therapies, group support, autogenic training, and spirituality. Certain mind-body intervention strategies listed here, such as group support for cancer survivors, are well integrated into conventional care and, while still considered mind-body interventions, are not considered to be complementary and alternative medicine.

The field views illness as an opportunity for personal growth and transformation and health care providers as catalysts and guides in this process.

Mind-body interventions constitute a major portion of the overall use of CAM by the public. In 2002, mind-body techniques, including relaxation techniques, meditation, guided imagery, biofeedback, and

465

hypnosis, were used by about 17 percent of the adult U.S. population. Prayer was used by 45 percent of the population for health reasons.[1]

Background

The concept that the mind is important in the treatment of illness is integral to the healing approaches of traditional Chinese and Ayurvedic medicine dating back more than 2,000 years. It was also noted by Hippocrates, who recognized the moral and spiritual aspects of healing, and believed that treatment could occur only with consideration of attitude, environmental influences, and natural remedies (circa 400 B.C.). While this integrated approach was maintained in traditional healing systems in the East, developments in the Western world by the 16th and 17th centuries led to a separation of human spiritual or emotional dimensions from the physical body. This separation began with the redirection of science, during the Renaissance and Enlightenment eras, to the purpose of enhancing humankind's control over nature. Technological advances (for example, microscopy, the stethoscope, the blood pressure cuff, and refined surgical techniques) demonstrated a cellular world that seemed far apart from the world of belief and emotion. The discovery of bacteria and, later, antibiotics further dispelled the notion of belief influencing health. Fixing or curing an illness became a matter of science and took precedence over, not a place beside, healing of the soul. As medicine separated the mind and the body, scientists of the mind (neurologists) formulated concepts, such as the unconscious, emotional impulses, and cognitive delusions, that solidified the perception that diseases of the mind were not real, that is, not based in physiology and biochemistry.

In the 1920s, Walter Cannon's work revealed the direct relationship between stress and neuroendocrine responses in animals.[2] Coining the phrase, fight or flight, Cannon described the primitive reflexes of sympathetic and adrenal activation in response to perceived danger and other environmental pressures (for example, cold and heat). Hans Selye further defined the deleterious effects of stress and distress on health.[3] At the same time, technological advances in medicine that could identify specific pathological changes, and new discoveries in pharmaceuticals, were occurring at a very rapid pace. The disease-based model, the search for a specific pathology, and the identification of external cures were paramount, even in psychiatry.

During World War II, the importance of belief reentered the web of health care. On the beaches of Anzio, morphine for the wounded soldiers was in short supply, and Henry Beecher, M.D., discovered that much of the pain could be controlled by saline injections. He coined the term placebo effect, and his subsequent research showed that up to 35 percent of a therapeutic response to any medical treatment could be the result of belief.[4] Investigation into the placebo effect and debate about it are ongoing.

Since the 1960s, mind-body interactions have become an extensively researched field. The evidence for benefits for certain indications from biofeedback, cognitive-behavioral interventions, and hypnosis is quite good, while there is emerging evidence regarding their physiological effects. Less research supports the use of CAM approaches like meditation and yoga. The following is a summary of relevant studies.

Mind-Body Interventions and Disease Outcomes

Over the past 20 years, mind-body medicine has provided considerable evidence that psychological factors can play a substantive role in the development and progression of coronary artery disease. There is evidence that mind-body interventions can be effective in the treatment of coronary artery disease, enhancing the effect of standard cardiac rehabilitation in reducing all-cause mortality and cardiac event recurrences for up to two years.[5]

Mind-body interventions have also been applied to various types of pain. Clinical trials indicate that these interventions may be a particularly effective adjunct in the management of arthritis, with reductions in pain maintained for up to four years and reductions in the number of physician visits.[6] When applied to more general acute and chronic pain management, headache, and low-back pain, mind-body interventions show some evidence of effects, although results vary based on the patient population and type of intervention studied.[7]

Evidence from multiple studies with various types of cancer patients suggests that mind-body interventions can improve mood, quality of life, and coping, as well as ameliorate disease—and treatment-related symptoms, such as chemotherapy-induced nausea, vomiting, and pain.[8] Some studies have suggested that mind-body interventions can alter various immune parameters, but it is unclear whether these alterations are of sufficient magnitude to have an impact on disease progression or prognosis.[9, 10]

Mind-Body Influences on Immunity

There is considerable evidence that emotional traits, both negative and positive, influence people's susceptibility to infection. Following systematic exposure to a respiratory virus in the laboratory, individuals who report higher levels of stress or negative moods have been shown to develop more severe illness than those who report less stress or more positive moods.[11] Recent studies suggest that the tendency to report positive, as opposed to negative, emotions may be associated with greater resistance to objectively verified colds. These laboratory studies are supported by longitudinal studies pointing to associations between psychological or emotional traits and the incidence of respiratory infections.[12]

Meditation and Imaging

Meditation, one of the most common mind-body interventions, is a conscious mental process that induces a set of integrated physiological changes termed the relaxation response. Functional magnetic resonance imaging (fMRI) has been used to identify and characterize the brain regions that are active during meditation. This research suggests that various parts of the brain known to be involved in attention and in the control of the autonomic nervous system are activated, providing a neurochemical and anatomical basis for the effects of meditation on various physiological activities.[13] Studies involving imaging are advancing the understanding of mind-body mechanisms. For example, meditation has been shown in one study to produce significant increases in left-sided anterior brain activity which is associated with positive emotional states. Moreover, in this same study, meditation was associated with increases in antibody titers to influenza vaccine, suggesting potential linkages among meditation, positive emotional states, localized brain responses, and improved immune function.[14]

Physiology of Expectancy (Placebo Response)

Placebo effects are believed to be mediated by both cognitive and conditioning mechanisms. Until recently, little was known about the role of these mechanisms in different circumstances. Now, research has shown that placebo responses are mediated by conditioning when unconscious physiological functions such as hormonal secretion are involved, whereas they are mediated by expectation when conscious physiological processes such as pain and motor performance come into play, even though a conditioning procedure is carried out.

Positron emission tomography (PET) scanning of the brain is providing evidence of the release of the endogenous neurotransmitter dopamine in the brain of Parkinson disease patients in response to placebo.[15] Evidence indicates that the placebo effect in these patients is powerful and is mediated through activation of the nigrostriatal dopamine system, the system that is damaged in Parkinson disease. This result suggests that the placebo response involves the secretion of dopamine, which is known to be important in a number of other reinforcing and rewarding conditions, and that there may be mind-body strategies that could be used in patients with Parkinson disease in lieu of, or in addition to, treatment with dopamine-releasing drugs.

Stress and Wound Healing

Individual differences in wound healing have long been recognized. Clinical observation has suggested that negative mood or stress is associated with slow wound healing. Basic mind-body research is now confirming this observation. Matrix metalloproteinases (MMP) and the tissue inhibitors of metalloproteinases (TIMP), whose expression can be controlled by cytokines, play a role in wound healing.[16] Using a blister chamber wound model on human forearm skin exposed to ultraviolet light, researchers have demonstrated that stress or a change in mood is sufficient to modulate MMP and TIMP expression and, presumably, wound healing.[17] Activation of the hypothalamic-pituitary-adrenal (HPA) and sympathetic-adrenal medullary (SAM) systems can modulate levels of MMP, providing a physiological link among mood, stress, hormones, and wound healing. This line of basic research suggests that activation of the HPA and SAM axes, even in individuals within the normal range of depressive symptoms, could alter MMP levels and change the course of wound healing in blister wounds.

Surgical Preparation

Mind-body interventions are being tested to determine whether they can help prepare patients for the stress associated with surgery. Initial randomized controlled trials—in which some patients received audiotapes with mind-body techniques (guided imagery, music, and instructions for improved outcomes) and some patients received control tapes—found that subjects receiving the mind-body intervention recovered more quickly and spent fewer days in the hospital.[18]

Behavioral interventions have been shown to be an efficient means of reducing discomfort and adverse effects during percutaneous vascular and renal procedures. Pain increased linearly with procedure time in a control group and in a group practicing structured attention, but remained flat in a group practicing a self-hypnosis technique. The self-administration of analgesic drugs was significantly higher in the control group than in the attention and hypnosis groups. Hypnosis also improved hemodynamic stability.[19]

Conclusion

Evidence from randomized controlled trials and, in many cases, systematic reviews of the literature, suggests that:

- Mechanisms may exist by which the brain and central nervous system influence immune, endocrine, and autonomic functioning, which is known to have an impact on health.

- Multicomponent mind-body interventions that include some combination of stress management, coping skills training, cognitive-behavioral interventions, and relaxation therapy may be appropriate adjunctive treatments for coronary artery disease and certain pain-related disorders, such as arthritis.

- Multimodal mind-body approaches, such as cognitive-behavioral therapy, particularly when combined with an educational/informational component, can be effective adjuncts in the management of a variety of chronic conditions.

- An array of mind-body therapies (for example, imagery, hypnosis, relaxation), when employed presurgically, may improve recovery time and reduce pain following surgical procedures.

- Neurochemical and anatomical bases may exist for some of the effects of mind-body approaches.

Mind-body approaches have potential benefits and advantages. In particular, the physical and emotional risks of using these interventions are minimal. Moreover, once tested and standardized, most mind-body interventions can be taught easily. Finally, future research focusing on basic mind-body mechanisms and individual differences in responses is likely to yield new insights that may enhance the effectiveness and individual tailoring of mind-body interventions. In the meantime, there is considerable evidence that mind-body interventions, even as they are being studied today, have positive effects on psychological functioning and quality of life, and may be particularly helpful for patients coping with chronic illness and in need of palliative care.

References

1. Barnes PM, Powell-Griner E, McFann K, Nahin RL. Complementary and alternative medicine use among adults: United States, 2002. *CDC Advance Data Report* #343. 2004.

2. Cannon WB. *The Wisdom of the Body*. New York, NY: Norton; 1932.

3. Selye H. *The Stress of Life*. New York, NY: McGraw-Hill; 1956.

4. Beecher H. *Measurement of Subjective Responses*. New York, NY: Oxford University Press; 1959.

5. Rutledge JC, Hyson DA, Garduno D, et al. Lifestyle modification program in management of patients with coronary artery disease: the clinical experience in a tertiary care hospital. *Journal of Cardiopulmonary Rehabilitation*. 1999;19(4):226–234.

6. Luskin FM, Newell KA, Griffith M, et al. A review of mind/body therapies in the treatment of musculoskeletal disorders with implications for the elderly. *Alternative Therapies in Health and Medicine*. 2000;6(2):46–56.

7. Astin JA, Shapiro SL, Eisenberg DM, et al. Mind-body medicine: state of the science, implications for practice. *Journal of the American Board of Family Practice*. 2003;16(2):131–147.

8. Mundy EA, DuHamel KN, Montgomery GH. The efficacy of behavioral interventions for cancer treatment-related side effects. *Seminars in Clinical Neuropsychiatry*. 2003;8(4):253–275.

9. Irwin MR, Pike JL, Cole JC, et al. Effects of a behavioral intervention, Tai Chi Chih, on varicella-zoster virus specific immunity and health functioning in older adults. *Psychosomatic Medicine*. 2003;65(5):824–830.

10. Kiecolt-Glaser JK, Marucha PT, Atkinson C, et al. Hypnosis as a modulator of cellular immune dysregulation during acute stress. *Journal of Consulting and Clinical Psychology*. 2001;69(4):674–682.

11. Cohen S, Doyle WJ, Turner RB, et al. Emotional style and susceptibility to the common cold. *Psychosomatic Medicine*. 2003;65(4):652–657.

12. Smith A, Nicholson K. Psychosocial factors, respiratory viruses and exacerbation of asthma. *Psychoneuroendocrinology*. 2001;26(4):411–420.

13. Lazar SW, Bush G, Gollub RL, et al. Functional brain mapping of the relaxation response and meditation. *Neuroreport*. 2000;11(7):1581–1585.

14. Davidson RJ, Kabat-Zinn J, Schumacher J, et al. Alterations in brain and immune function produced by mindfulness meditation. *Psychosomatic Medicine*. 2003;65(4):564–570.

15. Fuente-Fernandez R, Phillips AG, Zamburlini M, et al. Dopamine release in human ventral striatum and expectation of reward. *Behavioural Brain Research*. 2002;136(2):359–363.

16. Stamenkovic I. Extracellular matrix remodelling: the role of matrix metalloproteinases. *Journal of Pathology*. 2003;200(4): 448–464.

17. Yang EV, Bane CM, MacCallum RC, et al. Stress-related modulation of matrix metalloproteinase expression. *Journal of Neuroimmunology*. 2002;133(1-2):144–150.

18. Tusek DL, Church JM, Strong SA, et al. Guided imagery: a significant advance in the care of patients undergoing elective colorectal surgery. *Diseases of the Colon and Rectum*. 1997;40(2): 172–178.

19. Lang EV, Benotsch EG, Fick LJ, et al. Adjunctive non-pharmacological analgesia for invasive medical procedures: a randomised trial. *Lancet*. 2000;355(9214):1486–1490.

Section 62.4

Massage Therapy and Chiropractic Care

This section includes text from "Massage Therapy as CAM," National Center for Complementary and Alternative Medicine (NCCAM), NCCAM Publication No. D327, September 2006; and text from "An Introduction to Chiropractic," NCCAM Publication No. D403, November 2007.

What Massage Therapy Is

The term massage therapy (also called massage, for short; massage also refers to an individual treatment session) covers a group of practices and techniques. There are over 80 types of massage therapy. In all of them, therapists press, rub, and otherwise manipulate the muscles and other soft tissues of the body, often varying pressure and movement. They most often use their hands and fingers, but may use their forearms, elbows, or feet. Typically, the intent is to relax the soft tissues, increase delivery of blood and oxygen to the massaged areas, warm them, and decrease pain.

A few examples of popular massage therapies follow:

- In Swedish massage, the therapist uses long strokes, kneading, and friction on the muscles and moves the joints to aid flexibility.

- A therapist giving a deep tissue massage uses patterns of strokes and deep finger pressure on parts of the body where muscles are tight or knotted, focusing on layers of muscle deep under the skin.

- In trigger point massage (also called pressure point massage), the therapist uses a variety of strokes but applies deeper, more focused pressure on myofascial trigger points—knots that can form in the muscles, are painful when pressed, and cause symptoms elsewhere in the body as well.

- In shiatsu massage, the therapist applies varying, rhythmic pressure from the fingers on parts of the body that are believed to be important for the flow of a vital energy called qi. In traditional Chinese medicine, the vital energy or life force proposed to

473

regulate a person's spiritual, emotional, mental, and physical health, and to be influenced by the opposing forces of yin and yang.

Massage therapy (and, in general, the laying on of hands for health purposes) dates back thousands of years. References to massage have been found in ancient writings from many cultures, including those of Ancient Greece, Ancient Rome, Japan, China, Egypt, and the Indian subcontinent.

In the United States, massage therapy first became popular and was promoted for a variety of health purposes starting in the mid-1800s. In the 1930s and 1940s, however, massage fell out of favor, mostly because of scientific and technological advances in medical treatments. Interest in massage revived in the 1970s, especially among athletes.

More recently, a 2002 national survey on Americans' use of CAM (published in 2004) found that five percent of the 31,000 participants had used massage therapy in the preceding 12 months, and 9.3 percent had ever used it. According to recent reviews, people use massage for a wide variety of health-related intents: for example, to relieve pain (often from musculoskeletal conditions, but from other conditions as well); rehabilitate sports injuries; reduce stress; increase relaxation; address feelings of anxiety and depression; and aid general wellness.

What Massage Therapists Do in Treating Patients

Massage therapists work in a variety of settings, including private offices, hospitals, other clinical settings, nursing homes, studios, and sport and fitness facilities. Some also travel to patients' homes or workplaces to provide a massage.

Massage therapy treatments usually last for 30 to 60 minutes; less often, they are as short as 15 minutes or as long as 1.5–2 hours. For some conditions (especially chronic ones), therapists often advise a series of appointments. Therapists usually try to provide an environment that is as calm and soothing as possible (for example, by using dim lighting, soft music, and fragrances).

At the first appointment, a massage therapist will discuss your symptoms, medical history, the results you (and your health care provider, if applicable) desire, and possibly other factors such as your work and levels of stress. He or she will likely perform some evaluations through touch. If nothing is found that would make a massage inadvisable, he or she will proceed with the massage. At any time, you can bring up questions or concerns.

During treatment, you will lie on a special padded table or sit on a stool or chair. You might be fully clothed (for a chair massage) or partially or fully undressed (in which case you will be covered by a sheet or towel; only the parts of your body that the therapist is currently massaging are exposed). Oil or powder helps reduce friction on the skin. The therapist may use other aids, such as ice, heat, fragrances, or machines. The therapist may also provide recommendations for self-care, such as drinking fluids, learning better movement, and developing an awareness of your body.

Why People Use Massage Therapy

In the 2002 national survey on Americans' use of CAM, respondents who used a CAM therapy could choose from five reasons for using the therapy. The results for massage were as follows:

- They believed that massage combined with conventional medicine would help: 60 percent

- They thought massage would be interesting to try: 44 percent

- They believed that conventional medical treatments would not help: 34 percent

- Massage was suggested by a conventional medical professional: 33 percent

- They thought that conventional medicine was too expensive: 13 percent

Side Effects and Risks

Massage therapy appears to have few serious risks if appropriate cautions are followed. A very small number of serious injuries have been reported, and they appear to have occurred mostly because cautions were not followed or a massage was given by a person who was not properly trained.

Health care providers recommend that patients not have massage therapy if they have one or more of the following conditions:

- Deep vein thrombosis (a blood clot in a deep vein, usually in the legs)

- A bleeding disorder or are taking blood-thinning drugs such as warfarin

- Damaged blood vessels
- Weakened bones from osteoporosis, a recent fracture, or cancer
- A fever
- Any of the following in an area that would be massaged:
  - An open or healing wound
  - A tumor
  - Damaged nerves
  - An infection or acute inflammation
  - Inflammation from radiation treatment

If you have one or more of the following conditions, be sure to consult your health care provider before having massage:

- Pregnancy
- Cancer
- Fragile skin, as from diabetes or a healing scar
- Heart problems
- Dermatomyositis, a disease of the connective tissue
- A history of physical abuse

Side effects of massage therapy may include the following:

- Temporary pain or discomfort
- Bruising
- Swelling
- A sensitivity or allergy to massage oils

Some Other Points to Consider about Massage Therapy as CAM

- Massage therapy should not be used to replace your regular medical care or to delay seeing a doctor about a medical problem.
- Before you decide about having massage therapy, ask the therapist about the following:
  - Her training, experience, and any licenses or credentials

- Any medical conditions you have and whether the therapist has had any specialized training or experience with them

- The number of treatments that might be needed

- Cost

- Insurance coverage, if any

- If a massage therapist suggests using other CAM practices (such as herbs or other supplements, a special diet), discuss it first with your regular health care provider.

How Massage Therapy Might Work

Scientists are studying massage to understand what effects massage therapy has on patients, how it has those effects, and why. Some aspects of this are better understood than others. For example, it is known that:

- When certain forces are applied to the muscles, changes occur in the muscles (although those changes are not clearly understood or agreed upon).

- Massage therapy typically enhances relaxation and reduces stress. Stress makes some diseases and conditions worse.

There are many more aspects that are not yet known or well understood scientifically, however. Some of the proposed theories about what massage might do include the following:

- Provide stimulation that may help block pain signals sent to the brain (the "gate control theory" of pain reduction).

- Shift the patient's nervous system away from the sympathetic and toward the parasympathetic. The sympathetic nervous system helps mobilize the body for action. When a person is under stress, it produces the fight-or-flight response (the heart rate and breathing rate go up, for example; the blood vessels narrow; and muscles tighten). The parasympathetic nervous system creates what some call the rest and digest response (the heart rate and breathing rate slow down, for example; the blood vessels dilate; and activity increases in many parts of the digestive tract).

- Stimulate the release of certain chemicals in the body, such as serotonin or endorphins.

- Cause beneficial mechanical changes in the body—for example, by preventing fibrosis (the formation of scar-like tissue) or increasing the flow of lymph (a fluid that travels through the body's lymphatic system and carries cells that help fight disease).

- Improve sleep, which has a role in pain and healing.

- Provide some health benefit from the interaction between therapist and patient.

More well-designed studies are needed to understand and confirm these theories and other scientific aspects of massage.

An Introduction to Chiropractic Care

Chiropractic is a health care approach that focuses on the relationship between the body's structure—mainly the spine—and its functioning. Although practitioners may use a variety of treatment approaches, they primarily perform adjustments to the spine or other parts of the body with the goal of correcting alignment problems and supporting the body's natural ability to heal itself.

Overview and History

While some procedures associated with chiropractic care can be traced back to ancient times, the modern profession of chiropractic was founded by Daniel David Palmer in 1895 in Davenport, Iowa. Palmer, a self-taught healer, believed that the body has a natural healing ability. Misalignments of the spine can interfere with the flow of energy needed to support health, Palmer theorized, and the key to health is to normalize the function of the nervous system, especially the spinal cord.

Patterns of Use

A 2002 national survey on CAM use found that about 20 percent of American adults had received chiropractic care at some point during their lives. Chiropractic was one of the ten most commonly used CAM therapies. Those surveyed reported using chiropractic treatment for the following reasons:

- Combining chiropractic services with conventional medical treatments would help: 53 percent

- Conventional medicine would not help: 40 percent

- Chiropractic would be interesting to try: 32 percent

- Conventional medical professional suggested it: 20 percent

- Conventional medical treatments were too expensive: 10 percent

Many people who seek chiropractic care have chronic, pain-related health conditions. Low-back pain, neck pain, and headache are common conditions for which people seek chiropractic treatment.

What to Expect from Chiropractic Visits

During the initial visit, chiropractors typically take a health history and perform a physical examination, with a special emphasis on the spine. Other examinations or tests such as x-rays may also be performed. If chiropractic treatment is considered appropriate, a treatment plan will be developed.

During follow-up visits, practitioners may perform one or more of the many different types of adjustments used in chiropractic care. Given mainly to the spine, a chiropractic adjustment (sometimes referred to as a manipulation) involves using the hands or a device to apply a controlled, sudden force to a joint, moving it beyond its passive range of motion. The goal is to increase the range and quality of motion in the area being treated and to aid in restoring health. Other hands-on therapies such as mobilization (movement of a joint within its usual range of motion) also may be used.

Chiropractors may combine the use of spinal adjustments with several other treatments and approaches such as the following:

- Heat and ice

- Electrical stimulation

- Rest

- Rehabilitative exercise

- Counseling about diet, weight loss, and other lifestyle factors

- Dietary supplements

Side Effects and Risks

Side effects and risks depend on the specific type of chiropractic treatment used. For example, side effects from chiropractic adjustments can include temporary headaches, tiredness, or discomfort in parts of the body that were treated. The likelihood of serious complications, such as stroke, appears to be extremely low and related to the type of adjustment performed and the part of the body treated.

If dietary supplements are a part of the chiropractic treatment plan, they may interact with medicines and cause side effects. It is important that people inform their chiropractors of all medicines (whether prescription or over-the-counter) and supplements they are taking.

Regulation

Chiropractic is regulated individually by each state and the District of Columbia. Board examinations are required for licensing and include a mock patient encounter. Most states require chiropractors to earn annual continuing education credits to maintain their licenses. Chiropractors' scope of practice varies by state in areas such as laboratory tests or diagnostic procedures, the dispensing or selling of dietary supplements, and the use of other CAM therapies such as acupuncture or homeopathy.

Insurance Coverage

Compared with other CAM therapies, insurance coverage for chiropractic services is extensive. Many HMOs (health maintenance organizations) and private health care plans cover chiropractic treatment, as do all state workers' compensation systems. Chiropractors can bill Medicare, and many states cover chiropractic treatment under Medicaid. If you have health insurance, check whether chiropractic services are covered before you seek treatment.

References

1. Agency for Health Care Policy and Research. *Chiropractic in the United States: Training, Practice, and Research*. Rockville, MD: Agency for Health Care Policy and Research; 1997. AHCPR publication no. 98–N002.

2. Meeker WC, Haldeman S. Chiropractic: a profession at the crossroads of mainstream and alternative medicine. *Annals of Internal Medicine*. 2002;136(3):216–227.

3. Barnes PM, Powell-Griner E, McFann K, Nahin RL. Complementary and alternative medicine use among adults: United States, 2002. *CDC Advance Data Report #343*. 2004.

4. Coulter ID, Hurwitz EL, Adams AH, et al. Patients using chiropractors in North America: who are they, and why are they in chiropractic care? *Spine*. 2002;27(3):291–296.

5. The Council on Chiropractic Education. *Standards for Doctor of Chiropractic Programs and Requirements for Institutional Status January 2007*. The Council on Chiropractic Education website. June 28, 2007.

6. Dagenais S, Haldeman S. Chiropractic. *Primary Care*. 2002; 29(2):419–437.

7. Eisenberg DM, Cohen MH, Hrbek A, et al. Credentialing complementary and alternative medical providers. *Annals of Internal Medicine*. 2002;137(12):965–973.

8. Ernst, E, Pittler, MH, Wider, B, eds. *The Desktop Guide to Complementary and Alternative Medicine: An Evidence-Based Approach. 2nd ed*. St. Louis, MO: Mosby Elsevier; 2006.

9. Kaptchuk TJ, Eisenberg DM. Chiropractic: origins, controversies, and contributions. *Archives of Internal Medicine*. 1998; 158(20):2215–2224.

10. Senstad O, Leboeuf-Yde C, Borchgrevink C. Frequency and characteristics of side effects of spinal manipulative therapy. *Spine*. 1997;22(4):435–440.

Section 62.5

Glucosamine/Chondroitin Arthritis Intervention Trial (GAIT) Results

Excerpted from "Questions and Answers: NIH Glucosamine/Chondroitin Arthritis Intervention Trial (GAIT)," National Center for Complementary and Alternative Medicine (NCCAM), NCCAM Publication No. D310, updated April 2007.

What is the glucosamine/chondroitin arthritis intervention trial (GAIT)?

GAIT is the first large-scale, multicenter clinical trial in the United States to test the effects of the dietary supplements glucosamine hydrochloride (glucosamine) and sodium chondroitin sulfate (chondroitin sulfate) for the treatment of knee osteoarthritis. The study tested whether glucosamine and chondroitin sulfate used separately or in combination reduced pain in participants with knee osteoarthritis.

The University of Utah, School of Medicine coordinated this study, which was conducted at 16 rheumatology research centers across the United States. The National Center for Complementary and Alternative Medicine (NCCAM) and the National Institute of Arthritis and Musculoskeletal and Skin Diseases (NIAMS), two components of the National Institutes of Health (NIH), funded GAIT.

What was the purpose of the study?

Previous studies in the medical literature had conflicting results on the effectiveness of glucosamine and chondroitin sulfate as treatments for osteoarthritis. GAIT was designed to test the short-term (six months) effectiveness of glucosamine and chondroitin sulfate in reducing pain in a large number of participants with knee osteoarthritis.

What was the basic design of the study?

In GAIT, participants were randomly assigned to one of five treatment groups: (1) glucosamine alone, (2) chondroitin sulfate alone, (3) glucosamine and chondroitin sulfate in combination, (4) celecoxib, or (5) a placebo (an inactive substance that looks like the study substance). Glucosamine and chondroitin sulfate and their combination were compared with a placebo to evaluate whether these substances significantly improve joint pain. Celecoxib, which is a prescription drug effective in managing osteoarthritis pain, was also compared with placebo to validate the study design.

To reduce the chance of biased results, the study was double-blinded—neither the researchers nor the participants knew which of the five treatment groups the participants were in. Participants received treatment for 24 weeks. Participants were evaluated at the start of the study and at weeks 4, 8, 16, and 24 and closely monitored for improvement of their symptoms as well as for any possible adverse reactions to the study agents. X-rays documented each participant's diagnosis of osteoarthritis. Participants were also stratified into two pain subgroups—1,229 participants (78 percent) with mild pain and 354 participants (22 percent) with moderate-to-severe pain.

A positive response to treatment was defined as a 20 percent or greater reduction in pain at week 24 compared to the start of the study. All participants had the option to use up to 4000 milligrams (mg) of acetaminophen, as needed, to control pain from osteoarthritis throughout the study, except for the 24 hours prior to having their knee assessed. Acetaminophen use was low: on average, participants used fewer than two 500 mg tablets per day.

Study Background

More than 20 million adults in the United States live with osteoarthritis—the most common type of arthritis. Osteoarthritis, also called degenerative joint disease, is caused by the breakdown of cartilage, which is the connective tissue that cushions the ends of bones within the joint. Osteoarthritis is characterized by pain, joint damage, and limited motion. The disease generally occurs late in life, and most commonly affects the hands and large weight-bearing joints, such as the knees. Age, female gender, and obesity are risk factors for this condition.

What are glucosamine and chondroitin sulfate?

Glucosamine and chondroitin sulfate are natural substances found in and around the cells of cartilage. Glucosamine is an amino sugar that the body produces and distributes in cartilage and other connective tissue, and chondroitin sulfate is a complex carbohydrate that helps cartilage retain water. In the United States, glucosamine and chondroitin sulfate are sold as dietary supplements, which are regulated as foods rather than drugs.

What is celecoxib?

Celecoxib (brand name Celebrex) is a type of nonsteroidal anti-inflammatory drug (NSAID), called a COX-2 inhibitor. Like traditional NSAIDs, celecoxib blocks the COX-2 enzyme in the body that stimulates inflammation. Unlike traditional NSAIDs, however, celecoxib does not block the action of COX-1 enzyme, which is known to protect the stomach lining. As a result, celecoxib reduces joint pain and inflammation with reduced risk of gastrointestinal ulceration and bleeding. Recent reports have linked possible cardiovascular side effects to COX-2 inhibitors. Although GAIT was not designed to study the safety of celecoxib, participants were monitored for adverse events and no increase in such side effects was observed.

What doses were used for the various treatments?

The doses used in GAIT were based on the doses seen in the prevailing scientific literature:

- Glucosamine alone: 1500 mg daily given as 500 mg three times a day

- Chondroitin sulfate alone: 1200 mg daily given as 400 mg three times a day

- Glucosamine plus chondroitin sulfate combined: same doses— 1500 mg and 1200 mg daily

- Celecoxib: 200 mg daily

- Acetaminophen: participants were allowed to take up to 4000 mg (500 mg tablets) per day to control pain, except for the 24 hours before pain was assessed.

Key Results

Researchers found:

- Participants taking the positive control, celecoxib, experienced statistically significant pain relief versus placebo—about 70 percent of those taking celecoxib had a 20 percent or greater reduction in pain versus about 60 percent for placebo.

- Overall, there were no significant differences between the other treatments tested and placebo.

- For a subset of participants with moderate-to-severe pain, glucosamine combined with chondroitin sulfate provided statistically significant pain relief compared with placebo—about 79 percent had a 20 percent or greater reduction in pain versus about 54 percent for placebo. According to the researchers, because of the small size of this subgroup these findings should be considered preliminary and need to be confirmed in further studies.

- For participants in the mild pain subset, glucosamine and chondroitin sulfate together or alone did not provide statistically significant pain relief.

How many people participated in the study and who were they?

A total of 1,583 people participated in the study. People age 40 or older with knee pain and documented x-ray evidence of osteoarthritis were eligible to participate. Participants could not have used glucosamine for three months and chondroitin sulfate for six months prior to entering the study. Participants were about 59 years of age, on average, and nearly two-thirds of participants were women. Of the 1,583 study participants, 78 percent (1,229) were in the mild pain subgroup and 22 percent (354) were in the moderate-to-severe pain subgroup.

Were there any side effects from the treatments?

There were 77 reports of serious adverse effects during the study. Of those 77, only three were attributed to study treatments. Most side effects were mild, such as upset stomach, and were spread evenly across the different treatment groups. In addition, although GAIT was not designed to evaluate these risks, no change in glucose tolerance was seen for glucosamine nor was an increased incidence of cardiovascular events seen with celecoxib.

Consumer Information and Next Steps

Should people with osteoarthritis use glucosamine and chondroitin sulfate?

People with osteoarthritis should work with their health care provider to develop a comprehensive plan for managing their arthritis pain: eat right, exercise, lose excess weight, and use proven pain medications. If people have moderate-to-severe pain, they should talk with their health care provider about whether glucosamine plus chondroitin sulfate is an appropriate treatment option.

Can U.S. consumers get the glucosamine and chondroitin sulfate products used in GAIT?

Identical products may not be commercially available. GAIT was conducted under an Investigational New Drug application filed with the U.S. Food and Drug Administration (FDA). All of the products used in the study were developed for the study and subject to the FDA's pharmaceutical regulations. The glucosamine and chondroitin sulfate used were tested for purity, potency, quality, and consistency among batches. Products were retested for stability throughout the study.

Chapter 63

Placebo Effect and Pain Relief

What are placebos and their effects?

Catherine Stoney, Ph.D., National Center for Complementary and Alternative Medicine (NCCAM) program officer, defines a placebo response as one or more beneficial physical or psychological changes that occurs in response to a placebo—which can be defined in the following various ways:

- An inactive substance (for example, a sugar pill) designed to look like an active medication

- A "sham" procedure or device, such as a procedure designed to look like acupuncture but not to deliver treatment effects

- A "therapeutic encounter or symbol," such as:

  - an interaction with a health care provider

  - something symbolic in such an encounter (for example, the "white-coat effect" that some researchers have noted)

Placebos like inactive pills and sham procedures have a history of use in controlled experiments. They allow researchers to obtain a truer picture of the effects of the active treatment under study, above and

Excerpted from "Placebos: Sugar, Shams, Therapies, or All of the Above?" National Center for Complementary and Alternative Medicine (NCCAM), 2007.

beyond what might occur over time and due to the expectation of positive benefit. Placebos are also widely viewed as nuisances, however—producers of "noise" that complicate analysis of study data—because sometimes there are therapeutic responses to them.

Increasingly, scientists and clinicians have come to believe that the power of placebos, when harnessed, could potentially enhance health and health care. Studies of placebo effects could also provide insight into the mind's effects on the body and on practices in the complementary and alternative medicine (CAM) domain of mind-body medicine (such as meditation, hypnosis, and yoga).

"People Get Well in Ways We Don't Understand"

Ted Kaptchuk is an associate professor of medicine at Harvard Medical School, associate director of the Division for Research and Education in Complementary and Integrative Medical Therapies at Harvard's Osher Institute, and a member of NCCAM's Advisory Council. He received his training in Asian medicine in China. Professor Kaptchuk recalled that when he was working as director of a chronic pain unit at a chronic disease facility in the United States, he saw some improvements that led him to think, "People get well sometimes in ways that we don't understand. Practitioners usually credit their therapies. Sometimes, it seemed to me that relief and healing had nothing to do with the specific therapy—indeed, that important processes were going on underneath the official therapy. That's why I became interested in studying the placebo effect."

Professor Kaptchuk describes the placebo response in randomized, controlled trials as a "box" of many complex elements that he and his colleagues are seeking to "unpack." He described a few of his studies, including one published in 2006 in which he and his colleagues compared the effects of a sham device and an inactive pill with each other and with real treatments. His team was interested primarily in the placebos' effects. The participants were 270 adults with persistent arm pain from repetitive use.

Each participant was randomized into a so-called acupuncture group or amitriptyline (a type of medication) group. During the first two weeks, or "run-in period," all participants received either the sham acupuncture treatment or the inactive pill. Next, half of each group received the active treatment and the other half received the corresponding sham or placebo. Participants did not know at any time whether they were receiving active treatment or a sham/placebo. The team then looked at various pain outcomes.

Among their findings:

- The sham acupuncture device worked better than the placebo pill (except during the run-in period) on the primary measure of pain and on the severity of symptoms.

- A pain-relieving placebo effect persisted over time—not just for a short time—which is a commonly held belief about placebos.

- Placebo effects may relate to the expectations of participants and the information provided to them. As part of the standard informed-consent process, all participants had been told before the study started about possible side effects they might experience if they received an active treatment. Each group was told to expect different side effects. Interestingly, many participants who received only the sham device (about one-quarter) or inactive pill (about one-third) reported they experienced the side effects of the corresponding active treatment. This, said Professor Kaptchuk, also illustrates a strong "nocebo effect"—the flip side of the placebo effect. A person experiences negative, not positive, physical and psychological effects in response to a nocebo.

Professor Kaptchuk described a second study that also worked with participants' expectations about pain relief from an actual acupuncture treatment and that used a sham device. This controlled study used functional magnetic resonance imaging (fMRI) brain imaging to study participants' brain responses, literally shedding light on multiple pathways and mechanisms of the brain that may play an important role in placebo pain-relief effects. Another study examines various proposed components of the placebo effect both separately and together.

There Are Perfections in the Brain That Need to Be Exploited

Jon-Kar Zubieta, M.D., Ph.D., is a professor of psychiatry, radiology, and neurosciences at the University of Michigan Medical School and at the university's Molecular and Behavioral Neuroscience Institute. His training is in neuroimaging, nuclear medicine, and psychiatry.

Dr. Zubieta has been studying brain activity and responses to placebos in the context of pain and stress. He is interested in the operation of expectations and awareness in placebo effects and even more interested in resilience mechanisms—people's ability to mobilize a response, especially biologically, when they believe they are receiving or will receive a treatment that could be helpful. He and his team use positron-emission tomography (PET), to study the experiences of pain and pain relief (including from placebos) in the brain as they are occurring.

Dr. Zubieta highlighted some of his findings:

- He has seen an almost perfect match across people's responses to placebo treatment, between the release of substances called endogenous opioids (EO) and lessened sensitivity to pain over time. Endogenous opioids are chemicals that occur naturally in the body and have characteristics similar to those of drugs like morphine.

- In "executive areas" of the brain (areas that integrate information, and also reduce pain through the release of EO), there is "enormous individuality and variability" among study participants in terms of which regions are activated and how much.

- The brain chemical dopamine appears to be important in pain relief experienced from placebos. Dopamine and its pathways are known to be central in responses to reward and the prospect of reward. Dr. Zubieta thinks that they may also become activated by the prospect of pain relief, including from placebos. This, in turn, may drive systems like EO that reduce both the pain experience and its unpleasantness.

- Cognitive influences such as thoughts and beliefs, emotions, gender, hormones, and genetics all appear to play a role in how people experience pain, stress, and the placebo response. For example, in preliminary work, Dr. Zubieta found gender differences in how much people's EO respond to the administration of a placebo. He is trying to shed further light on this area by examining the influence of estrogen and progesterone.

When asked by an audience member, "Are there imperfections in the human brain that need to be remedied?" Dr. Zubieta answered, "There are perfections in the human brain that need to be exploited." Among other factors he hopes to study are individual variability in specific genes. "Then," he said, "our knowledge of the biology of the placebo effect can be examined in the context of disease states, including movement disorders, depression, and cardiovascular disease."

Chapter 64

Virtual Reality and Pain Reduction

The National Institutes on Health (NIH) Pain Consortium reports the following current uses of virtual reality (VR) for the treatment of pain.

- VR has been used to distract patients from various types of pain, including dental pain and burn wound treatment pain. In the treatment of burn wounds, a 76% reduction in perceived pain intensity was reported when using a VR world (South Pole Fantasy) versus controls. Measures of anxiety related to painful dental procedures were also significantly reduced. Further, in a pilot study, migraine headache, fibromyalgia, and chronic back pain were also reduced in a relaxing VR environment.

- VR produced a significant reduction in pain measures during burn wound care—both changing dressing and stretching the skin during physical therapy—compared to control subjects that were playing video games. These reductions in pain corresponded to changes in brain activity as measured by function magnetic resonance imaging (fMRI). Further, anxiety related to these procedures dropped dramatically. This resulted in less morphine being needed to treat patients that received VR treatment.

- VR was used in children who received venipuncture or wound care. Children who received VR had significantly less distress

"Virtual Reality and Pain Reduction Conference," National Institutes of Health (NIH) Pain Consortium, 2006.

compared to controls that were watching a movie. At this point in this study, both groups had similar pain ratings. During intravenous (IV) placement, VR was found to reduce pain in children, as indicated by both the child's and the parent's report of the child's pain. Anxiety of the children was also substantially reduced. Further, it was found that the caregivers were much more satisfied with the VR treatment than the control treatments.

Future Directions

The clinical use of VR in the treatment of disease is a new but rapidly growing field. In terms of pain treatment, many successes have recently been realized in the treatment of acute pain. However, there are likely many ways to extend and improve how VR is used in the treatment of acute pain, and to expand its use to the treatment of chronic pain.

In terms of acute pain, it was concluded that research that seeks to determine the characteristics of VR environments that work for distracting patients from various types of pain is of importance. For example, research is needed to determine if "cold" VR environments, including things like snow and penguins, works better on burn wound pain than other environments. In contrast, research is needed on whether other types of pain (for example, acute arthritis pain) respond better to a VR environment that depicts a warm scene. It may be the case that numerous VR worlds will be needed, each tailored to the specific types of pain being treated.

Further, VR worlds likely will prove to be more powerful if they are individualized to various patient characteristics. Factors like age, gender, and personal interests likely impact how effective various VR worlds are at producing distraction from pain. Designing and matching VR worlds to various patient characteristics would likely result in much greater pain distraction and patient acceptance.

Along these lines, basic research on general properties of the VR worlds and how these relate to their effectiveness is needed. This research could address if more realistic worlds produce more distraction or if simple cartoon-like graphics are sufficient or even superior. Various types of head mounted displays (HMD) are used to present VR visual stimuli. Research could help determine which types of displays are the most effective. A sense of "presences" in the VR is often sited as essential for the VR experience to be effective. Research on what this sense really is, how it can be produced, and if it impacts pain perception is also of importance.

It is also acknowledged that VR alone for acute pain in many cases may not suffice. Research on how VR can be used with other types of treatments may allow more effective treatment of acute pain, where lower amounts of drugs are needed in situations where pharmacotherapies are currently the treatments of choice.

While acute pain is a serious problem, approximately 50 million Americans suffer from chronic pain, and this type of pain can be debilitating, greatly reducing quality of life. The use of VR in the treatment of chronic pain is just beginning to be explored. Obviously, a person cannot be distracted from pain at all times by wearing a HMD. However, chronic pain typically varies over time. With the advent of less expensive VR equipment and software, it is possible for patients to use VR away from the clinic to treat bouts of pain. This may include a set-up where data about the treatments could be electronically forwarded to caregivers, who could monitor progress and change the treatment if needed. By treating bouts of chronic pain in this way, there also may be less "wind-up" pain, where a person's pain puts them in more of a hyperalgesic state. It may also reduce reliance on opioids, which is important because there is evidence that chronic opioid treatments can actually result in a hyperalgesic state (opioid-induced hyperalgesia).

Biobehavioral methods have efficacy in the treatment of chronic pain, where people learn to cope with their pain and are enabled to pursue more activities. VR is very suited for various biobehavioral treatments, and has been shown to be very effective at reinforcing various behavioral, social, and cognitive skills. Adapting VR protocols to promote a better quality of life in chronic pain patients is important. These protocols would likely include "serious games," where the patient plays a game in VR that teaches them about their pain conditions, and how to cope with and overcome their disease.

A further area of opportunity is the use of simulated VR people (avatars) to help teach pain treatment professionals. These simulated people can be programmed to present with various symptoms including pain. The clinician interacts with these avatars and establishes a diagnosis. This type of technology could be used in the pain treatment field as a means to allow clinicians to practice and improve their diagnosis skills. It could also be used to help train clinicians to be able to distinguish between people in pain and drug-addicted individuals faking painful symptoms in order to obtain opioids.

Chapter 65

Clinical Research Trials: Trying New Medications and Devices for Pain Relief

Choosing to participate in a clinical trial is an important personal decision. The following frequently asked questions provide detailed information about clinical trials. In addition, it is often helpful to talk to a physician, family members, or friends about deciding to join a trial. After identifying some trial options, the next step is to contact the study research staff and ask questions about specific trials.

What is a clinical trial?

Although there are many definitions of clinical trials, they are generally considered to be biomedical or health-related research studies in human beings that follow a pre-defined protocol. ClinicalTrials.gov includes both interventional and observational types of studies. Interventional studies are those in which the research subjects are assigned by the investigator to a treatment or other intervention, and their outcomes are measured. Observational studies are those in which individuals are observed and their outcomes are measured by the investigators.

Why participate in a clinical trial?

Participants in clinical trials can play a more active role in their own health care, gain access to new research treatments before they

This chapter includes excerpts from "Understanding Clinical Trials," National Institutes of Health (NIH), September 20, 2007; and the section titled "Information from ClinicalTrials.gov: Studies on Pain," is excerpted from a ClinicalTrials.gov online search of the topic "Pain," accessed March 5, 2008.

are widely available, and help others by contributing to medical research.

Who can participate in a clinical trial?

All clinical trials have guidelines about who can participate. Using inclusion and exclusion criteria is an important principle of medical research that helps to produce reliable results. The factors that allow someone to participate in a clinical trial are called inclusion criteria and those that disallow someone from participating are called exclusion criteria. These criteria are based on such factors as age, gender, the type and stage of a disease, previous treatment history, and other medical conditions. Before joining a clinical trial, a participant must qualify for the study. Some research studies seek participants with illnesses or conditions to be studied in the clinical trial, while others need healthy participants. It is important to note that inclusion and exclusion criteria are not used to reject people personally. Instead, the criteria are used to identify appropriate participants and keep them safe. The criteria help ensure that researchers will be able to answer the questions they plan to study.

What happens during a clinical trial?

The clinical trial process depends on the kind of trial being conducted. The clinical trial team includes doctors and nurses as well as social workers and other health care professionals. They check the health of the participant at the beginning of the trial, give specific instructions for participating in the trial, monitor the participant carefully during the trial, and stay in touch after the trial is completed.

Some clinical trials involve more tests and doctor visits than the participant would normally have for an illness or condition. For all types of trials, the participant works with a research team. Clinical trial participation is most successful when the protocol is carefully followed and there is frequent contact with the research staff.

What is informed consent?

Informed consent is the process of learning the key facts about a clinical trial before deciding whether or not to participate. It is also a continuing process throughout the study to provide information for participants. To help someone decide whether or not to participate, the doctors and nurses involved in the trial explain the details of the study. If the participant's native language is not English, translation assistance can be provided. Then the research team provides an informed consent document that includes details about the study, such as its purpose, duration, required procedures, and key contacts. Risks and potential benefits are explained in the informed consent document. The participant then decides whether or not to sign the document. Informed consent is not a contract, and the participant may withdraw from the trial at any time.

What are the benefits and risks of participating in a clinical trial?

Benefits

Clinical trials that are well-designed and well-executed are the best approach for eligible participants to:

- Play an active role in their own health care.

- Gain access to new research treatments before they are widely available.

- Obtain expert medical care at leading health care facilities during the trial.

- Help others by contributing to medical research.

Risks

There are risks to clinical trials.

- There may be unpleasant, serious, or even life-threatening side effects to experimental treatment.

- The experimental treatment may not be effective for the participant.

- The protocol may require more of their time and attention than would a non-protocol treatment, including trips to the study site, more treatments, hospital stays, or complex dosage requirements.

What are side effects and adverse reactions?

Side effects are any undesired actions or effects of the experimental drug or treatment. Negative or adverse effects may include headache, nausea, hair loss, skin irritation, or other physical problems.

Experimental treatments must be evaluated for both immediate and long-term side effects.

How is the safety of the participant protected?

The ethical and legal codes that govern medical practice also apply to clinical trials. In addition, most clinical research is federally regulated with built in safeguards to protect the participants. The trial follows a carefully controlled protocol, a study plan which details what researchers will do in the study. As a clinical trial progresses, researchers report the results of the trial at scientific meetings, to medical journals, and to various government agencies. Individual participants' names will remain secret and will not be mentioned in these reports.

What should people consider before participating in a trial?

People should know as much as possible about the clinical trial and feel comfortable asking the members of the health care team questions about it, the care expected while in a trial, and the cost of the trial. The following questions might be helpful for the participant to discuss with the health care team. Some of the answers to these questions are found in the informed consent document for the clinical trial being considered.

- What is the purpose of the study?
- Who is going to be in the study?
- Why do researchers believe the experimental treatment being tested may be effective? Has it been tested before?
- What kinds of tests and experimental treatments are involved?
- How do the possible risks, side effects, and benefits in the study compare with my current treatment?
- How might this trial affect my daily life?
- How long will the trial last?
- Will hospitalization be required?
- Who will pay for the experimental treatment?
- Will I be reimbursed for other expenses?
- What type of long-term follow up care is part of this study?

- How will I know that the experimental treatment is working? Will results of the trials be provided to me?

- Who will be in charge of my care?

What kind of preparation should a potential participant make for the meeting with the research coordinator or doctor?

- Plan ahead and write down possible questions to ask.

- Ask a friend or relative to come along for support and to hear the responses to the questions.

- Bring a tape recorder to record the discussion to replay later.

Every clinical trial in the U.S. must be approved and monitored by an Institutional Review Board (IRB) to make sure the risks are as low as possible and are worth any potential benefits. An IRB is an independent committee of physicians, statisticians, community advocates, and others that ensures that a clinical trial is ethical and the rights of study participants are protected. All institutions that conduct or support biomedical research involving people must, by federal regulation, have an IRB that initially approves and periodically reviews the research.

Does a participant continue to work with a primary health care provider while in a trial?

Yes. Most clinical trials provide short-term treatments related to a designated illness or condition, but do not provide extended or complete primary health care. In addition, by having the health care provider work with the research team, the participant can ensure that other medications or treatments will not conflict with the protocol.

Can a participant leave a clinical trial after it has begun?

Yes. A participant can leave a clinical trial, at any time. When withdrawing from the trial, the participant should let the research team know about it, and the reasons for leaving the study.

Where do the ideas for trials come from?

Ideas for clinical trials usually come from researchers. After researchers test new therapies or procedures in the laboratory and in animal studies, the experimental treatments with the most promising laboratory results are moved into clinical trials. During a trial, more and more information is gained about an experimental treatment, its risks and how well it may or may not work.

Who sponsors clinical trials?

Clinical trials are sponsored or funded by a variety of organizations or individuals such as physicians, medical institutions, foundations, voluntary groups, and pharmaceutical companies, in addition to federal agencies such as the National Institutes of Health (NIH), the Department of Defense (DOD), and the Department of Veteran's Affairs (VA). Trials can take place in a variety of locations, such as hospitals, universities, doctors' offices, or community clinics.

What is a protocol?

A protocol is a study plan on which all clinical trials are based. The plan is carefully designed to safeguard the health of the participants as well as answer specific research questions. A protocol describes what types of people may participate in the trial; the schedule of tests, procedures, medications, and dosages; and the length of the study. While in a clinical trial, participants following a protocol are seen regularly by the research staff to monitor their health and to determine the safety and effectiveness of their treatment.

What is a placebo?

A placebo is an inactive pill, liquid, or powder that has no treatment value. In clinical trials, experimental treatments are often compared with placebos to assess the experimental treatment's effectiveness. In some studies, the participants in the control group will receive a placebo instead of an active drug or experimental treatment.

What is a control or control group?

A control is the standard by which experimental observations are evaluated. In many clinical trials, one group of patients will be given an experimental drug or treatment while the control group is given either a standard treatment for the illness or a placebo.

What are the different types of clinical trials?

Treatment trials test experimental treatments, new combinations of drugs, or new approaches to surgery or radiation therapy.

Prevention trials look for better ways to prevent disease in people who have never had the disease or to prevent a disease from returning. These approaches may include medicines, vaccines, vitamins, minerals, or lifestyle changes.

Diagnostic trials are conducted to find better tests or procedures for diagnosing a particular disease or condition.

Screening trials test the best way to detect certain diseases or health conditions.

Quality of life trials (or supportive care trials) explore ways to improve comfort and the quality of life for individuals with a chronic illness.

What are the phases of clinical trials?

Clinical trials are conducted in phases. The trials at each phase have a different purpose and help scientists answer different questions:

Phase I trials: Researchers test an experimental drug or treatment in a small group of people (20–80) for the first time to evaluate its safety, determine a safe dosage range, and identify side effects.

Phase II trials: The experimental study drug or treatment is given to a larger group of people (100–300) to see if it is effective and to further evaluate its safety.

Phase III trials: The experimental study drug or treatment is given to large groups of people (1,000–3,000) to confirm its effectiveness, monitor side effects, compare it to commonly used treatments, and collect information that will allow the experimental drug or treatment to be used safely.

Phase IV trials: Post-marketing studies delineate additional information including the drug's risks, benefits, and optimal use.

Information from ClinicalTrials.gov: Studies on Pain

Following are some examples of clinical trials or studies seeking to improve the lives of people experiencing severe or chronic pain:

- "The Efficacy of Motor Cortex Stimulation for Pain Control," is a study which will test a motor cortex stimulation device as intervention for neuropathic pain, phantom limb pain, stump pain, brachial plexus avulsion, deafferentation pain, facial pain, or complex regional pain syndrome.

- "Effectiveness of Cognitive Behavioral Treatment and Mindfulness-Based Stress Reduction (MBSR) for Chronic Low Back Pain," is a study for those experiencing chronic low back pain which will study MBSR and cognitive behavioral treatment.

- "Proposal to Evaluate the Efficacy of the InterX 5000 in the Treatment of Chronic Neck and Shoulder Pain," is a study for people experiencing neck, shoulder, or cervical pain that will test if a device that provides electrical stimulation through a device, the InterX 5000, is effective.

- "Study on Magnetic Field Therapy to Improve Quality of Sleep and Reduction of Chronic Spine Pain," is using a magnetic sleep pad to determine if it is effective for individuals experiencing back or neck pain or sleep initiation and maintenance disorders.

To find detailed information about current studies on pain that are seeking participants, visit http://www.clinicaltrials.gov.

Part Four

Living With Pain

Chapter 66

Coping with Chronic Pain

Chronic pain is pain that lasts beyond the expected time for healing and interferes with normal life. The injury has healed, but the pain continues. The pain message may be triggered by muscle tension, stiffness, weakness, or spasms. Whatever the cause of chronic pain, feelings of frustration, anger, and fear can make the pain more intense. Chronic pain can affect all areas of your life and should be taken seriously.

The following information provides those who have chronic pain with an overview of different options for pain management. If you have chronic pain and need help managing it, you may wish to discuss these options with your doctor.

Coping Strategies: Physical Methods of Pain Management

Heat and ice: Heat, in the form of warm showers or hot packs, can relieve chronic pain or stiff muscles. Cold packs or ice packs provide pain relief by numbing the pain-sensing nerves in the affected area. Cold also helps reduce swelling and inflammation. Depending on which feels better, apply heat or cold for 15 to 20 minutes at a time to the area where you feel the pain. To protect your skin, place a towel

---

Excerpted from "Osteoporosis: Coping with Chronic Pain," National Institute of Arthritis and Musculoskeletal and Skin Diseases (NIAMS), March 2005.

between your skin and the source of the cold or heat. Some simple ways to make heat and ice packs:

- Warm towels or hot packs in the microwave for a quick source of heat. (Handle carefully.)

- Make instant cold packs from frozen juice cans or bags of frozen vegetables.

- Freeze a plastic, re-sealable bag filled with water to make a good ice bag.

Transcutaneous Electrical Nerve Stimulation (TENS): A TENS machine is a small device that sends electrical impulses to certain parts of the body to block pain signals. Two electrodes are placed on the body where you are experiencing pain. The electrical current that is produced is very mild, but it can prevent pain messages from being transmitted to the brain. Pain relief can last for several hours. Some people may use a small, portable TENS unit that hooks onto a belt for more continuous relief. TENS machines should only be used under the supervision of a physician or physical therapist. They can be purchased or rented from hospital supply or surgical supply houses; however, a prescription is necessary for insurance reimbursement.

Braces and supports: Spinal supports or braces reduce pain and inflammation by restricting movement. Following a vertebral fracture, a back brace or support will relieve pain and allow you to resume normal activities while the fracture heals. However, continuous use of a back support can weaken back muscles. For this reason, exercises to strengthen the muscles in the back should be started as soon as possible.

Exercise and physical therapy: Prolonged inactivity increases weakness and causes loss of muscle mass and strength. A regular exercise program and physical therapy can help you regain strength, energy, and a more positive outlook on life. Because exercise raises the body's level of endorphins—natural pain killers produced by the brain—it will relieve pain somewhat. Exercise also relieves tension, increases flexibility, strengthens muscles, and reduces fatigue.

A physical therapist can help you reorganize your home or work environment to avoid further injuries. Physical therapists also teach proper posture and exercises to strengthen the back and abdominal muscles without injuring a weakened spine. Water therapy in a pool, for example, is one of the best exercise techniques for gently improving back muscle strength and reducing pain.

Acupuncture and acupressure: Acupuncture is the use of special needles that are inserted into the body at certain points. These needles stimulate nerve endings and cause the brain to release endorphins. It may take several acupuncture sessions before the pain is relieved. Acupuncture has been used for centuries in China and other parts of Asia to treat many types of pain.

Acupressure is direct pressure applied to areas that trigger pain. This technique can be self-administered after training with an instructor.

Massage therapy: Massage therapy can be a light, slow, circular motion with the fingertips or a deep, kneading motion that moves from the center of the body outward toward the fingers or toes. Massage relieves pain, relaxes stiff muscles, and smoothes out muscle knots by increasing the blood supply to the affected area and warming it. The person doing the massage uses oil or powder so that her or his hands slide smoothly over the skin. Massage can also include gentle pressure over the affected areas or hard pressure over trigger points in muscle knots.

Note: Deep muscle massage should not be done near the spine of a person who has spinal osteoporosis. Light, circular massage with fingers or the palm of the hand is best in this case.

Coping Strategies: Psychological Methods of Pain Management

Relaxation training: Relaxation involves concentration and slow, deep breathing to release tension from muscles and relieve pain. Learning to relax takes practice, but relaxation training can focus attention away from pain and release tension from all muscles. Relaxation tapes are widely available to help you learn these skills.

Biofeedback: Biofeedback is taught by a professional who uses special machines to help you learn to control bodily functions, such as heart rate and muscle tension. As you learn to release muscle tension, the machine immediately indicates success. Biofeedback can be used to reinforce relaxation training. Once the technique is mastered, it can be practiced without the use of the machine.

Visual imagery and distraction: Imagery involves concentrating on mental pictures of pleasant scenes or events or mentally repeating positive words or phrases to reduce pain. Tapes are also available to help you learn visual imagery skills.

Distraction techniques focus your attention away from negative or painful images to positive mental thoughts. This may include activities as simple as watching television or a favorite movie, reading a book, listening to a book on tape, listening to music, or talking to a friend.

Hypnosis: Hypnosis can be used in two ways to reduce your perception of pain. Some people are hypnotized by a therapist and given a post-hypnotic suggestion that reduces the pain they feel. Others are taught self-hypnosis and can hypnotize themselves when pain interrupts their ability to function. Self-hypnosis is a form of relaxation training.

Individual, group, or family therapy: These forms of psychotherapy may be useful for those whose pain has not responded to physical methods. People who suffer from chronic pain often experience emotional stress and depression. Therapy can help you cope with these feelings, making it easier to manage your pain.

Coping Strategies: Medication for Pain Management

Medications are the most popular way to manage pain. Commonly used medications include aspirin, acetaminophen, and ibuprofen. Although these are probably the safest pain relievers available, they sometimes cause stomach irritation and bleeding.

Narcotic drugs may be prescribed for short-term acute pain. These drugs should not be used for long periods because they are addictive and can affect your ability to think clearly. They also have other side effects, such as constipation.

Many people with persistent pain that has not responded to other forms of pain relief are treated with antidepressant medication. These drugs may work in a different way when used for treatment of unyielding pain. The body's internal pain suppression system may depend upon the concentrations of various chemicals in the brain. These concentrations are increased by the use of antidepressants.

Chapter 67

Choosing a Multidisciplinary Pain Program

To regain control of your life, it is important to learn how to cope with chronic pain. Although your pain may never go away, it is possible to reduce pain levels and, more importantly, to improve the quality of your life. To do so, you may need a multidisciplinary approach to chronic pain. While many people with pain have tried every available medical intervention without great success, sometimes these therapies are most effective when performed together in a controlled setting.

A multidisciplinary pain program can provide you with the necessary skills, medical intervention, and direction to effectively cope with chronic pain. Here is advice on how to locate a pain management program in your area, what to look for in a well-defined pain program, and what other issues to consider.

Consumer Guidelines to Selecting a Pain Unit

Make Sure You Locate a Legitimate Program

- Hospitals and rehabilitation centers are more likely to offer comprehensive treatment than are "stand alone" programs.

- Facilities that offer pain management should include several specific components:

- The Commission on Accreditation of Rehabilitation Facilities (CARF), online at http://www.carf.org or telephone: 888-281-6531, can provide you with a listing of accredited pain programs in your area (your health insurance may require that the unit be CARF accredited in order for you to receive reimbursement).

- You can also contact the American Pain Society, an organization for health care providers, at http://www.ampainsoc.org or 847-375-4715, for additional information about pain units in your area.

Choose a Good Program That Is Convenient for You and Your Family

- Most pain management programs are part of a hospital or rehabilitation center. The program should be housed in a separate unit designed for pain management.

- Many pain management programs do not offer inpatient care. Choosing a program close to your home will enable you to commute to the program each day.

Learn Something about the People Who Run the Program

Try to meet several of the staff members to get a sense of the people you will be dealing with while on the unit. The program should have a complete medical staff trained in pain management techniques including:

- Physician (a neurologist, psychiatrist, physiatrist, or anesthesiologist with expertise in pain management)
- Registered nurse
- Psychiatrist or psychologist
- Physical therapist
- Occupational therapist
- Biofeedback therapist
- Family counselor
- Vocational counselor
- Massage therapy
- Other personnel trained in pain management intervention

Make Sure the Program Includes Most of the Following Features

- Biofeedback training

- Group therapy

- Counseling

- Occupational therapy

- Family counseling

- Assertiveness training

- Transcutaneous Electrical Nerve Stimulation (TENS) units

- Regional anesthesia (nerve blocks)

- Physical therapy (for example, exercise and body mechanics training, not massage, whirlpool)

- Relaxation training and stress management

- Educational program covering medications and other aspects of pain and its management

- Aftercare (follow-up support once you have left the unit)

Be Sure Your Family Can Be Involved in Your Care

- Family members should be required to be involved in your treatment.

- The program should provide special educational sessions for family members.

- Joint counseling for you and your family should also be available.

Consider These Additional Factors

- What services will your medical insurance reimburse and what will you be expected to cover?

- Will you need a primary care physician (PCP) referral?

- What is the unit's physical set-up (is it in a patient care area or in an area by itself)?

- What is the program's length of stay?

- Is the program inpatient or outpatient (when going through medication detoxification, inpatient care is recommended)?

- If you choose an out-of-town unit, can your family be involved in your care?

- Do you understand what will be required of you during your stay (for example, length of time you will be on unit, responsibility to take care of personal needs)?

- Does the unit provide any type of job retraining?

Make sure that, before accepting you, the unit reviews your medical records and gives you a complete physical evaluation to be sure you can participate in the program. Obtain copies of your recent medical records to prevent duplicate testing.

Try to talk with both present and past program participants to get their feedback about their stay on the unit.

Pain programs are difficult, but pain management can make a significant difference in your life. You must realize, however, that much of what you gain from your stay will be up to you.

For More Information

American Chronic Pain Association
P.O. Box 850
Rocklin, CA 95677
Toll-Free: 800-533-3231
Fax: 916-632-3208
Website: http://www.theacpa.org
E-mail: ACPA@pacbell.net

Chapter 68

Managing Breakthrough Pain

Do you feel that your daily pain is fairly well controlled, yet still find there are times when you experience a sudden flare of pain that breaks through? These flares are called breakthrough pain or BTP.

What is BTP?

Breakthrough pain is an intense increase in pain that occurs suddenly even when pain-control medication is being used. Breakthrough pain can happen spontaneously or in relation to a specific activity. BTP can start and become severe in as little as three to five minutes and last an average of 30 to 60 minutes. Most people with BTP report that it happens three to four times a day. Sixty-four percent of people treated for chronic pain associated with cancer and seventy-four percent of people treated for other chronic pain conditions will experience BTP.

What causes it?

BTP can hit unexpectedly at any time or place and it may be hard to identify what triggers it. A cough or rolling over in bed can cause BTP. Or, it can happen when a dose of your persistent pain medicine wears off before it is time to take another dose.

The Impact of Untreated BTP

Even when persistent pain is well controlled, BTP can be devastating for you and your family or caregivers. Untreated BTP can:

- make you feel depressed and irritable;

- cause you to you avoid people, even those you love;

- make you isolate yourself and prevent you from enjoying normal activities;

- keep you from getting a goods night's sleep;

- interfere with doing a good job at work or even keeping a job;

- make it more difficult to relieve your persistent pain;

- increase the number of visits to your doctors and to emergency departments.

Understanding Your BTP

The first step to coping with your BTP is to learn more about it. Keep a log of when it occurs and what you were doing at the time. Note your stress levels and state of mind, as well.

Review your log every week to see if there are certain times of the day that BTP occurs. You also may find that certain activities or feelings trigger your BTP. When you know more about what causes BTP, you can begin to manage it better.

Always take your log with you to your doctor appointments. Talk to your health care provider about your concerns and fears. When your health care provider understands your issues, he or she can work with you to find a solution.

Getting the Right Treatment for Your Pain

The key to relieving breakthrough pain is to learn why these flares of pain are different from the pain you feel all day. You can:

- Talk with your doctor about medication that might help during BTP episodes. When using pain medications for BTP, the goal should always be improved pain relief and improved function.

- Ask your doctor about biofeedback training or stress management classes. Reducing stress may help you reduce the number of episodes of BTP you have or lessen their severity.

- Understand what activities create BTP. Then you can pace your activities so you don't push yourself beyond your limits.

- Learn about the pain management skills offered through the American Chronic Pain Association (ACPA).

- Involve your family in your treatment plans.

For many people with moderate-to-severe chronic pain who also experience BTP, a logical treatment plan includes a pain medicine that can be taken at regular times around-the-clock to treat persistent pain, plus a short-acting medicine to take when you need to relieve the rapid onset of a BTP flare. In addition, you can get involved in managing your pain by practicing relaxation techniques, setting more realistic goals, pacing yourself, and asking for help when you need it to avoid triggering flares.

Managing BTP is a group effort. Work with your health care team to find the overall treatment plan that's right for you.

Prepare for Your Next Doctor Visit

- Note if there is a regular time during the day when your persistent pain medicine doesn't last until you can take another dose.

- List methods of pain relief you have tried, such as exercise, meditation, or stress reduction, and how they work.

- List all the pain medicine you are taking, including over-the-counter medications, vitamins, and herbal supplements. Include a list of all medications or other treatments you take for any other reason, as well.

- List treatable conditions (for example, persistent cough, nausea, constipation) that you feel might be a source of BTP.

- Take your pain log with you.

- Talk about activities your pain interferes with or the impact it has on your life.

Like all pain, BTP can be managed but you must play an active role in the recovery process by becoming part of the treatment team. Working with your health care team, taking part in a peer support group, and learning as much as you can, will help you make the transition from patient to person.

For More Information on Pain Management and BTP

American Cancer Society
National Home Office
250 Williams St. N.W.
Atlanta, GA 30303
Toll-Free: 800-ACS-2345 (227-2345)
Website: http://www.cancer.org

American Chronic Pain Association
P.O. Box 850
Rocklin, CA 95677
Toll-Free: 800-533-3231
Phone: 916-632-0922
Fax: 916-632-3208
Website: http://www.theacpa.org
E-mail: ACPA@pacbell.net

American Pain Society
4700 W. Lake Ave.
Glenview, IL 60025-1485
Phone: 847-375-4715
Fax: 877-734-8758
Website: http://www.ampainsoc.org
E-mail: info@ampainsoc.org

OncoLink
Abramson Cancer Center of the University of Pennsylvania
3400 Spruce St., 2 Donner
Philadelphia, PA 19104-4283
Fax: 215-349-5445
Website: http://www.oncolink.com

Chapter 69

Palliative Care: Symptom Management and End-of-Life Care

Chapter Contents

Section 69.1

Palliative Care at Home

Management of Pain

Assess the patient for pain:

- Determine the cause of the pain by history and examination (for new pain and any change in pain).

- Determine the type of pain—is it common pain (such as bone or mouth pain) or special pain (such as shooting nerve pain, zoster, colic, or muscle spasms)?

- Is there a psychological or spiritual component?

- Grade the pain with a pain scale or with your hand (with zero being no pain, one finger very mild pain, and five fingers the worst possible pain). Record your findings.

Treat pain, according to whether it is a common or a special pain problem or both with the following:

- analgesics

- medications to control special pain problems, as appropriate; explain reason for treatment and side effects; always take into account patient preference

- non-medical treatments

Reassess need for pain medication and other interventions frequently. Repeat grading of the pain. Investigate any new problems.

Treat Chronic Pain

By mouth:

- If possible, give by mouth (rectal is an alternative—avoid intramuscular).

By the clock:

- Give pain killers at fixed time intervals (by clock, radio, or sun).
- Start with small dose, then titrate dose against patient's pain, until the patient is comfortable.
- Next dose should happen before effect of previous dose wears off.
- For breakthrough pain, give an extra "rescue" dose (same dosing of the 4-hourly dose) in addition to the regular schedule.

By the individual:

- Link first and last dose with waking and sleeping times.
- Write out drug regimen in full or present in a drawing.
- Teach its use.
- Check to be sure patient and family or assistant at home understand it.
- Ensure that pain does not return and patient is as alert as possible.

Give Medications to Control Special Pain Problems

There are nerve injury pains and pains from special conditions which can be relieved by specific medication. Ask your health care provider about medication for special pain problems such as burning pains, muscle spasms in end-of-life care, herpes zoster pain, gastrointestinal pain, bone pain, or other nerve or persistent pain.

Teach patient and family how to give pain medications—this applies to all pain medications:

- Explain frequency and importance of giving regularly—do not wait for the pain to return. The next dose should be given before the previous dose wears off—usually every four hours.
- The aim of pain treatment is that the pain will not come back and the patient is as alert as possible.
- Write out instructions clearly.

Table 69.1. Respond to Side Effects of Morphine or Other Opioids

If patient has this side effect:	Then manage as follows:
Constipation	Increase fluids and bulk. Give stool softener (docusate) at time of prescribing plus stimulant (senna). Prevent by prophylaxis (unless diarrhea).
Nausea or vomiting	Give an antiemetic (metoclopramide, haloperidol, or chlorpromazine). Usually resolves in several days. May need round-the-clock dosing.
Respiratory depression (rare when oral morphine is increased step by step for pain)	If severe, consider withholding next opioid dose, then halve dose.
Confusion or drowsiness (if due to opioid); Decreased alertness; Trouble with decisions	Usually occurs at start of treatment or dose is increased. Usually resolves within few days. Can occur at end of life with renal failure. Halve dose or increase time between doses. Or provide time with less analgesia when patient wants to be more fully alert to make decisions.
Twitching (myoclonus— if severe or bothers patient during waking hours)	If on high dose, consider reducing dose or changing opioids (consult or refer). Re-assess the pain and its treatment.
Somnolence (excessively sleepy)	Extended sleep can be from exhaustion due to pain. If persists more than two days after starting, reduce the dose by half.
Itching	May occur with normal dose. If present for more than a few days and hard to tolerate, give chlorpheniramine.
Urinary retention	Pass urinary catheter if trained—in and out since it usually does not recur.

Reduce morphine when cause of pain is controlled:

- If used only for a short time, stop or rapidly reduce.
- If used for weeks, reduce gradually to avoid withdrawal symptoms.

Advise Family on Additional Methods for Pain Control

Combine these with pain medications if patient agrees and it helps (for local adaptation):

- Emotional support

- Physical methods of touch (stroking, massage, rocking, vibration), ice or heat, or deep breathing

- Cognitive methods such as distraction with radio, music, imagining a pleasant scene

- Prayer (respect patient's practice)

- Traditional practices which are helpful and not harmful

Teach Family to Give Oral Morphine

Oral morphine is a strong pain killer. It should be given to the sick person, by mouth, and by the clock (regularly, approximately every four hours).

Help the caregiver manage side effects:

- Nausea—this usually goes away after a few days of morphine and does not usually come again

- Constipation—offer water, fruit

- Dry mouth—give sips of water

- Drowsiness—this usually goes away after a few days of morphine; if it persists or gets worse, halve the dose and inform the health worker

- Sweating or muscle jerks—tell the health worker

If the pain is getting worse, inform the health worker as the dose may be increased.

If the pain is getting better, the dose may be reduced by half. Inform the health worker, but do not stop the drug suddenly.

Preventive Interventions for All Patients

Preventive Oral Care for All Patients

Instruct all patients in oral care:

- Use soft toothbrush to gently brush teeth, tongue, palate, and gums to remove debris.

- Use diluted sodium bicarbonate (baking soda) or toothpaste.

- Rinse mouth with diluted salt water after eating and at bedtime (usually 3–4 times daily).

Prevent Bedsores in All Bedridden Patients

Remember that prevention of bedsores is better than cure:

- Help the bedridden patient to sit in a chair from time to time if possible.

- Lift the sick person up the bed—do not drag as it breaks the skin.

- Encourage the sick person to move his or her body in bed if able.

- Change the sick person's position on the bed often, if possible every one or two hours—use pillows or cushions to keep the position.

- Keep the beddings clean and dry.

- Look for damaged skin (change of color) on the back, shoulders, and hips every day.

- Put extra soft material such as a soft cotton towel under the sick person.

Instructions for Bathing

- Provide privacy during bathing.

- Dry the skin after bath gently with a soft towel.

- Oil the skin with cream, body oil, lanolin, or vegetable oil.

- Use plastic sheets under the bed sheets to keep the bed dry when one cannot control urine or feces.

- Massage the back and hips, elbows, and ankles with petroleum jelly.

- If there is leakage of urine or stool, protect skin with petroleum jelly applied around private parts, back, hips, ankles, and elbows.

- Support the sick person over the container when passing urine or stool, so as to avoid wetting the bed and injury.

Prevent Pain, Stiffness, and Contractures in Muscles and Joints

- Encourage mobilization.
- If patient is immobile, do simple range of motion exercises:
  - Exercise limbs and joints at least twice daily.
  - Protect the joint by holding the limb above and below it and support as much as you can.
  - Bend, straighten, and move joints as far as they normally go; be gentle and move slowly without causing pain.
  - Stretch joints by holding as before but with firm, steady pressure.
  - Let the patient do it as far as they can and help the rest of the way.
  - Massage.

Exercises to Help Prevent Pain Stiffness and Contractures

- Exercise the elbow by gently bringing the hand as close as possible to the shoulder.
- Exercise the wrist doing the full ROM (range of motion).
- Exercise the shoulder by lifting the arm up and bringing it behind the head and laterally as far as possible.
- Exercise the knee by lifting the thigh up and bringing it close to the chest and laterally as far as possible.

Moving the Bedridden Patient

The following instructions are for a single caregiver. If the patient is unconscious or unable to cooperate, it is better to have two people help with moving.

1. Roll the patient on one side.

2. Move the patient to the side of the bed. Ask the patient to bend legs and to prop on the same side elbow.

3. Hold your hands on the patient's pelvis, ask to raise their buttocks. Sit patient on the edge of the bed with feet flat on the floor.

4. Stand in front of the patient and hold both shoulders. Keep patient's feet flat on the floor.

5. Help patient raise bottom from the bed and rotate patient towards the chair.

6. Transfer from bed to chair. Hold patient under their shoulders and with your knees.

Remember if you lose your balance, it is better to help the patient fall gently rather than hurting yourself.

Manage Key Symptoms: Home Care

Treat Weight Loss

- Encourage the sick person to eat, but do not use force as the body may not be able to accept it, and he or she may vomit.

- Offer smaller meals frequently of what the sick person likes.

- Let the sick person choose the foods he or she wants to eat from what is available.

- Accept that intake will reduce as patient gets sicker and during end-of-life care.

Seek help from a trained health worker if you notice rapid weight loss, or if the sick person consistently refuses to eat any food, or is not able to swallow.

Control Nausea and Vomiting

If the sick person feels like vomiting:

- Seek locally available foods which patient likes (tastes may change with illness) and which cause less nausea.

- Frequently offer small amounts of foods such as roasted potatoes, cassava, or rice.

- Offer the drinks the sick person likes, such as water, juice, or tea; ginger drinks can help.

- Take drinks slowly and more frequently.

- Avoid cooking close to the sick person.

- Use effective and safe local remedies.

Seek help from a trained health worker for vomiting of more than one day, dry tongue, passing little urine, or abdominal pain.

For Painful Mouth Ulcers or Pain when Swallowing

- Remove bits of food stuck in the mouth with cotton wool, gauze, or soft cloth soaked in salt water.
- Rinse the mouth with diluted salt water (a finger pinch of salt or ½ teaspoon sodium bicarbonate in a glass of water) after eating and at bedtime.
- Mix two tablets of aspirin in water and rinse the mouth up to four times a day.

Diet

- Give a soft diet such as yogurt to decrease discomfort, depending on what the sick person feels is helpful.
- Give more textured foods and fluids that may be swallowed more easily than fluids.
- Avoid extremely hot, cold, or spicy foods.

Seek help from a health worker for persistent sores, smelly mouth, white patches, or difficult swallowing.

Treat Dry Mouth

- Encourage frequent sips of drinks.
- Moisten his or her mouth regularly with water.
- Let the sick person suck on fruits such as pineapple, oranges, or passion fruit.

Seek help from a health worker if dry mouth persists.

Prevent and Treat Constipation

- Offer drinks often.
- Encourage any fruits, vegetables, porridge, or locally available high-fiber foods.

- Use local herbal treatment, for example, crush some dried paw-paw seeds and mix half a teaspoon full of water and give to the sick person to drink.

- Take a tablespoon of vegetable oil before breakfast.

- If impacted, gently put petroleum jelly or soapy solution into the rectum. If the patient cannot do it, the caregiver can help—always use hand gloves.

Seek help from a trained worker if stool causes pain or no stool is passed in five days.

Incontinence of Urine

- Regularly change cloth or disposable pads.

- Keep patient dry.

- Protect skin with petroleum jelly.

Vaginal Discharge from Cervical Cancer

- Sit in basin of water with pinch of salt. If this is comfortable, do twice daily.

Incontinence of Stool

- Use cotton cloth or disposable pads and plastic or rubber pants.

- Keep patient clean—change cloth or disposable pads as needed.

Rectal Tenderness

Special care for the rectal area:

- After the sick person has passed stool clean with toilet or soft tissue paper; wash the rectal area when necessary with soap and water; and apply petroleum jelly around the rectal area.

- Sit in basin of water with pinch of salt. If this is comfortable do twice daily.

Manage Diarrhea

- Increase fluid intake:

- Encourage patient to drink plenty of fluids to replace lost water.

- Give the sick person drinks frequently in small amounts, such as rice soup, porridge, water (with food), other soups, or oral rehydration solution (ORS), but avoid sweet drinks.

- Continue eating.

Seek help from a health worker for the following situations:

- Vomiting with fever

- Blood in the stool

- Diarrhea that continues more than five days

- If patient becomes even weaker

- If there is broken skin around the rectal area

Manage Persistent Diarrhea

For persistent diarrhea, suggest a supportive diet.

- Carrot soup helps to replace vitamins and minerals. Carrot soup contains pectin. It soothes the bowels and stimulates the appetite.

- Foods that may help reduce diarrhea are rice and potatoes.

- Eat bananas and tomatoes (for their potassium).

- Eat 5–6 small meals rather than three large ones.

- Add nutmeg to food.

Avoid the following:

- Coffee, strong tea, and alcohol

- Raw foods, cold foods, high-fiber foods, food containing much fat

- Test the benefit of avoiding milk and cheese (yogurt is better tolerated)

Help with Worries

- Take time to listen to the sick person.

- Discuss the problem in confidence.

- Providing soft music or massage may help the sick person to relax.

- Pray together if requested.

For Trouble Sleeping

- Listen to the sick person's fears that may be keeping them awake; answer their fears.

- Reduce noise where possible.

- Do not give the sick person strong tea or coffee late in the evening.

- Treat pain if present.

Care for Patient Experiencing Confusion (Dementia or Delirium)

Patients with confusion will show the following signs:

- forgetful

- lacks concentration

- trouble speaking or thinking

- frequently changing mood

- unacceptable behavior, such as going naked and using bad language

What to Do

- As far as possible, keep patient in a familiar environment.

- Keep things in the same place—easy to reach and see.

- Keep familiar schedules for the day's activities.

- Remove dangerous objects.

- Speak in simple sentences, one person at a time.

- Keep other noises down (such as television, radio).

- Make sure somebody they trust is present to look after the sick person and supervises.

Detect and Treat Depression

- Provide support.

- If at suicide risk, do not leave alone. Also advise caregiver to gradually take more control of medications.

Treat Itching

You can help the sick person get some relief by trying any of the following:

- If dry skin, moisturize with aqueous cream or petroleum jelly mixed with water.

- Put one tablespoon of vegetable oil in a gallon of water when washing the sick person.

- Rub the itchy skin with local remedies (examples: effective and safe herbs, cucumber, wet tea bags, or tea leaves put in a clean piece of cloth and soaked in hot water).

- Use water for bathing that is at a comfortable temperature for the patient.

Seek help from a trained health worker for painful blisters or extensive skin infection.

Treat Bedsores

You can do the following to soothe the pain of bedsores and quicken healing:

- For small sores, clean gently with salty water and allow to dry.

- Apply ripe paw-paw flesh to bedsores that are not deep and leave the wound open to the air.

- If painful, give pain killers such as acetaminophen, ibuprofen, or aspirin regularly.

- For deep or large sores, every day clean gently with diluted salt water, fill the bedsore area with pure honey or ripe paw-paw flesh, and cover with a clean light dressing to encourage healing.

Seek help from a trained health worker for any discolored skin or bedsores getting worse.

Section 69.2

Helping Cancer Patients Help Themselves

Text in this section is from "Pain Control," National Cancer Institute (NCI),
January 24, 2008.

Cancer Pain Can Be Managed

Having cancer doesn't mean that you'll have pain. But if you do, you can manage most of your pain with medicine and other treatments. People who have cancer don't always have pain. Everyone is different. But if you do have cancer pain, you should know that you don't have to accept it. Cancer pain can almost always be relieved.

Cancer pain can be reduced so that you can enjoy your normal routines and sleep better. It may help to talk with a pain specialist. These may be oncologists, anesthesiologists, neurologists, surgeons, other doctors, nurses, or pharmacists. If you have a pain control team, it may also include psychologists and social workers.

Pain and palliative care specialists are experts in pain control. Palliative care specialists treat the symptoms, side effects, and emotional problems of both cancer and its treatment. They will work with you to find the best way to manage your pain. Ask your doctor or nurse to suggest someone. Or contact one of the following for help finding a pain specialist in your area:

- Cancer center

- Your local hospital or medical center

- Your primary care provider

- People who belong to pain support groups in your area

- The Center to Advance Palliative Care, available online at http://www.getpalliativecare.org (for lists of providers in each state)

When cancer pain is not treated properly, you may be:

- tired,

- depressed,

- angry,

- worried,

- lonely, or

- stressed.

When cancer pain is managed properly, you can do the following:

- Enjoy being active

- Sleep better

- Enjoy family and friends

- Improve your appetite

- Enjoy sexual intimacy

- Prevent depression

Types and Causes of Cancer Pain

Cancer pain can range from mild to very severe. Some days it can be worse than others. It can be caused by the cancer itself, the treatment, or both.

You may also have pain that has nothing to do with your cancer. Some people have other health issues or headaches and muscle strains. But always check with your doctor before taking any over-the-counter medicine to relieve everyday aches and pains.

Controlling pain is a key part of your overall cancer treatment. The most important member of the team is you. You're the only one who knows what your pain feels like. Talking about pain is important. It gives your health care team the feedback they need to make you feel better.

Tell your health care team if you are:

- taking any medicine to treat other health problems;

- taking more or less of the pain medicine than prescribed;

- allergic to certain drugs; or

- using any over-the-counter medicines, home remedies, or herbal or alternative therapies.

This information could affect the pain control plan your doctor suggests for you.

If you feel uneasy talking about your pain, ask a family member or friend to speak for you. Or let your loved one take notes and ask questions. Remember, open communication between you, your loved ones, and your health care team will lead to better pain control.

Talking about Your Pain

The first step in getting your pain under control is talking honestly about it. Try to talk with your health care team and your loved ones about what you are feeling. This means telling them the following:

- Where you have pain

- What it feels like (sharp, dull, throbbing, constant, burning, or shooting)

- How strong your pain is

- How long it lasts

- What lessens your pain or makes it worse

- When it happens (what time of day, what you're doing, and what's going on)

- If it gets in the way of daily activities

Describe and Rate Your Pain

No matter how you or your doctor keep track of your pain, make sure that you do it the same way each time. You also need to talk about any new pain you feel.

It may help to keep a record of your pain. Some people use a pain notebook or journal. Others create a list or a computer spreadsheet. Choose the way that works best for you.

Your record could list the following:

- When you take pain medicine

- Name and dose of the medicine you're taking

- Any side effects you have

- How long the pain medicine works

- Other pain relief methods you use to control your pain

- Any activity that is affected by pain, or makes it better or worse

- Things that you cannot do at all because of the pain

Share your record with your health care team. It can help them figure out how helpful your pain medicines are, or if they need to change your pain control plan.

Make Your Pain Control Plan Work for You

Your pain control plan will be designed for you and your body. Everyone has a different pain control plan. Even if you have the same type of cancer as someone else, your plan may be different.

Take your pain medicine dose on schedule to keep the pain from starting or getting worse. This is one of the best ways to stay on top of your pain. Do not skip doses. Once you feel pain, it is harder to control and may take longer to get better.

Here are some other things you can do:

- Bring your list of medicines to each visit.

- If you are seeing more than one doctor, make sure each one sees your list of medicines, especially if he or she is going to change or prescribe medicine.

- Never take someone else's medicine. What helped a friend or relative may not help you. Do not get medicine from other countries or the internet without telling your doctor.

- Do not wait for the pain to get worse.

- Ask your doctor to change your pain control plan if it isn't working.

Do not wait until the pain gets bad or unbearable before taking your medicine. Pain is easier to control when it is mild. And you need to take pain medicine often enough to stay ahead of your pain. Follow the dose schedule your doctor gives you. Do not try to hold off between doses.

- Your pain could get worse.

- It may take longer for the pain to get better or go away.

- You may need larger doses to bring the pain under control.

Your Feelings and Pain

Having pain and cancer affects every part of your life. It can affect not only your body, but your thoughts and feelings as well. Whether you have a lot of pain or a little, if it is constant, you may feel like you are not able to focus on anything else. It may keep you from doing things and seeing people that you normally do. This can be upsetting and may feel like a cycle that never seems to end.

Sometimes things that people used to take for granted are not as easy anymore. These may include cooking, getting dressed, or just moving around. Some people cannot work because of the pain or have to cut back on their hours. They may worry about money. Limits on work and everyday life may also make people less social, wanting to see others less often.

Research shows that people in pain may feel sad or anxious and may get depressed more often. At other times they may feel angry and frustrated. And they can feel lonely, even if they have others around them.

A common result of having cancer and being in pain is fear. For many, pain and fear together feel like suffering. People get upset worrying about the future. They focus their thoughts on things that may or may not happen. You may feel fear about many things, such as fear of the following:

- The cancer getting worse
- The pain being too much to handle
- Your job or daily tasks becoming too hard to do
- Not being able to attend special trips or events
- Loss of control

This roller coaster of feelings often makes people look for the meaning that cancer and pain have in their life. Some question why this could happen to them. They wonder what they did to deserve it. Others may turn to religion or explore their spirituality more, asking for guidance and strength.

If you have feelings like these, know that you're not alone. Many people with cancer pain have had these kinds of feelings. Having negative thoughts is normal. And some people have positive thoughts, too, finding benefits in facing cancer. But if your negative thoughts overwhelm you, don't ignore your feelings. Help is there for you if you're distressed about your future.

Finding Support

There are many people who can help you. You can talk with oncology social workers, health psychologists, or other mental health experts at your hospital or clinic. Your health care team can help you find a counselor who is trained to help people with long-term illnesses. These people can help you talk about what you are going through and find answers to your concerns. They may suggest medicine that will help you feel better if you need it.

Many people say that they regain a sense of control and well-being after talking with people in their spiritual or religious community. A leader from one of these groups may be able to offer support, too. Many are trained to help people cope with illness. Also, many hospitals have a staff chaplain who can counsel people of all faiths.

You can also talk with friends or others in your community. Some join a support group. Cancer support groups are made up of people who share their feelings about coping with cancer. They can meet in person, by phone, or over the internet. They may help you gain new insights and ideas on how to cope. To find a support group for you, talk with your doctor, nurse, or oncology social worker.

Talking with Family Members

You may want to let family members and friends know how you are feeling. For some, this can be hard or awkward. Some people say that they want to avoid upsetting those closest to them. Others say that they do not want to seem negative. But open and honest communication can help everyone. Letting others know about your pain may help them understand what you are going through. They can then look for ways to help you. Your loved ones may also feel better knowing that they are helping to make you feel more comfortable.

Family Problems before Your Cancer

Any problems your family had before you got cancer are likely to be more intense now. Or maybe your family just does not communicate very well. If this is the case, you can ask a social worker to set up a family meeting for you. During these meetings, the doctor can explain treatment goals and issues. And you and your family members can state your wishes for care. These meetings can also give everyone a chance to express their feelings in the open. Remember, there are many people you can turn to at this time.

Chapter 70

Pain Affects Sleep: What You Can Do

When Pain and Sleep Problems Arise

When you have aches and pains, you are also likely to lose a lot of sleep. When pain disrupts sleep, it may lead to difficulty maintaining alertness, lack of energy, impaired mood, and trouble handling stress. Lack of sleep can also put you at risk for injury, poor health, workplace accidents, and motor vehicle crashes.

Pain and Sleep: A Two-Way Street

Pain can cause difficulty falling asleep, nighttime awakenings, or waking too early in the morning. Hence, people who suffer from pain during sleep often find it difficult to function at their best.

In fact, studies have shown that sleep loss can make a person more sensitive to pain. One study found that the kind of sleep deprivation caused by continuous sleep disturbances throughout the night, in particular, caused an increase in spontaneous pain and impaired the body's ability to process and cope with painful stimuli.

Understanding Your Pain and Your Sleep

What's keeping you awake? Whether it's back pain, headaches, arthritis, or other health problems, you can work with your doctor to identify the cause and find a treatment to improve your symptoms and your sleep.

When preparing to talk with your doctor, ask yourself:

1. How often does the pain occur? Is it sudden and acute, or is it chronic?

2. Have you noticed any triggers that seem to cause the pain or make it worse?

3. When you have pain, do you also have difficulty falling asleep, staying asleep, or waking earlier than you'd like?

4. How many hours of sleep do you normally get?

5. How often do you have problems sleeping?

6. Are you sleepy during the day, when you drive, or during other activities?

It may be helpful to keep a sleep diary for two weeks to record your sleep and health habits, and share this with your doctor during your next visit.

Back Pain

Back pain's cost to society is high—it is estimated to exceed $100 billion each year, mostly due to lost wages and reduced productivity. The personal cost is all too familiar to back pain sufferers, and often includes difficulty sleeping. Your doctor or a specialist can provide information on medications, exercises, acupuncture, or other behavioral changes that may help. Some medications may alter sleep patterns and make sleeping more difficult, so it is important to talk with your doctor to find the best treatment to manage both pain and sleep.

Headaches

Headaches can interfere with sleep, and changes in your sleep schedule or sleep problems can trigger or worsen headaches. Research shows that sleep disorders, such as sleep apnea and insomnia, are associated with chronic morning headaches, as well as cluster, tension, and migraine headaches. Managing sleep disorders such as sleep apnea or insomnia can improve headache symptoms, so it is important to talk with your doctor if you suspect you have a sleep disorder.

Among migraine sufferers, 50% report that sleep disturbances trigger migraines, and many report sleep problems such as insomnia. In one study, individuals who slept only six hours per night reported more frequent and more severe headaches than those who slept longer. Of the migraine sufferers in the study, 71% also reported that migraines awakened them from sleep.

People with migraines report an intense, throbbing pain in one area of the head, and often have nausea, fatigue, and sensitivity to light and sound. The attack may be preceded by an aura—visual disturbances such as flashing lights, zigzag lines, blind spots, or blurred vision. Migraine sufferers tend to have recurring episodes triggered by physical or mental stress, missed meals, alcohol, bright lights, hormonal fluctuations, or changes in sleep patterns. Sleep problems, lack of sleep, oversleeping to make up for lost sleep, or changing the sleep and wake schedule may contribute to migraines. Prescription medications are available to prevent and treat migraine attacks. It is also important to keep track of personal migraine triggers and to make sleep a priority.

Fibromyalgia

Sleep problems are common in fibromyalgia, a medical syndrome that includes widespread pain and stiffness, chronic fatigue, and many tender points throughout the body. Fibromyalgia can affect both sexes and people of all ages, but is most commonly diagnosed in middle-aged women. The cause is unknown, and researchers believe several factors may be involved, such as repetitive injuries, illness, automobile crashes, or other traumatic events. People with rheumatoid arthritis and other autoimmune diseases, such as lupus, are more likely to develop fibromyalgia.

The combination of pain and sleep disturbance can be a double-edged sword, since pain disturbs sleep, and sleep loss makes pain worse. Some research also suggests that people with fibromyalgia are more vulnerable to internal and environmental sleep disturbances since they may be more sensitive to sensory stimuli. Studies have also shown that people with fibromyalgia may lose deep sleep due to alpha wave interrupted sleep pattern, in which deep sleep is interrupted by bursts of brain activity similar to wakefulness. Restless legs syndrome, which causes unpleasant feelings in the limbs that tend to worsen at night and are relieved by movement, is also common in fibromyalgia and can interfere with sleep. Other symptoms of fibromyalgia can include headaches, numbness or tingling, irritable bowel syndrome, temperature sensitivity, cognitive and memory problems, and mood disturbances such as depression or anxiety.

There is no cure for fibromyalgia yet, and the best treatment often requires a team approach. This may involve your doctor, a physical therapist, a sleep specialist, or a pain or rheumatology clinic. Ways to cope include prioritizing sleep; low-impact exercises, such as walking, yoga, or swimming; and relaxation techniques, such as gentle massage and deep breathing. The drug pregabalin, recently approved by the Food and Drug Administration, can improve fibromyalgia symptoms by reducing pain. Medications used for other disorders may also help with fibromyalgia symptoms by alleviating pain and improving sleep, so it is important to talk with your doctor to find a treatment plan that is tailored to your needs. It is not uncommon to try several different therapy combinations before finding the one that works best for you.

Arthritis and Other Medical Conditions

Many people with rheumatic or arthritic disorders—for example, osteoarthritis, rheumatoid arthritis, and autoimmune diseases such as lupus—tend to have lighter or more restless sleep due to pain and stiffness. Doctors can provide information on exercises, diet, splints or braces, heat or cold therapies, and relaxation techniques that may lessen pain and promote sleep. While most rheumatic and arthritic diseases cannot be cured, there are medications that may help by targeting pain and inflammation or by slowing or preventing damage to joints and other tissues. By working with your doctor to manage your symptoms, you can improve your sleep quality which can lead to better health and quality of life.

In general, there is a high prevalence of sleep problems related to various medical conditions. For example, gastrointestinal problems, such as heartburn, ulcers, and irritable bowel syndrome often bring discomfort and lead to difficulty obtaining a good night's sleep. Medical conditions may also be associated with psychological distress which also contributes to poor, inadequate sleep. These sleep problems, in turn, can further aggravate medical conditions.

Managing Pain and Sleep Problems

To find a treatment plan tailored to your needs, it is important to talk with your doctor. He or she may recommend a combination of treatments that includes medication, lifestyle changes, or other therapies, such as exercises, relaxation techniques, dietary changes, or learning to control muscle tension or other body functions. You may also consider visiting a pain specialist.

Be sure to include sleep in your discussion with your doctor. It can help to share a complete description of your sleep experiences, including the following:

- The number of hours you usually sleep each night

- Whether you snore and how loudly

- Whether you gasp for breath or stop breathing during sleep

- Whether you have unpleasant tingling or crawling sensations in your legs that are relieved by movement

- How often you have difficulty falling asleep or staying asleep

- Whether you feel sleepy during the day or fall asleep when reading, watching television, or driving

- Whether you keep a regular bed and wake time

- Your use and timing of alcohol or tobacco products

- The time of day you use caffeinated products, exercise, and eat your last meal

- Whether you experience nighttime heartburn, pain, or the need to urinate

- Your level of stress and whether you have experienced lifestyle changes recently

- Whether you are an evening, night, or rotating shift worker

You may also want to bring results from your sleep diary, as well as medications or supplements you are taking. You may wish to speak with your physician about a referral to a sleep specialist who can also help with diagnosing and treating sleep disorders that may be aggravating your pain or medical condition.

What You Can Do to Get Good Sleep

Practicing healthy sleep habits can help improve the quality of your sleep.

Steps to Better Sleep

- Keep a regular bed and wake time schedule, including weekends. Exposing yourself to enough bright light during the day can also help you keep a consistent sleep schedule.

- Establish a relaxing bedtime routine such as listening to soft music, reading a book, or taking a warm bath. Avoid alerting activities or exposure to bright light before bedtime.

- Create a sleep-conducive environment that is cool, quiet, and dark. Block out unwanted noise with earplugs or use white noise such as a fan or air conditioner.

- Sleep on a mattress and pillows that are comfortable and supportive—choose the kind that suits you best.

- Use your bedroom only for sleep and sex.

- Avoid heavy meals or feeling hungry before bed. Finish eating meals at least 2–3 hours before bedtime. If you are hungry, a light, healthy snack is best.

- Exercise regularly, but finish at least a few hours before bedtime. A low-impact fitness program (for example, walking, swimming, stationary bicycle, yoga) carried out on a regular basis can be helpful for managing pain and stiffness and improving sleep.

- Avoid caffeine (coffee, tea, soda, or chocolate) in the afternoon and in the evening.

- Avoid alcohol close to bedtime since it disrupts sleep and causes nighttime awakenings.

- Avoid nicotine (cigarettes, tobacco products) which makes you more alert and causes withdrawal symptoms that disrupt sleep.

- Sleeping in the afternoon can interfere with nighttime sleep. If you need to take a nap, do so by mid-afternoon and for 15–30 minutes only.

- Talk with your doctor about other therapies or medications that may help.

Medications

Depending on your medical history and symptoms, your doctor may include medication as part of your treatment program. Work with your doctor to be sure any medication selected will not interact with others you are taking or cause sleep problems, since healthy sleep is an important part of any treatment plan.

Treating the Pain

Analgesics are medications designed specifically to relieve pain and include over-the-counter (OTC) products, such as acetaminophen, as well as prescription narcotics. To relieve both inflammation and pain, medications such as ibuprofen, aspirin, naproxen sodium, and ketoprofen are also available at your local drug store. Prescription-strength drugs that relieve pain and inflammation are also available from your doctor. Side effects can include stomach irritation and digestive problems, so it is important to work with your doctor to choose the medication that is safest and most effective for you.

Some prescription drugs used to treat other disorders, such as antidepressants, may be effective for controlling pain when used in a lower dose. For example, tricyclic medications and selective serotonin reuptake inhibitors (SSRIs) may be effective for some people. Some antidepressants can cause or worsen insomnia, however, so it is important to talk with your doctor about potential sleep effects of any medications you are taking.

When Pain Is Accompanied by Sleeplessness

When pain and sleeplessness strike at the same time, a combination of treatments may be recommended. Prescription drugs that promote sleep, called hypnotics, include drugs such as benzodiazepine agonists and ramelteon, and are proven to be effective and safe when used properly. Studies have shown that prescription hypnotics are effective and reliable for shortening the time it takes to fall asleep, increasing total sleep time, decreasing the number of awakenings during the night, and improving overall sleep quality. Over-the-counter sleep aids are also available, but it is important to use these medications carefully, since they tend to be longer-acting and may cause drowsiness the next day. With any type of sleep aid, it is important to follow instructions on proper dosage to ensure that it does not interfere with driving or other daytime activities. As with any medication, alcohol and other drugs can interact with sleep aids. Your doctor will be able to provide information on sleep aids and whether they should be part of your treatment plan.

For More Information

National Sleep Foundation
1522 K Street, N.W., Suite 500
Washington, DC 20005

Phone: 202-347-3471
Fax: 202-347-3472
Website: http://www.sleepfoundation.org
E-mail: nsf@sleepfoundation.org

Chapter 71

Positive Thinking Impacts the Pain Experience

While the theory that "mind over matter" exists is an ancient belief, the scientific studies to support this idea have remained elusive.
A new study provides brain imaging evidence that positive thinking
interacts with and shapes the sensory experience of pain. This study
suggests that decreasing the expectation of pain can reduce both the
pain-related brain activity and perception of pain intensity. This
knowledge may lead to new and effective ways to manage chronic pain.

"Our data shows that what you think really changes what you experience," says Robert Coghill, Ph.D. of Wake Forest University School
of Medicine in Winston-Salem, North Carolina. "Positive thinking
could be an important adjunct to managing chronic pain. The most
effective treatment for patients suffering from chronic pain may be a
combination of medicinal and psychological therapies." The study was
funded by the National Institute of Neurological Disorders and Stroke
(NINDS), a component of the National Institutes of Health (NIH), and
appeared in the September 6, 2005 issue of *Proceedings of the National
Academy of Sciences*.[1]

When expecting pain, we first form an active mental picture of the
event that is about to happen. This picture is composed by incorporating past experiences with the current situation and what we believe will happen. Secondly, brain regions that are involved with the

"Expectations of Pain: I Think, Therefore I Am," by Michelle D. Jones-Lon-
don, Ph.D., National Institute of Neurological Disorders and Stroke (NINDS),
January 31, 2007.

mental picture interact with the brain areas responsible for processing pain. As a result, the brain regions supporting the experience of pain are modulated by these predetermined expectations.

The new study focuses on this modulation of pain that is controlled by our expectations. The study uses functional magnetic resonance imaging (fMRI), a technology that shows which areas of the brain are activated during a task, to reveal the brain regions involved in the expectation of pain and the resulting experience. This is one of the first studies to look at pain perception through brain imaging techniques.

In the experiment, subjects participated in several sessions using a computer-controlled miniature heat pump to stimulate the sensation of pain. Researchers taught participants to expect three different levels of painful heat after different timed intervals. A seven-second interval signaled a heat level that caused mild pain, a 15-second interval signaled a heat level that produced moderate pain, and a 30-second interval signaled a heat level that produced severe pain. The heat stimuli were on for only 20 seconds and did not produce enough heat to cause burns or damage to the skin.

One or two days after training, participants underwent the fMRI testing during 30 different heat trials. During testing the researchers unexpectedly mixed the signals for the pain levels, so that participants were expecting one temperature, but actually received either a higher or lower temperature about 30 percent of the time. The researchers were able to see that levels of pain reported were reflected in the fMRI scans of the brain. People with decreased expectations for pain reported less pain. At the same time, activity decreased in areas of the brain important to both sensory and emotional processing of pain. These areas included the primary somatosensory cortex, the insular cortex, and the anterior cingulate cortex. These lower expectations reduced reports of pain by more than 28 percent. "Expectations about pain can affect its intensity at a level of pain reduction that is comparable to that of a normal dose of the painkiller morphine," says Dr. Coghill.

Many factors change the way that pain is perceived, and pain can be viewed as more intense or less intense depending on the situation. Different factors that can alter perception specifically when it comes to pain include how much attention is focused on the symptom. People also have different pain thresholds at which sensory nerves that carry pain information will send those signals. Some people need only a little stimulation in order for their nerves to send pain signals while others need a much greater amount of stimulation. Future research in the lab will examine the brains of people with these different thresholds for pain.

This study shows that the nature of pain perception is different in each individual. Not only are there individual differences in the nervous system, but also individual experiences contribute to how pain is perceived. The researchers are planning to use the fMRI technique to examine the effect of different personality types on pain perception. The study will examine how optimistic versus pessimistic personality types influence how people deal with pain and modulate pain processes in the brain.

"Pain needs to be treated with more than just pills," says Dr. Robert Coghill. "The brain can powerfully shape pain, and we need to exploit its power."

Reference

1. Koyama T, McHaffie JG, Laurienti PJ, Coghill RC. "The subjective experience of pain: Where expectations become reality." *Proceedings of the National Academy of Sciences*, September 6, 2005, Vol.102, pp.12950–12955.

Chapter 72

Managing Stress to Help Manage Pain

Stress can arise for a variety of reasons. Stress can be brought about by a traumatic accident, death, or emergency situation. Stress can also be a side effect of a serious illness or disease. There is also stress associated with daily life, the workplace, and family responsibilities.

Stress can take on many different forms and can contribute to symptoms of illness. Common symptoms include headache, sleep disorders, difficulty concentrating, short-temper, upset stomach, job dissatisfaction, low morale, depression, and anxiety.

How does stress affect my body and my health?

Everyone has stress. We have short-term stress, like getting lost while driving or missing the bus. Even everyday events, such as planning a meal or making time for errands, can be stressful. This kind of stress can make us feel worried or anxious.

Other times, we face long-term stress, such as racial discrimination, a life-threatening illness, or divorce. These stressful events also affect your health on many levels. Long-term stress is real and can increase your risk for some health problems, like depression.

Both short- and long-term stress can have effects on your body. Research is starting to show the serious effects of stress on our bodies. Stress triggers changes in our bodies and makes us more likely

---

Excerpted from "Stress and Your Health," U.S. Department of Health and Human Services (HHS), August 1, 2005.

to get sick. It can also make problems we already have worse. It can play a part in these problems:

- trouble sleeping
- headaches
- constipation
- diarrhea
- irritability
- lack of energy
- lack of concentration
- eating too much or not at all
- anger
- sadness
- higher risk of asthma and arthritis flare-ups
- tension
- stomach cramping
- stomach bloating
- skin problems, like hives
- depression
- anxiety
- weight gain or loss
- heart problems
- high blood pressure
- irritable bowel syndrome
- diabetes
- neck and/or back pain
- less sexual desire
- harder to get pregnant

What is post-traumatic stress disorder (PTSD)?

Post-traumatic stress disorder (PTSD) can be a debilitating condition that can occur after exposure to a terrifying event or ordeal in which grave physical harm occurred or was threatened. Traumatic events that can trigger PTSD include, violent personal assaults such as rape or mugging, natural or human-caused disasters, accidents, or military combat.

Most people who are exposed to a traumatic, stressful event have some symptoms of PTSD in the days and weeks following the event, but the symptoms generally disappear. However, about 8% of men and 20% of women go on to develop PTSD, and roughly 30% of these people develop a chronic, or long-lasting, form that persists throughout their lives.

How can I help handle my stress?

Do not let stress make you sick. Listen to your body, so that you know when stress is affecting your health. Here are ways to help you handle your stress.

- **Relax:** It is important to unwind. Each person has his or her own way to relax. Some ways include deep breathing, yoga, meditation, and massage therapy. If you cannot do these things, take a few minutes to sit, listen to soothing music, or read a book.

- **Make time for yourself:** It is important to care for yourself. Think of this as an order from your doctor, so you do not feel guilty. No matter how busy you are, you can try to set aside at least 15 minutes each day in your schedule to do something for yourself, like taking a bubble bath, going for a walk, or calling a friend.

- **Sleep:** Sleeping is a great way to help both your body and mind. Your stress could get worse if you do not get enough sleep. You also cannot fight off sickness as well when you sleep poorly. With enough sleep, you can tackle your problems better and lower your risk for illness. Try to get seven to nine hours of sleep every night.

- **Eat right:** Try to fuel up with fruits, vegetables, and proteins. Good sources of protein can be peanut butter, chicken, or tuna salad. Eat whole-grains, such as wheat breads and wheat crackers. Do not be fooled by the jolt you get from caffeine or sugar. Your energy will wear off.

- **Get moving:** Believe it or not, getting physical activity not only helps relieve your tense muscles, but helps your mood too. Your body makes certain chemicals, called endorphins, before and after you work out. They relieve stress and improve your mood.

- **Talk to friends:** Talk to your friends to help you work through your stress. Friends are good listeners. Finding someone who will let you talk freely about your problems and feelings, without judging you, does a world of good. It also helps to hear a different point of view. Friends will remind you that you are not alone.

- **Get help from a professional if you need it:** Talk to a therapist. A therapist can help you work through stress and find better ways to deal with problems. For more serious stress-related disorders, like PTSD, therapy can be helpful. There also are medications that can help ease symptoms of depression and anxiety and help promote sleep.

- **Compromise:** Sometimes, it is not always worth the stress to argue. Give in once in awhile.

- **Write down your thoughts:** Have you ever typed an e-mail to a friend about your lousy day and felt better afterward? Why not grab a pen and paper and write down what is going on in your life? Keeping a journal can be a great way to get things off your chest and work through issues. Later, you can go back and read through your journal and see how you have made progress.

- **Help others:** Helping someone else can help you. Help your neighbor, or volunteer in your community.

- **Get a hobby:** Find something you enjoy. Make sure to give yourself time to explore your interests.

- **Set limits:** When it comes to things like work and family, figure out what you can really do. There are only so many hours in the day. Set limits with yourself and others. Do not be afraid to say no to requests for your time and energy.

- **Plan your time:** Think ahead about how you are going to spend your time. Write a list. Figure out what is most important to do.

- **Do not deal with stress in unhealthy ways:** This includes drinking too much alcohol, using drugs, smoking, or overeating.

Deep breathing is a good way to relax. Try it a couple of times every day. Here is how to do it.

1. Lie down or sit in a chair.

2. Rest your hands on your stomach.

3. Slowly count to four and inhale through your nose. Feel your stomach rise. Hold it for a second.

4. Slowly count to four while you exhale through your mouth. To control how fast you exhale, purse your lips like you are going to whistle. Your stomach will slowly fall.

5. Repeat five to ten times.

Does stress cause ulcers?

Doctors used to think that ulcers were caused by stress and spicy foods. Now, we know that stress does not cause ulcers, it just irritates them. Ulcers are actually caused by a bacterium (germ) called *H. pylori*. Researchers do not yet know for sure how people get it. They think people might get it through food or water. It is treated with a combination of antibiotics and other drugs.

Chapter 73

Avoid Mixing Alcohol with Pain Medicines

Mixing alcohol with certain medications can cause nausea and vomiting, headaches, drowsiness, fainting, or loss of coordination. It also can put you at risk for internal bleeding, heart problems, and difficulties in breathing. In addition to these dangers, alcohol can make a medication less effective or even useless, or it may make the medication harmful or toxic to your body.

Some medicines that you might never have suspected can react with alcohol, including many medications which can be purchased over-the-counter—that is, without a prescription. Even some herbal remedies can have harmful effects when combined with alcohol.

This chapter lists medications for pain relief that can cause harm when taken with alcohol and describes the effects that can result. The list gives the brand name by which each medicine is commonly known (for example, Benadryl®) and its generic name or active ingredient (in Benadryl®, this is diphenhydramine). The list presented here does not include all the medicines that may interact harmfully with alcohol. Most important, the list does not include all the ingredients in every medication.

Medications are safe and effective when used appropriately. Your pharmacist or other health care provider can help you determine which medications interact harmfully with alcohol.

_____

Excerpted from "Harmful Interactions: Mixing Alcohol with Medicines," National Institute on Alcohol Abuse and Alcoholism (NIAAA), NIH Publication No. 03–5329, revised 2007.

Did You Know?

Mixing alcohol and medicines can be harmful. Alcohol, like some medicines, can make you sleepy, drowsy, or lightheaded. Drinking alcohol while taking medicines can intensify these effects. You may have trouble concentrating or performing mechanical skills. Small amounts of alcohol can make it dangerous to drive, and when you mix alcohol with certain medicines, you put yourself at even greater risk. Combining alcohol with some medicines can lead to falls and serious injuries, especially among older people.

Medicines May Have Many Ingredients

Some medications—including many popular painkillers and cough, cold, and allergy remedies—contain more than one ingredient that can react with alcohol. Read the label on the medication bottle to find out exactly what ingredients a medicine contains. Ask your pharmacist if you have any questions about how alcohol might interact with a drug you are taking.

Some Medicines Contain Alcohol

Certain medicines contain up to ten percent alcohol. Cough syrup and laxatives may have some of the highest alcohol concentrations.

Alcohol Affects Women Differently Than Men

Women, in general, have a higher risk for problems than men. When a woman drinks, the alcohol in her bloodstream typically reaches a higher level than a man's even if both are drinking the same amount. This is because women's bodies generally have less water than men's bodies. Because alcohol mixes with body water, a given amount of alcohol is more concentrated in a woman's body than in a man's. As a result, women are more susceptible to alcohol-related damage to organs such as the liver.

Older People Face Greater Risk

Older people are at particularly high risk for harmful alcohol-medication interactions. Aging slows the body's ability to break down alcohol, so alcohol remains in a person's system longer. Older people also are more likely to take a medication that interacts with alcohol—in fact, they often need to take more than one of these medications.

Table 73.1. Commonly Used Medicines (Both Prescription and Over-the-Counter) That Interact with Alcohol

Symptoms/ Disorders	Medication (Brand Name)	Medication (Generic Name)	Some possible reactions with alcohol
Angina (chest pain), coronary heart disease	Isordil®	Nitroglycerin Isosorbide	Rapid heartbeat, (chest pain), sudden changes in blood pressure, dizziness, fainting
Arthritis	Celebrex® Naprosyn® Voltaren®	Celecoxib Naproxen Diclofenac	Ulcers, stomach bleeding, liver problems
Heartburn, indigestion, sour stomach	Axid® Reglan® Tagamet® Zantac®	Nizatidine Metoclopramide Cimetidine Ranitidine	Rapid heartbeat, sudden changes in blood pressure (metoclopramide); increased alcohol effect
Muscle pain	Flexeril® Soma®	Cyclobenzaprine Carisoprodol	Drowsiness, dizziness; increased risk of seizures; increased risk for overdose; slowed or difficulty breathing; impaired motor control; unusual behavior; memory problems
Pain (such as headache, muscle ache, minor arthritis pain), fever, inflammation	Advil® Aleve® Excedrin® Motrin® Tylenol®	Ibuprofen Naproxen Aspirin, Acetaminophen Ibuprofen Acetaminophen	Stomach upset, bleeding and ulcers; liver damage (acetaminophen); rapid heartbeat
Severe pain from injury, postsurgical care, oral surgery, migraines	Darvocet–N® Demerol® Fiorinal® with codeine Percocet® Vicodin®	Propoxyphene Meperidine Butalbital plus codeine Oxycodone Hydrocodone	Drowsiness, dizziness; increased risk for overdose; slowed or difficulty breathing; impaired motor control; unusual behavior; memory problems

Timing Is Important

Alcohol and medicines can interact harmfully even if they are not taken at the same time.

557

Remember

Mixing alcohol and medicines puts you at risk for dangerous reactions. Protect yourself by avoiding alcohol if you are taking a medication and do not know its effect. To learn more about a medicine and whether it will interact with alcohol, talk to your pharmacist or other health care provider.

Chapter 74

Exercise Benefits for People with Chronic Pain

Chapter Contents

Section 74.1

Physical Activity

"Physical Exercise," by Richard W. Hanson, Ph.D., *Self-Management of Chronic Pain: Patient Handbook*, April 2007, Chronic Pain Management Program, Long Beach VA Healthcare System. Reprinted with permission.

One of the important goals of pain self-management is to develop and maintain a healthy physical activity level. Many persons with chronic pain become overly inactive and sedentary. Some doctors contribute to the problem by recommending bed rest and inactivity as a response to chronic pain. Unfortunately, this often makes the chronic pain syndrome worse by promoting physical deconditioning, excessive disability, and increased depression.

Physical Deconditioning and Disuse Syndrome

Following are some potential adverse medical consequences of prolonged physical inactivity and immobilization:

1. Muscle deterioration (atrophy).

2. Stiffening of joints.

3. Loss of calcium from the bone making them more brittle.

4. Impairments in the functioning of the heart and blood pressure system.

5. Loss of red blood cells.

6. Decrease in sex hormones and the impaired development of sperm.

7. Decreased resistance to infection.

8. Increased proportion of body fat in relation to muscle tissue and development of obesity.

9. Decreased catecholamine secretion leading to chemical changes in the brain which result in increased depression.

Physical Reconditioning

The obvious solution to the deconditioning and disuse syndrome is developing a physical reconditioning exercise program. The basic goals of physical exercise include:

1. Increase joint flexibility.

2. Improve muscle tone and strengthen weak muscles.

3. Increase aerobic and cardiovascular fitness.

4. Decrease excessive body fat.

Developing a Personalized Exercise Program

A very important self-management goal for most chronic pain sufferers is the development of a regular physical exercise program. Although it is beyond the scope of this section to specify what that exercise program should consist of, it may be noted that several of chronic pain self-management books include descriptions of some basic physical exercises which you may find useful. Ideally, your personal exercise program should be developed under the initial guidance of a properly trained professional such as a physical therapist. In particular, it is important that the professional be familiar with the special requirements of those with chronic pain conditions.

Following are some basic principles and guidelines which apply to physical exercise programs.

- Prior to undertaking a physical exercise program, it is always wise to first obtain clearance from your physician. Some chronic pain sufferers have other medical conditions (for example, heart disease, elevated blood pressure, respiratory conditions) which must be considered in developing a physical exercise program.

- Physical exercise programs are more likely to be successful if you start slowly and make gradual increments in whatever it is you are trying to do. We recommend use of the quota system which is described in section 74.2 of this chapter.

- The experience of some pain and discomfort when doing physical exercise is not necessarily a bad thing. The key issue here is to distinguish hurt from harm. Just because you experience some hurt while exercising does not automatically mean that the activity is dangerous or that you are harming yourself. The old cliché, "no pain, no gain" applies to many chronic pain conditions.

- Increased joint flexibility can be developed through appropriate range of motion (stretching) exercises. Important target areas include the legs, trunk, neck, shoulders, and arms. It is much easier to stretch muscles and joints when the muscles are relaxed. Many chronic pain sufferers also find it easier to do these exercises when submerged in warm water.

- Increased muscle tone can be developed through muscle resistance including static isometric and moving isotonic exercises (for example, use of weights and stretch bands).

- Increased aerobic fitness can be developed through exercises which elevate your heart rate for extended periods of time (usually a minimum of 20 minutes). These exercises may include walking, use of treadmills, bicycling, use of stationary bicycles, and swimming. It is typically recommended that aerobic exercises be carried out a minimum of three times per week in order to be beneficial.

- Decreased body fat can be developed through a combination of aerobic exercise, muscle toning exercise, and decreased dietary consumption of high caloric foods.

- No physical exercise program or weight loss program will be effective unless it is carried out and maintained consistently. Exercise and proper nutrition have to become life-long habits in order for you to keep realizing the benefits.

Benefits of Physical Exercise

Regular physical exercise is beneficial to many chronic pain sufferers for the following reasons:

- Properly paced exercise can promote healing in injured body tissue.

- Exercise can prevent or slow down further deterioration in many degenerative arthritic conditions.

- Exercise can prevent the occurrence of many painful physical injuries.

- Exercise promotes the development of endorphins, your body's natural pain killers.

- Exercise can increase your tolerance for physical activity.

- Exercise promotes not only improved physical functioning, but increased psychological well-being as well. That is, regular physical exercise can enhance self-esteem, counteract depression, and serve as a healthy outlet for frustration and anger.

Section 74.2

Self-Management of Daily Physical Activities

"Self-Management of Daily Physical Activities," by Richard W. Hanson, Ph.D., *Self-Management of Chronic Pain Patient Handbook*, April 2007, Chronic Pain Management Program, Long Beach VA Healthcare System. Reprinted with permission.

If your pain intensity is affected by your physical activity the following self-management principles apply to you.

Basic Principles

1. Discover your true physical limitations.

2. Improve activity tolerance through systematic retraining.

3. Learn to live within your limitations on a day-by-day basis.

4. Work on better accepting yourself in spite of having physical limitations.

Discover Your True Physical Limitations

Many persons with chronic pain have become more physically limited than they really need to be. This means that their physical activity level has become less than is really required by their disabling pain condition. They have developed what we call "excess disability." Following are some common causes of excess disability.

Sources of Excess Disability

Physical Deconditioning Syndrome

People who respond to pain by significantly curtailing their daily physical activities, may develop a deconditioning syndrome. In other words, they "get out of shape." Joints become stiff, muscles become flabby, endurance decreases, and some put on excess weight. Unfortunately, the deconditioning syndrome leads to decreased pain tolerance.

Solution: Develop and maintain a regular physical exercise program that is individually tailored to your needs.

Physical Compensation (Overuse) Syndrome

Many attempt to compensate for pain in one body part by overusing another body part. For example, if it hurts to walk on the right leg, one may compensate by overusing the left leg. This in turn can put excess strain on the overused body part and new pain problems can develop. Another common form of physical compensation is called bracing. This occurs when one tries to compensate for painful movement either by making the painful area stiff (for example, tensing the muscles so it becomes like a brace), or actually wearing some kind of external brace (such as a neck collar). Excessive bracing and limiting movement can over time lead to additional deterioration and decreased pain tolerance.

Solution: Learn ways to make your body movements as normal as possible.

Excessive Muscle Strain Syndrome

A very common reaction to pain is elevated muscle tension. People also respond to emotional stress with elevated muscle tension. The combination of chronic pain and chronic stress can easily lead to chronically tense muscles. When muscles are held in a state of contraction for prolonged periods of time, pain results. This fact provides another explanation why persons with chronic pain in one area of the body often develop pain in other areas as well. Suppose, for example, a person named Fred develops chronic low back pain. If Fred responds to his low back pain and other stressors in his life with chronically elevated tension in his neck and shoulder muscles, he may eventually develop pain in these areas as well. The elevated tension in his upper body may also travel up the back of his head causing the development of tension headaches.

Solution: Learn how to decrease excess muscle tension through use of deep muscle relaxation exercises and other appropriate physical exercises

Fear and Avoidance

Many persons with chronic pain become afraid of doing certain activities, and therefore, avoid doing them. Usually, this means that at some time in the past they have experienced an increase in pain while doing these activities. Some develop a condition known as kinesophobia which means fear of movement. They may hold themselves rigidly or move in a very slow, guarded, and deliberate manner. Most often this is based on misunderstandings regarding the relationship between "hurt" and "harm." It is the mistaken belief that if you experience hurt by doing something you are actually causing harm or damage to your body. People with this fear often view their bodies as being extremely fragile. For example, they may fear that their spines will break, nerves will become damaged, or they will end up even more impaired (for example, confined to bed or wheelchair).

Solution: Consult your doctor or physical therapist and get their input. Increased pain intensity while doing certain activities does not necessarily mean that you are damaging your body. Hurt does not mean harm. Reduce risk of damage by increasing your physical activity level gradually.

Depression

It is common for persons with chronic pain to become depressed. Common symptoms of depression are decreased energy, loss of motivation and initiative, and withdrawal from people and activities. People who are depressed may use their pain as an excuse to avoid certain activities. Unfortunately, people who are depressed become even more preoccupied by their pain and misery.

Solution: Work on ways to overcome your depression.

Distorted, "All or Nothing" Thinking

Some persons with chronic pain approach certain physical activities with an "all or none" attitude which says, "either I do it the way I used to do it, or I won't do it at all." Rather than making modifications

565

and compromises in how they go about doing certain tasks, they avoid doing them all together.

Solution: Learn how to make modifications in the way you approach and complete certain physical chores and activities. Learn how to pace yourself, take rest breaks, find short cuts, or ask for assistance.

Pain Payoffs

Pain payoffs occur when people avoid doing certain activities, not because they can't do them, but rather because they really don't want to do them. Pain can become a very convenient excuse to get out of doing certain chores and responsibilities that you really would rather not do. Although it is certainly possible to fool other people, it is also possible to fool yourself. Rather than admit to yourself that you really don't want to do certain jobs or tasks, you tell yourself that you are not capable of doing them because of your pain condition.

Solution: Begin with an honest self-examination. All of us have to do certain chores and responsibilities that we would prefer not to do. Don't use your pain as an excuse.

Discover your true physical limitations on your own. Don't put all the responsibility on doctors to determine what you can and cannot do. All they can do is make educated guesses. Let your own experience be your guide. Discover for yourself, on a trial-and-error basis, what you can and what you cannot do. While you are discovering your capabilities, use good common sense and approach physical activities cautiously and gradually.

- Which of the above factors may have resulted in excessive disability for you?
- What can you do about it?

Improving Activity Tolerance: The Quota System

Some physical activities which have been limited as a result of your pain condition can be improved by following a systematic procedure sometimes referred to as the quota system. Two examples will be offered here: intolerance for prolonged sitting, and intolerance for walking extended distances.

Establishing a Baseline

The first step is to establish a baseline of your current tolerance level for the specific activity. This means actually measuring the extent to which you can engage in the activity without being overwhelmed with pain. The unit of measurement which you use will depend on the activity in question. In the case of sitting intolerance, the obvious choice would be time. Thus, you would measure how long you can sit in a particular chair before the pain becomes too uncomfortable. In the case of walking intolerance, you might choose distance as the measure. That is, how far can you walk (in feet or yards) on a particular terrain before it becomes too uncomfortable? Since it is likely that there will be some variability, you may have to take several measures (say four or five) and then compute an average. This will be your baseline or starting point. Please note that the baseline should not be the point where the pain becomes excruciating. Rather, it should be at that point where it starts becoming noticeably uncomfortable.

Establishing Activity Quotas

Once you have established your baseline or starting point, the goal is to gradually and systematically increase your tolerance by setting quotas. The quota refers the activity level you are aiming for (length of time sitting, or distance walked). The activity quota should begin with a very small increase over your baseline. For example, let's say that your baseline sitting tolerance is 30 minutes. You may want to begin your first quota with 35 minutes, or even less if you think that the five minute increase is too much. In the case of walking distance, let's say for example that your baseline is 50 yards. You may then want to set your first quota increase to 55 yards. It is very important that you set your quota at a level that will enable you to experience success. Once you feel comfortable at a particular quota level, you should increase it again and again. If at any point during the training process you are unable to reach your quota, you should either lower the quota or stay at the previous quota level until you feel ready to increase it once again.

You find it very helpful to make use of mental pain coping techniques (for example, distraction, or positive self-statements) while you are doing the target activity. Some like to reward themselves with a special treat when they reach a particular quota. Most people also find it very useful to make a graph or chart of their progress. This can serve as a visual indication of the progress you have made. Obviously, at some point you will reach an upper limit as to how far you can go with the quota increases. That's okay. Remember in pain self-management, we always view improvement as relative. Any improvement is better than no improvement at all.

Living within Your Limitations on a Day-by-Day Basis

Knowing your physical limitations and putting this knowledge into practice are two different things. Although some persons know better, they find themselves frequently overdoing it and exceeding their physical limitations. Keep the following principles in mind:

Maintain a Balanced, Healthy, Activity Level

Avoid the extremes of underactivity and overactivity. Watch out for the overactivity—crash and burn cycles. Discover an activity balance that is right for you.

Use Good Pacing Procedures

Pacing is probably the most important principle to master. You should plan in advance how you want to approach certain physical tasks. Break the activity down into smaller chunks. Depending on the nature of your pain condition, you may need to avoid staying in one position too long or avoid specific repetitive movements for extended periods of time. Vary your routine. Take rest breaks before your pain significantly increases. Monitor your distorted thinking and challenge yourself by asking, "What is the rush?" or "Who says I must complete this job all at once?" Think about completing tasks in a parallel manner (working on several tasks simultaneously) rather than serially (moving to a new task only after you have completed the previous task).

Use Good Body Mechanics

Be aware of your posture and body position while you do certain activities like bending, lifting, pushing, pulling, or carrying things. Avoid excessive and unnecessary strain.

Do Warm-up Exercises

Before athletes begin their sporting activities they do warm-up exercises. If you are planning to do some activity that is likely to put a strain on your pain area, you might benefit from some stretching and limbering up exercises first. For example, if you suffer from chronic low back pain and plan to do an activity or chore which might put a strain on your back, you can do some pelvic tilts or other back exercises before you start the activity.

Use Caution during Danger Times

Many persons tend to overdo it and exceed their physical limitations during certain danger times. Here are some common examples of danger times:

1. **Days when you feel good:** Many of you have good days and bad days. Good days occur when you are feeling good and are not feeling as much pain. Be careful that you don't turn a good day into a bad day by becoming careless and overconfident in your physical activities.

2. **While doing some physical activity that you enjoy:** Enjoyable physical activities are wonderful ways to distract your attention away from pain. Unfortunately, they can also distract your attention from using good pacing techniques. Be careful that you don't become so engrossed in an enjoyable activity that you forget to pace yourself.

3. **While competing with other people:** Competition is a great motivator, but it can also get you into trouble. Don't let competition trick you into exceeding your physical limitations.

4. **While trying to please other people:** It is nice to please others, but don't let this lead to neglecting your own need to stay within your limits.

5. **When you are feeling rushed, pressured, or emotionally upset:** These are times when you can become careless and forget to use good judgment while doing physical activities.

Increasing Self-Acceptance

Unfortunately, many persons with a disabling chronic pain condition suffer a significant blow to their self-esteem. Inability to accept yourself because of having physical limitations can really get you into trouble. It can lead to dependency, depression, or chronic frustration, anger, and bitterness. Following are some general guidelines for improving your self-acceptance and self-esteem:

Remember That Physical Limitations Do Not Make You a Less Valuable or Worthwhile Person

Who says that a person's worth is determined by their physical capabilities? When you really think about it, just about everyone has some physical limitations. Also, everyone develops more physical limitations as they get older. Just because you can't do all of the physical tasks you did when you were in your late teens and early twenties, doesn't make you a less valuable person. Some have pointed out that a very destructive irrational belief is the tendency to equate one's worth as a person with his or her physical accomplishments. People who are severely disabled have no less worth as a human being than an able-bodied person.

Focus on What You Can Do Rather than on What You Can No Longer Do

Rather than dwelling on those activities you can no longer do as before, try to focus instead on all those things you still can do. Try to promote an attitude of gratitude for what you have, rather than an attitude of regret for what you no longer have. Think of the severely disabled spinal cord injured person who considered it a great achievement when he learned to feed himself on his own (something the rest of us take for granted).

Develop New Knowledge and Skills

It will become easier to focus on your positive abilities if you direct your energy to developing new knowledge and skills that are not as physically demanding. In our society, the people who earn the most money are those who have special knowledge and skills rather than those who have the biggest muscles and strongest backs.

What Really Counts Is Doing the Best You Can with Your Abilities

Build your self-esteem on making the best use of your knowledge, skills, and abilities. It doesn't matter what others can do or what you used to do. What really matters is that you do your best today.

Find Ways to Be a Better Person

All of us have room for self-improvement. Self-improvement does not necessarily require physical achievements. There are many ways to be a better person, like working on your character. Developing more positive attitudes, healthier ways of living, improving your social relationships, giving of yourself to other people, and spiritual growth, are all ways to become a better person.

What can you do to improve your own self-esteem and self-acceptance?

Chapter 75

Pain and Travel

Pain-Free Tips for Travel

The summer is in full swing, and many Americans are packing their cars and booking flights to head to the beach or visit family and friends for barbecues and other fun outdoor activities. For people living with chronic pain, traveling can be especially challenging. Many worry about the possibility of flare-ups in a new environment. The American Pain Foundation (APF) recently surveyed more than 1,700 people with pain about travel. Here are some highlights:

- Most people have traveled for work or pleasure within the last two years.

- Four out of five people who traveled by car said that unexpected problems on the road worsened their pain. Those who chose to travel by bus or train were less likely to report challenges that led to increased pain.

- Of those who took flights, half said the security screening process increased their pain.

- More than one-third of those surveyed said they had difficulty taking medication as prescribed while traveling. Of these, three out of four people believe this increased their pain.

No matter where you are headed this summer, there are steps you can take to ensure you and your family will have an enjoyable time.

1. Get organized and plan ahead. Making last-minute travel arrangements, or trying to pack and get everything at home in order in the final hours leading up to your trip, can be stressful. And stress can trigger flare-ups of pain.

2. Be true to yourself. Choose destinations where you know you'll feel comfortable traveling.

3. Stretch out and stay active. Sitting in one position for too long will cause you to become stiff, increasing your pain. Whether you're traveling by car, rail, bus, or plane, wear comfortable, loose clothing and try to move and stretch as much as possible to keep your blood flowing and to reduce muscle tension.

4. When booking hotel reservations, call the hotel directly rather than using the 800 number. This way you can ask specific questions about the actual facility where you'll be staying (for example, preferred room location, access to local sites).

5. Always pack needed medications in your carry-on bag. Be sure to ask your health care provider if you need to adjust dosages if your eating and sleeping schedules change due to time changes. Bring your provider's contact information and a list of prescribed medications and your medical conditions with you.

6. Know your limits. Don't try to do and see everything. You can always plan a return visit.

7. Call ahead to your airline if you need extra assistance or a wheelchair.

8. Pack lightly. Traveling while negotiating overly packed luggage can make things more difficult, not to mention the added strain on your back and muscles. When lifting your bags, maintain good posture and keep the weight close to your body.

9. Set expectations for fellow travelers. Sit down before your trip to talk about what activities you think you may or may not be able to do.

10. Get plenty of sleep, eat healthful meals, and stay hydrated. Make sure to take advantage of opportunities to rest throughout the day. You may want to bring a pillow and a favorite blanket for added comfort.

Make sure your travels go smoothly by planning ahead. It's also important to talk about measures you and those you are traveling with can take to ease your pain so you can enjoy the ride.

Helpful Travel Resources

Transportation Security Administration (TSA)
Website: http://www.tsa.gov/travelers/index.shtm

Society for Accessible Travel and Hospitality (SATH)
Website: http://www.sath.org

Centers for Disease Control and Prevention
Website: http://wwwn.cdc.gov/travel/default.aspx

Chapter 76

Using Ergonomics to Avoid Pain

Chapter Contents

Section 76.1

Computer Workstation Guidelines

Excerpted from "Ergonomics for Computer Workstations,"
National Institutes of Health (NIH).

Computer Monitors

With regard to the computer monitor, one must take into consideration how the placement and maintenance of the monitor can affect both the eyes and the musculoskeletal system. The following suggestions can help prevent the development of eye strain, neck pain, and shoulder fatigue while using your computer workstation:

- Make sure the surface of the viewing screen is clean.

- Adjust brightness and contrast to optimum comfort.

- Position the monitor directly in front of user to avoid excessive twisting of the neck.

- Position the monitor approximately 20–26 inches (arm's length) from user.

- Tilt top of the monitor back 10 to 20 degrees.

- Position monitors at right angles from windows to reduce glare.

- Position monitors away from direct lighting which creates excessive glare or use a glare filter over the monitor to reduce glare.

- The top of the viewing screen should be at eye level when the user is sitting in an upright position (Note: Bifocal and trifocal wearers may need to lower monitor a couple of inches).

Adjusting Your Chair

Contrary to popular belief, sitting, which most people believe is relaxing, is hard on the back. Sitting for long periods of time can cause increased pressure on the intervertebral discs—the springy, shock-absorbing part of the spine. Sitting is also hard on the feet and legs. Gravity tends to pool blood in the legs and feet and create a sluggish return to the heart.

The following recommendations can help increase comfort for computer users:

- Dynamic sitting, don't stay in one static position for extended periods of time.

- When performing daily tasks, alternate between sitting and standing.

- Adjust height of backrest to support the natural inward curvature of the lower back.

  - It may be useful to use a rolled towel or lumbar pad to support the lower back.

  - Set the backrest angle so that your hip-torso angle is 90 degrees or greater.

- Adjust height of chair so feet rest flat on floor (use footrest if necessary).

  - Sit upright in the chair with the lower back against the backrest and the shoulders touching the backrest.

  - Thighs should be parallel to the floor and knees at about the same level as the hips.

  - Back of knees should not come in direct contact with the edge of the seat (there should be 2–3 inches between the edge of the seat and the back of the knee).

- Do not use armrests to slouch.

- Adjust height and width of armrests so they allow the user to rest arms at their sides and relax or drop their shoulders while keyboarding.

- Where armrests are used, elbows and lower arms should rest lightly so as not to cause circulatory or nerve problems.

Desktops for Computer Workstations

If you are like many computer users, your computer, keyboard, and mouse are resting on your desk or a portable computer workstation.

There is no specific height recommended for your desktop; however, the working height of your desk should be approximately elbow height for light duty desk work.

To allow for proper alignment of your arms your keyboard should be approximately one inch to two inches above your thighs. Most times this requires a desk which is 25 inches to 29 inches in height (depending upon size of individual) or the use of an articulating keyboard tray. The area underneath the desk should always be clean to accommodate the user's legs and allow for stretching.

The desktop should be organized so frequently used objects are close to the user to avoid excessive extended reaching. If a document holder is used, it should be placed at approximately the same height as the monitor and at the same distance from the eyes to prevent frequent eye shifts between the screen and reference materials.

Keyboard and Mouse

Many ergonomic problems associated with computer workstations occur in the forearm, wrist, and hand. Continuous work on the computer exposes soft tissues in these areas to repetition, awkward postures, and forceful exertions.

The following adjustments should be made to your workstation to help prevent the development of an ergonomic problem in the upper extremities:

- Adjust keyboard height so shoulders can relax and allow arms to rest at sides (an articulating keyboard tray is often necessary to accommodate proper height and distance).

- Keyboard should be close to the user to avoid excessive extended reaching.

- Forearms parallel to the floor (approximately 90 degree angle at elbow).

- Mouse should be placed adjacent to keyboard and at the same height as the keyboard (use articulating keyboard tray if necessary).

- Avoid extended and elevated reaching for keyboard and mouse. Wrist should be in neutral position (not excessively flexed or extended).

- Do not rest the hand on the mouse when you are not using it. Rest hands in your lap when not entering data.

Lighting for Computer Workstations

Lighting not suited to working with a video display terminal is a major contributing factor in visual discomforts including eyestrain, burning or itching eyes, and blurred or double vision. Typical office environments have illumination levels of 75 to 100 foot-candles, but according to the American National Standards Institute (ANSI), computer workstations require only 18 to 46 foot-candles.

Use the following recommendations to reduce eyestrain and eye fatigue:

- Close drapes and blinds to reduce glare. Adjust lighting to avoid glare on screen (light source should come at a 90 degree angle, with low-watt lights rather than high.) Place monitor at 90 degree angle to windows (where possible). Reduce overhead lighting (where possible). Use indirect or shielded lighting where possible. Walls should be painted medium or dark color and not have reflective finish.

- Use a glare screen to reduce glare (alternatively, place a large manila folder on top of the monitor and let it hang over the monitor 2–3 inches to reduce glare from overhead lighting).

Section 76.2

Maintaining a Healthy Back

Excerpted from "Industrial and Shops Ergonomics,"
National Institutes of Health (NIH).

Lifting with Proper Posture

Lifting is strenuous—it requires proper training and technique. By lifting with your large, strong, leg muscles instead of the small muscles of the back, you can prevent back injuries and reduce lower back pain. There are five steps to follow when lifting an object:

1. **Get close to the load:** Get as close to the load as possible—as if you are hugging the object. Having the object close to your body put less force on your lower back.

2. **Maintain your curves:** Keep yourself in an upright position while squatting to pick up.

3. **Tighten your stomach muscles:** Tightening the stomach helps support the spine. Don't hold your breath while tightening the muscles.

4. **Lift with your legs:** Your legs are the strongest muscles in your body—so use them.

5. **Pivot, do not twist:** Turn with your feet, not your back. It is not built for twisting from side to side.

Large or heavy loads: If a load is too heavy to lift alone, ask for help. Pick one person to coach the lift—this way you lift and lower at the same time.

Overhead loads: If a load is above your shoulders, use a step stool to elevate yourself until the load is at least chest level—preferably waist height. Pull the object close to your body and then lift. Remember to maintain your curves—use your arms and legs to do the work.

Maintain a Healthy Back

The muscles in the back are unlike many other muscles in your body—they are almost always in use. They hold your torso in an upright position throughout your day. They assist you every time you pick something up, whether it is a pen or a concrete block. They support posture while you sit in your chair, and they even work at night when you sleep.

In order for you to understand what is good posture and what is bad posture—let's take a look at how your back is designed.

Three curves of your back: Your back is composed of three natural curves that form an S-shape. When your three natural curves are properly aligned, your ears, shoulders, and hips are in a straight line. Without support from strong, flexible muscles, your back loses its three natural curves. Poor posture can lead to pain and serious injury.

When you use good posture, your back is aligned in three natural curves supported by strong, flexible muscles. Good posture helps prevent back strain and pain.

Maintaining a Healthy Back with Exercise and Rest

It does not take much time to improve the strength and flexibility of your back. In just ten minutes a day, you can perform a few exercises which can prevent a lifetime of lower back pain.

Partial Sit-Ups

This exercise strengthens your stomach muscles:

- Lie on your back with both knees bent and your feet flat on the floor. Slowly raise your head and shoulders off the floor, keeping your hands across your chest.
- Work up to 30 repetitions.

Bridge

This exercise strengthens your lower back:

- Lie on your back with both knees bent and your feet flat on the floor.
- With arms lying at your sides, tighten stomach muscles, squeeze buttocks, and slowly raise your hips into the air. Hold

583

for five seconds, and then slowly bring the buttocks back to the floor.

- Repeat 20 times.

Wall Slide

This exercise strengthens your back and leg muscles:

- Stand with your back against a wall and your feet slightly apart.
- Slide into a half-sit. Hold as long as you can; slide back up.
- Repeat five times.

Aerobic Exercise

Aerobic exercise also stretches and strengthens the muscles that support your lower back which combined with healthy eating can also help you maintain your ideal weight. If you are overweight, the extra pounds add to the strain on your lower back. Aerobic exercise, like walking, can help you lose weight.

Proper Rest

The best position for resting the back muscles is lying on your back on your living room floor with a pillow under your knees and a rolled up towel under your neck. You can also lie on your side in the fetal position—bend the knees to reduce strain on the lower back and put a pillow between your knees, and under your head and neck to keep them level.

Chapter 77

Guidelines for Caregivers of Adults Needing Pain Relief

Understanding the Problem

Some people think that pain is natural with aging, or that when older people are not clear in explaining the cause or nature of their pain that they are just complaining. Both of these views are wrong. There is almost always a real problem behind pain.

Arthritis is said to be the most common cause of pain in people over the age of 65. Circulatory problems, shingles, and other types of nerve damage, certain bowel diseases, and cancer are other common reasons for pain in older people.

Muscle pain is also quite common. Conditions that contribute to muscle pain in older people are fibromyalgia (especially in older women) and myofascial pain (which can result from trauma, nerve damage, and arthritis). These conditions are treated differently than other types of pain, and may get better without taking any medicine at all (that is, they may be best treated with physical therapy).

Pain can lead to other problems such as losing the ability to move around and do everyday activities. The sufferer may have trouble sleeping, experience bad moods, and develop a poor self-image. In addition, people with pain often become anxious or depressed. They may be at greater risk for falls, weight loss, poor concentration, and difficulties with relationships.

On the positive side, most pain can improve with treatment that usually consists of a combination of medicine and non-medicine strategies. Treatments such as physical therapy, massage, application of heat and/or cold, exercise, and relaxation may be tried first. If these treatments are not successful alone, pain pills should be prescribed along with them and the person closely observed for side effects. Since all medicines have side effects, pain pills should be prescribed with care.

Non-Medication Strategies for Pain Relief

There are a number of ways to control pain without medicines. These include the following:

- Physical therapy, such as exercise, muscle stretching and strengthening, as well as heat, cold, and massage
- TENS (transcutaneous electrical nerve stimulation)
- Biofeedback
- Hypnosis
- Medicine

Often these strategies alone will relieve pain and the use of pain medicine can sometimes be avoided. If your doctor prescribes a medicine for pain, you should ask him or her whether other treatments are also available.

Medicines for Pain Relief

The medicines used to relieve pain are called analgesics. There are many types of analgesics:

- Aspirin, Motrin™, and Advil™ are examples of medicines called non-steroidal anti-inflammatory drugs (NSAIDs). These medicines are often used to relieve arthritis pain and, while effective, most of them can also cause unwanted side effects, such as gastrointestinal bleeding, if taken at high doses for long periods of time.
- Newer arthritic medicines called COX-2 drugs may be less harmful to the gastrointestinal tract, but like the other NSAIDs, they can be harmful to the kidneys and may elevate blood pressure.

- Another type of arthritis medicine, called non-acetylated salicylates (for example, Disalcid™, Trilisate™), is relatively easy on the stomach and generally does not harm the kidneys or elevate the blood pressure.

These medicines are worth discussing with your doctor.

Strong pain medicines called opioids (narcotics) may be very effective in treating more severe types of pain, but they also have a variety of side effects. Examples of opioids include Vicodin™, Percocet™, and morphine. Some opioids can be given via a patch applied to the skin every three days. Side effects of these types of medicine include tiredness, constipation, and confusion. These side effects may be treated by decreasing the dose of the medicine or by treating the side effect directly, such as by adding high-fiber foods and exercise to treat constipation.

Opioids can sometimes be habit forming if used over a long period of time, but this does not occur very often. It is more important to treat the pain than to withhold medicine because of fear of causing addiction.

Believe the person you are caring for. If people with pain think that others do not believe them, they become upset and may stop reporting their pain accurately. This makes controlling the pain more difficult. People with pain are the only ones who know how much pain they are feeling. Pain is whatever a person says it is and exists whenever he or she says it does.

Every person has the right to good pain control. Your job as a caregiver is to make sure that good pain control is provided. Tell the doctor or nurse if pain does not lessen with treatment and ask the doctor to try new treatments until the pain is controlled. It is important to also recognize that while most pain can improve with treatment complete pain relief may not be possible in every case.

Your goals are to:

- help evaluate and relieve pain; and

- keep your doctor or nurse informed about pain levels and responses to pain treatments.

When to Get Professional Help

Call the doctor or nurse immediately or go to the emergency room if any of the following symptoms occur (A good rule of thumb is that all pain deserves to be treated, so inform the doctor or nurse of any pain so that the patient does not suffer needlessly.):

- **There is a sudden change in the ability to walk or carry out other important activities because of pain.** Sudden changes in activity level often mean that the person is having significant pain and that the condition causing the pain has changed. Sometimes people can break a hip without having fallen. The only way to determine whether this has occurred is to do an x-ray. On the other hand, the confused older person may become frightened because of pain, and because of this fear, he or she may refuse to walk or move even though there is nothing serious causing the pain. The best way to sort out this sometimes complicated situation is for the person with pain to be evaluated by a medical professional.

- **There is new pain that is severe.** Whenever this occurs, seek help immediately.

- **There is new pain that is not severe, but it is causing the person significant distress.** The new occurrence of chest discomfort, for example, may indicate a heart attack. Often this pain is not severe. The person may be experiencing a sensation of heaviness or pressure. Another example is abdominal pain. If the person has abdominal pain along with fever or vomiting, help should be sought immediately. There are many other pain situations that warrant immediate medical attention. If you are concerned about pain, call the doctor.

- **There is talk about not wanting to live any more.** When pain is severe and lasts a long time (especially certain kinds of pain related to nerve damage), older people may want to escape from the pain. If they feel that help is not available, they may talk about suicide. This should be taken very seriously. If older people have thoughts about wanting to harm themselves, this should be considered an emergency.

Call the doctor or nurse during office hours to discuss the following problems:

- **No relief after taking pain medication as prescribed.** The doctor may change the amount of medicine, how often it is taken, or the type of pain medicine, or he or she might want to do a physical examination.

- **Some pain relief, but there is still a lot of pain one or two days after starting the medicine.** In this case, the doctor or nurse needs to reevaluate the amount or type of pain medicine prescribed.

- **New or different pain.** New pain may need to be evaluated before the next regularly scheduled office visit. If in doubt, call and speak with the doctor or nurse.

- **Adverse side effects of pain medications.** If the patient cannot tolerate a particular pain medicine, let the doctor know so that something different can be prescribed. Don't wait until the next scheduled appointment. There is no need to suffer pain when it can be treated.

- **Changes in sleep.** Getting good sleep is very important in the treatment of pain. If a person does not sleep well, it becomes more difficult for him or her to tolerate pain. Many things can cause difficulty sleeping, for example, depression, anxiety, sleep apnea, certain medicines, or the pain itself. The treatment depends upon the cause. If the person you are caring for is having difficulty sleeping, be sure to let the doctor know so that this important problem can be addressed.

- **Difficulty coping with pain.** Pain that persists for a long time may take a toll on a person's emotions. He or she may become anxious, depressed, or irritable. These problems should be taken very seriously. They usually respond well to treatment with medicines and other strategies.

Know the answers to the following questions before calling the doctor.

Describe the Pain

- How long has the pain been a problem?

- Is it a new pain or has it happened before?

- Where is it located? Is it in more than one area? If so, which location is most bothersome? Does it move from one place to another?

- How severe is the pain? Ask the person whether it is mild, moderate, severe, or unbearable.

- Is the pain sharp and stabbing, dull and aching, burning, or does it feel like an electric shock?

- Is there any numbness, tingling, or new weakness in the pain area?

- How does the pain interfere with doing normal activities? What activities or conditions make the pain worse?

- What has been tried to relieve the pain?

- What medicines are being taken? Are the medicines taken at set times or just when the person you are caring for needs them? Is he or she allergic or sensitive to any pain medicine?

Here is an example of what you might say when calling for help: "This is Margaret Smith, John Smith's daughter. My father is a patient of Dr. Troy. This morning he refused to get out of bed because his leg hurt so badly near the hip, and it hurts even if he tries to move just a little in bed. He said his pain is sharp. At 6:00 a.m. he took two Percocet™ but didn't feel any better. The next time for his medicine isn't until noon. We tried a heating pad, but it didn't help."

What You Can Do to Help

Evaluate Pain

- **Ask about the pain.** The best way to find out if a person is in pain is to ask. No medical test can give you this information. It is also very important to be sure that the older person knows that you believe him or her.

- **Listen for words other than "pain."** Older people may use different words to describe their pain, such as discomfort, soreness, ache, or heaviness.

- **Look for behavior or body language that looks like a response to pain.** An older person may be unwilling to report pain or be unable to communicate about pain in words. Behaviors or body language to look for include facial expressions such as the following:

  - Tears

  - Eyes that are closed tightly

  - Knitted eyebrows

  - Wrinkled forehead (grimacing)

  - Groaning when moved

- Clenched fists
- A stiffened upper or lower body that is held rigidly and moved slowly
- Decreased activity level
- Trouble sleeping
- Poor appetite

Other signs may include rubbing certain parts of the body, slouched or bent posture, avoiding sitting or standing.

Everyone expresses pain differently. As the caregiver you are in the best position to know when the person you are caring for is in pain because you know him or her better than anyone.

Keeping track of pain is difficult. Severity of pain can change over time or it can come and go. Sometimes it can be difficult to get information about the pain from the person who has it. And sometimes it can be hard to tell the difference between old pain and new pain. It is important that you do the best that you can and keep a record of the pain.

Improve Chances for Obtaining Good Pain Relief

- **Use pain medicines as prescribed.** If the prescription says to take the medicine at certain times or at certain time intervals (for example, every six hours), make sure the person you are caring for does so. Do not wait until the pain comes back to give the medicine. This will cause needless suffering. One of the important ways that pain medicine works is that it helps to prevent episodes of severe pain. In order to do this, there has to be a certain amount of medicine in the blood. This is why the doctor prescribes taking the medicine at regular intervals—to be sure that the blood level stays high enough.

- **Don't withhold medicine for fear of addiction.** Addiction is very rare in patients who have real pain and who take pain medicine under a doctor's supervision. Also, do not withhold medicine for fear the medicine will become less effective over time. The amount or type of medicine can always be changed.

- **Insist on good pain control.** Pain generally tends to be undertreated. Make sure the doctor knows there is a pain problem, and let him or her know if treatment is not meeting the needs of the person you are caring for.

591

- **Ask about pain clinics.** If your doctor cannot control the pain, ask for a referral to a pain clinic that has a team of people (doctors, nurses, physical and occupational therapists, psychologists) that specialize in pain treatment. Universities and large hospitals often have these types of clinics.

Help to Reduce Pain

- **Use warm showers, baths, hot water bottles, or warm washcloths.** Heat relaxes muscles; this can help reduce pain and give a sense of comfort. Do not set heating pads on high because they can burn the skin. Also, try massaging sore spots, such as neck and shoulders. Check with the doctor about how long to apply heat since prolonged exposure to heat can cause tissue damage.

- **Use cool cloths.** Cooling the skin and muscles can soothe pain, especially pain that comes from inflammation or swelling. For example, many people find that using a cool washcloth on their forehead reduces pain when they have a headache. Check with the doctor about how long to apply cold since prolonged exposure to cold can cause tissue damage.

- **Position the person carefully with pillows and soft seat cushions.**

- **Encourage relaxation.** Breathing slowly and quietly helps the mind and body to relax and helps decrease pain. Simple relaxation methods can be learned from books on relaxation techniques which are available at most bookstores. Relaxation audiotapes can also be purchased through most bookstores.

- **Provide pleasant activities.** Being active takes the mind off the pain. Distractions such as pleasant visits with friends and grandchildren should be encouraged. Watching television, reading, and listening to music may also decrease a person's awareness of pain.

- **Avoid stressful events when possible.** Emotional stress and anxiety increase pain. Try to minimize these types of situations.

Carrying Out and Adjusting Your Plan

Problems You Might Have Carrying Out Your Plan

Problem: "If I tell the doctor about my pain she'll think I'm a complainer."

Response: It is the doctor and nurse's job to work out the best way to control pain. To do this, they rely on you to tell them about the pain of the person you are caring for. They can't do their job unless you do yours.

Problem: "Of course she has aches and pains. She's old."

Response: Pain is not a normal part of growing old. Pain in older adults, just like pain in any other age group, is a signal that something is wrong. You and the person you are caring for need to talk about this with a doctor so the problem can be treated.

Problem: "My father is confused. What he says doesn't make sense, so I can't tell whether he's in pain or not."

Response: Even when people are confused, oftentimes they can let you know when they are in pain. It may be helpful to look for changes in mood, activity level, body language, and facial expressions as discussed in the previous section, "What You Can Do to Help."

Problem: "I'm afraid of addiction."

Response: It is very unusual for people who have pain to become addicted to pain medicines. They are taking the medicines for a good reason, to relieve their pain, not to get high. People who have pain need to be treated, so concerns about addiction, in most cases, should not enter into the doctor's decision to prescribe these medicines.

There is a difference between addiction, which is a psychological craving for medicine, and physical dependence. People who need opioids (narcotics) for only a period of time may develop a physical dependence on the medicine, with uncomfortable symptoms, such as sweating, chills, and nausea, if the medicine is stopped suddenly. This is only a temporary situation that can be prevented by slowly reducing the medicine over a few days or a few weeks.

Think of Other Problems You Might Have Carrying Out Your Plan

What other problems could get in the way of doing the things suggested in this chapter? For example, will the older person cooperate? Will other people help? How will you explain your needs to other people? Do you have the time and energy to carry out this plan?

You need to make plans for solving these problems.

Checking on Progress

Ask about pain regularly and keep notes. Adjusting pain medicines to fit each patient takes time so change may be slow. Keep the doctor or nurse informed about changes in pain.

What to Do If Your Plan Isn't Working

If, after a reasonable time, pain is still a problem, ask for a referral to a pain clinic. Relief from pain is possible in most cases. It is also important to recognize that most pain that has gone on for a long time cannot be totally relieved, but people can be taught how to live better lives with their pain. Remember that help is available, but persistence on your part is important in order to get the relief that the person you are caring for deserves.

Part Five

Additional Help
and Information

Chapter 78

Glossary of Terms Related to Pain

acetaminophen: A drug that reduces pain and fever (but not inflammation). It belongs to the family of drugs called analgesics. [1]

acupuncture: The technique of inserting thin needles through the skin at specific points on the body to control pain and other symptoms. It is a type of complementary and alternative medicine. [1]

addiction: Uncontrollable craving, seeking, and use of a substance such as a drug or alcohol. [1]

anesthetic: A substance that causes loss of feeling or awareness. Local anesthetics cause loss of feeling in a part of the body. General anesthetics put the person to sleep. [1]

angiography: An imaging technique that provides a picture, called an angiogram, of blood vessels. [2]

anti-inflammatory: Having to do with reducing inflammation. [1]

anticonvulsant: A drug or other substance used to prevent or stop seizures or convulsions. Also called an antiepileptic. [1]

Terms in this chapter marked [1] are excerpted from PDQ® Cancer Information Summary. National Cancer Institute: Bethesda, MD. Pain (PDQ®): Supportive Care–Patient. Updated 03/2008. Available at: http://cancer.gov. Accessed March 2008. Terms marked [2] are excerpted from "Headache: Hope through Research," National Institute of Neurological Disease and Stroke (NINDS), NIH Publication No. 02–158, updated January 2008.

antidepressant: A drug used to treat depression. [1]

anxiety: Feelings of fear, dread, and uneasiness that may occur as a reaction to stress. A person with anxiety may sweat, feel restless and tense, and have a rapid heart beat. Extreme anxiety that happens often over time may be a sign of an anxiety disorder. [1]

aspirin: A drug that reduces pain, fever, inflammation, and blood clotting. Aspirin belongs to the family of drugs called nonsteroidal anti-inflammatory agents. [1]

assessment: In health care, a process used to learn about a patient's condition. This may include a complete medical history, medical tests, a physical exam, a test of learning skills, tests to find out if the patient is able to carry out the tasks of daily living, a mental health evaluation, and a review of social support and community resources available to the patient. [1]

barrier: Something that blocks, prevents, separates, or limits. [1]

biofeedback: A technique in which patients are trained to gain some voluntary control over certain physiological conditions, such as blood pressure and muscle tension, to promote relaxation. Thermal biofeedback helps patients consciously raise hand temperature, which can sometimes reduce the number and intensity of migraines. [2]

bisphosphonate: A type of drug used to treat osteoporosis and the bone pain caused by some types of cancer. Also called diphosphonate. [1]

blood vessel: A tube through which the blood circulates in the body. Blood vessels include a network of arteries, arterioles, capillaries, venules, and veins. [1]

cancer: A term for diseases in which abnormal cells divide without control. Cancer cells can invade nearby tissues and can spread to other parts of the body through the blood and lymph systems. There are several main types of cancer. [1]

central nervous system (CNS): The brain and spinal cord. [1]

chemotherapy: Treatment with drugs that kill cancer cells. [1]

chronic: A disease or condition that persists or progresses over a long period of time. [1]

clinical: Having to do with the examination and treatment of patients. [1]

clinical trial: A type of research study that tests how well new medical approaches work in people. These studies test new methods of screening, prevention, diagnosis, or treatment of a disease. Also called a clinical study. [1]

computer tomography (CT): An imaging technique that uses x-rays and computer analysis to provide a picture of body tissues and structures. [2]

constipation: A condition in which stool becomes hard, dry, and difficult to pass, and bowel movements do not happen very often. Other symptoms may include painful bowel movements, and feeling bloated, uncomfortable, and sluggish. [1]

cope: To adjust to new situations and overcome problems. [1]

coping skills: The methods a person uses to deal with stressful situations. These may help a person face a situation, take action, and be flexible and persistent in solving problems. [1]

corticosteroid: Any steroid hormone made in the adrenal cortex (the outer part of the adrenal gland). They are also made in the laboratory. Corticosteroids have many different effects in the body, and are used to treat many different conditions. They may be used as hormone replacement, to suppress the immune system, and to treat some side effects of cancer and its treatment. [1]

counseling: The process by which a professional counselor helps a person cope with mental or emotional distress, and understand and solve personal problems. [1]

depression: A mental condition marked by ongoing feelings of sadness, despair, loss of energy, and difficulty dealing with normal daily life. Other symptoms of depression include feelings of worthlessness and hopelessness, loss of pleasure in activities, changes in eating or sleeping habits, and thoughts of death or suicide. Depression can affect anyone, and can be successfully treated. Depression affects 15–25% of cancer patients. [1]

diagnosis: The process of identifying a disease by the signs and symptoms. [1]

diagnostic procedure: A method used to identify a disease. [1]

disorder: In medicine, a disturbance of normal functioning of the mind or body. Disorders may be caused by genetic factors, disease, or trauma. [1]

dose: The amount of medicine taken, or radiation given, at one time. [1]

drug: Any substance, other than food, that is used to prevent, diagnose, treat or relieve symptoms of a disease or abnormal condition. Also refers to a substance that alters mood or body function, or that can be habit-forming or addictive, especially a narcotic. [1]

drug abuse: The use of illegal drugs or the use of prescription or over-the-counter drugs for purposes other than those for which they are meant to be used, or in large amounts. Drug abuse may lead to social, physical, emotional, and job-related problems. [1]

drug tolerance: A condition that occurs when the body gets used to a medicine so that either more medicine is needed or different medicine is needed. [1]

electrode: In medicine, a device such as a small metal plate or needle that carries electricity from an instrument to a patient for treatment or surgery. Electrodes can also carry electrical signals from muscles, brain, heart, skin, or other body parts to recording devices to help diagnose certain conditions. [1]

electroencephalogram (EEG): A technique for recording electrical activity in the brain. [2]

electromyography (EMG): A special recording technique that detects electric activity in muscle. Patients are sometimes offered a type of biofeedback called EMG training, in which they learn to control muscle tension in the face, neck, and shoulders. [2]

endorphins: Naturally occurring painkilling chemicals. Some scientists theorize that people who suffer from severe headache have lower levels of endorphins than people who are generally pain free. [2]

fatigue: A condition marked by extreme tiredness and inability to function due lack of energy. Fatigue may be acute or chronic. [1]

fentanyl: A narcotic opioid drug that is used in the treatment of pain. [1]

hydromorphone: A drug used to relieve pain. [1]

hypnosis: A trance-like state in which a person becomes more aware and focused and is more open to suggestion. [1]

imagery: A technique in which the person focuses on positive images in his or her mind. [1]

impairment: A loss of part or all of a physical or mental ability, such as the ability to see, walk, or learn. [1]

implant: A substance or object that is put in the body as a prosthesis, or for treatment or diagnosis. [1]

infusion: A method of putting fluids, including drugs, into the bloodstream. Also called intravenous infusion. [1]

injection: Use of a syringe and needle to push fluids or drugs into the body; often called a shot. [1]

intervention: In medicine, a treatment or action taken to prevent or treat disease, or improve health in other ways. [1]

intestine: The long, tube-shaped organ in the abdomen that completes the process of digestion. The intestine has two parts, the small intestine and the large intestine. Also called the bowel. [1]

intravenous (IV): Into or within a vein. Intravenous usually refers to a way of giving a drug or other substance through a needle or tube inserted into a vein. [1]

invasive procedure: A medical procedure that invades (enters) the body, usually by cutting or puncturing the skin or by inserting instruments into the body. [1]

kidney: One of a pair of organs in the abdomen. Kidneys remove waste from the blood (as urine), produce erythropoietin (a substance that stimulates red blood cell production), and play a role in blood pressure regulation. [1]

laxative: A substance that promotes bowel movements. [1]

lubricant: An oily or slippery substance. [1]

magnetic resonance imaging (MRI): An imaging technique that uses radio waves, magnetic fields, and computer analysis to provide a picture of body tissues and structures. [2]

massage therapy: A treatment in which the soft tissues of the body are kneaded, rubbed, tapped, and stroked. Massage therapy may help people relax, relieve stress and pain, lower blood pressure, and improve circulation. It is being studied in the treatment of symptoms such as lack of energy, pain, swelling, and depression. [1]

methadone: A morphine-like drug used to treat severe pain and to prevent withdrawal symptoms in patients who are addicted to heroin or other opiates. It may also be used to treat severe coughing in lung cancer patients. Methadone belongs to the family of drugs called opioid analgesics. [1]

migraine: A vascular headache believed to be caused by blood flow changes and certain chemical changes in the brain leading to a cascade of events—including constriction of arteries supplying blood to the brain and the release of certain brain chemicals—that result in severe head pain, stomach upset, and visual disturbances. [2]

morphine: A narcotic drug used in the treatment of pain. [1]

nausea: A feeling of sickness or discomfort in the stomach that may come with an urge to vomit. Nausea is a side effect of some types of cancer therapy. [1]

nerve: A bundle of fibers that receives and sends messages between the body and the brain. The messages are sent by chemical and electrical changes in the cells that make up the nerves. [1]

nerve block: A procedure in which medicine is injected directly into or around a nerve or into the spine to block pain. [1]

nociceptors: The endings of pain-sensitive nerves that, when stimulated by stress, muscular tension, dilated blood vessels, or other triggers, send messages up the nerve fibers to nerve cells in the brain, signaling that a part of the body hurts. [2]

noninvasive: In medicine, it describes a procedure that does not require inserting an instrument through the skin or into a body opening. In cancer, it describes disease that has not spread outside the tissue in which it began. [1]

nonsteroidal anti-inflammatory drug (NSAID): A drug that decreases fever, swelling, pain, and redness. [1]

obstruction: Blockage of a passageway. [1]

opioid: A drug used to treat moderate to severe pain. Opioids are similar to opiates such as morphine and codeine, but they do not contain and are not made from opium. [1]

oral: By or having to do with the mouth. [1]

oxycodone: A morphine-like drug used to treat medium to severe pain. It belongs to the family of drugs called opioid analgesics and may be habit-forming. [1]

patient-controlled analgesia (PCA): A method of pain relief in which the patient controls the amount of pain medicine that is used. When pain relief is needed, the person can receive a preset dose of pain medicine by pressing a button on a computerized pump that is connected to a small tube in the body. [1]

prescription: A doctor's order for medicine or another intervention. [1]

prevention: In medicine, action taken to decrease the chance of getting a disease or condition. For example, cancer prevention includes avoiding risk factors (such as smoking, obesity, lack of exercise, and radiation exposure) and increasing protective factors (such as getting regular physical activity, staying at a healthy weight, and having a healthy diet). [1]

prognosis: The likely outcome or course of a disease; the chance of recovery or recurrence. [1]

prostaglandins: Naturally occurring pain-producing substances thought to be implicated in migraine attacks. Their release is triggered by the dilation of arteries. Prostaglandins are extremely potent chemicals involved in a diverse group of physiological processes. [2]

psychiatrist: A medical doctor who specializes in the prevention, diagnosis, and treatment of mental, emotional, and behavioral disorders. [1]

psychological: Having to do with how the mind works and how thoughts and feelings affect behavior. [1]

pump: A device that is used to give a controlled amount of a liquid at a specific rate. For example, pumps are used to give drugs (such as chemotherapy or pain medicine) or nutrients. [1]

quality of life: The overall enjoyment of life. Many clinical trials assess the effects of treatments for pain and cancer on the quality of life. These studies measure aspects of an individual's sense of well-being and ability to carry out various activities. [1]

radiation therapy: The use of high-energy radiation from x-rays, gamma rays, neutrons, protons, and other sources to kill cancer cells and shrink tumors. Radiation may come from a machine outside the body (external-beam radiation therapy), or it may come from radioactive material placed in the body near cancer cells (internal radiation therapy). Systemic radiation therapy uses a radioactive substance, such as a radiolabeled monoclonal antibody, that travels in the blood to tissues throughout the body. Also called radiotherapy and irradiation. [1]

radioactive: Giving off radiation. [1]

radiofrequency ablation: The use of electrodes to heat and destroy abnormal tissue. [1]

rectal: By or having to do with the rectum. The rectum is the last several inches of the large intestine and ends at the anus. [1]

regimen: A treatment plan that specifies the dosage, the schedule, and the duration of treatment. [1]

relaxation technique: A method used to reduce tension and anxiety, and control pain. [1]

sedative: A drug or substance used to calm a person down, relieve anxiety, or help a person sleep. [1]

serotonin: A key neurotransmitter that acts as a powerful constrictor of arteries, reducing the blood supply to the brain and contributing to the pain of headache. [2]

side effect: A problem that occurs when treatment affects healthy tissues or organs. Some common side effects of cancer treatment are fatigue, pain, nausea, vomiting, decreased blood cell counts, hair loss, and mouth sores. [1]

social support: A network of family, friends, neighbors, and community members that is available in times of need to give psychological, physical, and financial help. [1]

spine: The bones, muscles, tendons, and other tissues that reach from the base of the skull to the tailbone. The spine encloses the spinal cord and the fluid surrounding the spinal cord. Also called backbone, spinal column, and vertebral column. [1]

spirituality: Having to do with deep, often religious, feelings and beliefs, including a person's sense of peace, purpose, connection to others, and beliefs about the meaning of life. [1]

stimulant: In medicine, a family of drugs used to treat depression, attention deficit disorder (a common disorder in which children are inattentive, impulsive, and/or over-active), and narcolepsy (a sleep disorder that causes uncontrollable sleepiness). Stimulants increase brain activity, alertness, attention, and energy. They also raise blood pressure and increase heart rate and breathing rate. [1]

stool: The material in a bowel movement. Stool is made up of food that was not digested, bacteria, mucus, and cells from the intestines. Also called feces. [1]

support group: A group of people with similar disease who meet to discuss how better to cope with their disease and treatment. [1]

supportive care: Care given to improve the quality of life of patients who have a serious or life-threatening disease. The goal of supportive care is to prevent or treat as early as possible the symptoms of a disease, side effects caused by treatment of a disease, and psychological, social, and spiritual problems related to a disease or its treatment. Also called palliative care, comfort care, and symptom management. [1]

symptom: An indication that a person has a condition or disease. Some examples of symptoms are headache, fever, fatigue, nausea, vomiting, and pain. [1]

therapy: Treatment. [1]

trigger: In medicine, a specific event that starts a process or that causes a particular outcome. For example, chemotherapy, painful treatments, or the smells, sounds, and sights that go with them may trigger anxiety and fear in a patient who has cancer. In allergies, exposure to mold, pollen or dust may trigger sneezing, watery eyes, and coughing. [1]

vomit: To eject some or all of the contents of the stomach through the mouth. [1]

Chapter 79

Additional Resources for Information about Pain

American Academy of Orthopaedic Surgeons
6300 N. River Rd.
Rosemont, IL 60018-4262
Phone: 847-823-7186
Fax: 847-823-8125
Website: http://www.aaos.org
E-mail: custserv@aaos.org

American Burn Association
625 N. Michigan Ave., Suite 2550
Chicago, IL 60611
Toll-Free: 800-548-2876
Phone: 312-642-9260
Fax: 312-642-9130
Website: http://www.ameriburn.org
E-mail: info@ameriburn.org

American Cancer Society
National Home Office
250 Williams St. N.W.
Atlanta, GA 30303
Toll-Free: 800-ACS-2345 (227-2345)
Website: http://www.cancer.org

American Chiropractic Association
1701 Clarendon Blvd.
Arlington, VA 22209
Toll-Free: 800-986-4636
Phone: 703-276-8800
Fax: 703-243-2593
Website: http://www.acatoday.org

Information in this chapter was compiled from many sources deemed reliable; inclusion does not constitute endorsement and omission does not imply objection. All contact information was updated and verified in March 2008.

**American Chronic Pain
Association (ACPA)**
P.O. Box 850
Rocklin, CA 95677-0850
Toll-Free: 800-533-3231
Phone: 916-632-0922
Fax: 916-632-3208
Website: http://
www.theacpa.org
E-mail: ACPA@pacbell.net

**American College of
Gastroenterology**
P.O. Box 342260
Bethesda, MD 20827-2260
Phone: 301-263-9000
Website: http://www.acg.gi.org

**American College of
Rheumatology (ACR)**
1800 Century Place
Suite 250
Atlanta, GA 30345-4300
Phone: 404-633-3777
Fax: 404-633-1870
Website: http://
www.rheumatology.org

**American Council for
Headache Education**
19 Mantua Road
Mt. Royal, NJ 08061
Toll-Free: 800-255-ACHE
(255-2243)
Phone: 856-423-0258
Fax: 856-423-0082
Website: http://www.achenet.org
E-mail: achehq@talley.com

**American Diabetes
Association**
1701 N. Beauregard St.
Alexandria, VA 22311
Toll-Free: 800-342-2383
Fax: 703-549-6995
Website: http://www.diabetes.org
E-mail: askada@diabetes.org

**American
Gastroenterological
Association**
National Office
4930 Del Ray Avenue
Bethesda, MD 20814
Phone: 301-654-2055
Fax: 301-654-5920
Website: http://www.gastro.org
E-mail: member@gastro.org

**American Osteopathic
Association**
142 E. Ontario St.
Chicago, IL 60611
Toll-Free: 800-621-1773
Phone: 312-202-8000
Fax: 312-202-8200
Website: http://
www.osteopathic.org

American Pain Foundation
201 N. Charles St., Suite 710
Baltimore, MD 21201-4111
Toll-Free: 888-615-PAIN (7246)
Fax: 410-385-1832
Website: http://
www.painfoundation.org
E-mail: info@painfoundation.org

*American Podiatric
Medical Association*
9312 Old Georgetown Rd.
Bethesda, MD 20814-1698
Toll-Free: 800-366-8227
Phone: 301-571-9200
Fax: 301-530-2752
Website: http://www.apma.org
E-mail: askapma@apma.org

*American RSDHope
Organization*
P.O. Box 875
Harrison, ME 04040-0875
Phone: 207-583-4589
Website: http://www.rsdhope.org
E-mail: rsdhope@roadrunner.com

*American Society for
Surgery of the Hand*
6300 N. River Rd.
Suite 600
Rosemont, IL 60018-4256
Phone: 847-384-8300
Fax: 847-384-1435
Website: http://www.assh.org
E-mail: info@assh.org

*American Urological
Association Foundation*
1000 Corporate Blvd.
Suite 410
Linthicum, MD 21090
Toll-Free: 866-746-4282
Phone: 410-689-3700
Fax: 410-689-3800
Website: http://
www.auafoundation.org
E-mail: patienteducation
@auafoundation.org

Arthritis Foundation
P.O. Box 7669
Atlanta, GA 30357-0669
Toll-Free: 800-283-7800
Phone: 404-872-7100
Website: http://
www.arthritis.org

*Brain Resources and
Information Network
(BRAIN)*
P.O. Box 5801
Bethesda, MD 20824
Toll-Free: 800-352-9424
Website: http://
www.ninds.nih.gov

*Centers for Disease Control
and Prevention (CDC)*
1600 Clifton Road, N.E.
Atlanta, GA 30333
Toll-Free: 800-311-3435
Phone: 404-639-3311
Fax: 404-639-3543
Website: http://
www.cdc.gov
E-mail: cdcinfo@cdc.gov

Family Caregiver Alliance
180 Montgomery St., Ste. 1100
San Francisco, CA 94104
Toll-Free: 800-445-8106
Phone: 415-434-3388
Fax: 415-434-3508
Website: http://
www.caregiver.org
E-mail: info@caregiver.org

609

Fibromyalgia Network
P.O. Box 31750
Tucson, AZ 85751-1750
Toll-Free: 800-853-2929
Phone: 520-290-5508
Fax: 520-290-5550
Website: http://
www.fmnetnews.com
E-mail: inquiry@fmnetnews.com

**International Foundation
for Functional
Gastrointestinal Disorders**
P.O. Box 170864
Milwaukee, WI 53217-8076
Toll-Free: 888-964-2001
Phone: 414-964-1799
Fax: 414-964-7176
Website: http://www.iffgd.org
E-mail: iffgd@iffgd.org

**International Radio
Surgery Association**
3002 N. 2nd Street
Harrisburg, PA 17110
Phone: 717-260-9808
Fax: 717-260-9809
Website: http://www.irsa.org
E-mail: office1@irsa.org

**International Research
Foundation for RSD/CRPS**
7612 Woodbridge Blvd.
Tampa, FL 33615
Phone: 813-907-2312
Fax: 813-830-7446
Website: http://
www.rsdfoundation.org
E-mail: info@rsdfoundation.org

**Interstitial Cystitis
Association of America**
110 N. Washington St.
Suite 340
Rockville, MD 20850
Toll-Free: 800-435-7422
Fax: 301-610-5308
Website: http://www.ichelp.org
E-mail: icamail@ichelp.org

**Lower Extremity
Amputation Prevention
Program**
Bureau of Primary Health Care
Health Resources and Services
Administration
U.S. Department of Health and
Human Services
1770 Physicians Park Dr.
Baton Rouge, LA 70816
Toll-Free: 888-275-4772
Website: http://
www.bphc.hrsa.gov/leap

MedWatch
Office of the Center Director
Center for Drug Evaluation
and Research
5515 Security Lane
Suite 5100
Rockville, MD 20852
Toll-Free: 800-332-1088
Fax: 800-332-0178
Website: http://www.fda.gov/
medwatch

**National Cancer
Institute (NCI)**
Cancer Information Service
6116 Executive Blvd.
Room 3036A
Bethesda, MD 20892-8322
Toll-Free: 800-4-CANCER
(422-6237)
TTY Toll-Free: 800-332-8615
Website: http://www.cancer.gov
E-mail:
cancergovstaff@mail.nih.gov

**National Center for
Complementary and
Alternative Medicine
(NCCAM)**
P.O. Box 7923
Gaithersburg, MD 20898-7923
Toll-Free: 888-644-6226
TTY Toll-Free: 866-464-3615
Phone: 301-519-3153
Fax: 866-464-3616
Website: http://nccam.nih.gov
E-mail: info@nccam.nih.gov

**National Diabetes
Education Program**
1 Diabetes Way
Bethesda, MD 20814-9692
Toll-Free: 800-438-5383
Phone: 301-496-3583
Website: http://www.ndep.nih
.gov
E-mail: ndep@mail.nih.gov

**National Digestive Diseases
Information Clearinghouse**
2 Information Way
Bethesda, MD 20892-3570
Toll-Free: 800-891-5389
Fax: 703-738-4929
Website: http://
www.digestive.niddk.nih.gov
E-mail:nddic@info.niddk.nih.gov

**National Eye Institute
(NEI)**
National Institutes of Health
31 Center Drive MSC 2510
Bethesda, MD 20892-2510
Toll-Free: 800-869-2020
Phone: 301-496-5248
Website: http://www.nei.nih.gov
E-mail: 2020@nei.nih.gov

**National Family
Caregivers Association**
10400 Connecticut Ave.
Suite 500
Kensington, MD 20895-3944
Toll-Free: 800-896-3650
Phone: 301-942-6430
Fax: 301-942-2302
Website: http://ww.nfcacares.org
E-mail:
info@thefamilycaregiver.org

**National Fibromyalgia
Association**
2200 N. Glassell St., Suite A
Orange, CA 92865
Phone: 714-921-0150
Fax: 714-921-6920
Website: http://www.fmaware.org
E-mail: nfa@fmaware.org

National Fibromyalgia Partnership, Inc.
P.O. Box 160
Linden, VA 22642-0160
Toll-Free: 866-725-4404
Fax: 866-666-2727
Website: http://
www.fmpartnership.org
E-mail:
mail@fmpartnership.org

National Foundation for the Treatment of Pain
P.O. Box 70045
Houston, TX 77270
Phone: 713-862-9332
Fax: 713-862-9346
Website: http://
www.paincare.org
E-mail: NFTPain@cwo.com

National Headache Foundation
820 N. Orleans
Suite 217
Chicago, IL 60610-3132
Toll-Free: 888-NHF-5552
(643-5552)
Phone: 312-274-2650
Fax: 312-640-9049
Website: http://
www.headaches.org
E-mail: info@headaches.org

National Institute of Arthritis and Musculoskeletal and Skin Diseases (NIAMS)
Information Clearinghouse
1 AMS Circle
Bethesda, MD 20892-3675
Toll-Free: 877-22-NIAMS
(226-4267)
Phone: 301-495-4484
TTY: 301-565-2966
Fax: 301-718-6366
Website: http://
www.niams.nih.gov
E-mail:
NIAMSinfo@mail.nih.gov

National Institute of Diabetes and Digestive and Kidney Diseases (NIDDK)
Building 31, Room 9A06
31 Center Drive, MSC 2560
Bethesda, MD 20892-2560
Phone: 301-496-3583
Website: http://
www.niddk.nih.gov
E-mail:
dkwebmaster@extra.niddk.nih.gov

National Institute of Neurological Disorders and Stroke (NINDS)
NIH Neurological Institute
P.O. Box 5801
Bethesda, MD 20824
Toll-Free: 800-352-9424
Phone: 301-496-5751
TTY: 301-468-5981
Website: http://
www.ninds.nih.gov
E-mail: braininfo@ninds.nih.gov

National Kidney and Urologic Diseases Information Clearinghouse
3 Information Way
Bethesda, MD 20892-3580
Toll-Free: 800-891-5390
Fax: 703-738-4929
Website: http://
www.kidney.niddk.nih.gov
E-mail:
nkudic@info.niddk.nih.gov

National Kidney Foundation, Inc.
30 East 33rd St.
New York, NY 10016
Toll-Free: 800-622-9010
Phone: 212-889-2210
Fax: 212-689-9261
Website: http://www.kidney.org

National Osteonecrosis Foundation
Good Samaritan
Professional Bldg.
5601 Loch Raven Blvd.
Suite 201
Baltimore, MD 21239
Phone: 410-532-5985
Fax: 410-532-5908
Website: http://www.nonf.org

Neuropathy Association
60 East 42nd St., Suite 942
New York, NY 10165-0999
Phone: 212-692-0662
Fax: 212-692-0668
Website: http://
www.neuropathy.org
E-mail: info@neuropathy.org

NIH Osteoporosis and Related Bone Diseases ~ National Resource Center
2 AMS Circle
Bethesda, MD 20892-3676
Toll-Free: 800-624-BONE (2663)
Phone: 202-223-0344
TTY: 202-466-4315
Fax: 202-466-4315
Website: http://
www.niams.nih.gov/
Health_Info/bone/default.asp
E-mail:
NIAMSBoneInfo@mail.nih.gov

North American Spine Society (part of AAOS)
7075 Veterans Blvd.
Burr Ridge, IL 60527
Phone: 630-230-3600
Fax: 630-230-3742
Website: http://www.spine.org
E-mail: info@spine.org

North American Society for Pediatric Gastroenterology, Hepatology, and Nutrition
P.O. Box 6
Flourtown, PA 19031
Phone: 215-233-0808
Fax: 215-233-3918
Website: http://
www.naspghan.org
E-mail:
naspghan@naspghan.org

Occupational Safety and Health Administration
U.S. Department of Labor
200 Constitution Ave., N.W.
Washington, DC 20210
Toll-Free: 800-321-OSHA (6742)
Website: http://www.osha.gov

Oxalosis and Hyperoxaluria Foundation
201 East 19th St.
Suite 12E
New York, NY 10003
Toll-Free: 800-643-8699
Phone: 212-777-0470
Fax: 212-777-0471
Website: http://www.ohf.org

Paget Foundation
120 Wall St., Suite 1602
New York, NY 10005-4001
Toll-Free: 800-23-PAGET (72438)
Phone: 212-509-5335
Fax: 212-509-8492
Website: http://www.paget.org
E-mail: pagetfdn@aol.com

Pediatric/Adolescent Gastroesophageal Reflux Association, Inc. (PAGER)
P.O. Box 486
Buckeystown, MD 21717-0486
Phone: 301-601-9541
(message center, checked daily)
Website: http://www.reflux.org
E-mail: gergroup@aol.com

Pedorthic Footwear Association
7150 Columbia Gateway Dr.
Suite G
Columbia, MD 21046-1151
Toll-Free: 800-673-8447
Phone: 410-381-7278
Fax: 410-381-1167
Website: http://www.pedorthics.org

Phoenix Society for Burn Survivors, Inc.
1835 R W Berends Dr. S.W.
Grand Rapids, MI 49519-4955
Toll-Free: 800-888-2876
Phone: 616-458-2773
Fax: 616-458-2831
Website: http://www.phoenix-society.org
E-mail: info@phoenix-society.org

Reflex Sympathetic Dystrophy Syndrome Association (RSDSA)
P.O. Box 502
Milford, CT 06460
Toll-Free: 877-662-7737
Phone: 203-877-3790
Fax: 203-882-8362
Website: http://www.rsds.org
E-mail: info@rsds.org

Trigeminal Neuralgia Association
925 N.W. 56th Terrace, Suite C
Gainesville, FL 32605-6402
Toll-Free: 800-923-3608
Phone: 352-331-7009
Fax: 352-331-7078
Website: http://
www.endthepain.org
E-mail: info@fpa-support.org

U.S. Food and Drug Administration (FDA)
Office of Consumer Affairs
5600 Fishers Lane, HFE-50
Rockville, MD 20857
Toll-Free: 888-463-6332
(888-INFO-FDA)
Phone: 301-827-4420
Fax: 301-443-9767
Website: http://www.fda.gov

VZV Research Foundation
Research on Varicella Zoster
1202 Lexington Ave., Suite 204
New York, NY 10028
Phone: 212-222-3390
Fax: 212-222-8627
Website: http://
www.vzvfoundation.org
E-mail: vzv@vzvfoundation.org

Index

Index

M

Health Reference Series
COMPLETE CATALOG
List price $87 per volume. **School and library price $78 per volume.**

Adolescent Health Sourcebook, 2nd Edition

Basic Consumer Health Information about the Physical, Mental, and Emotional Growth and Development of Adolescents, Including Medical Care, Nutritional and Physical Activity Requirements, Puberty, Sexual Activity, Acne, Tanning, Body Piercing, Common Physical Illnesses and Disorders, Eating Disorders, Attention Deficit Hyperactivity Disorder, Depression, Bullying, Hazing, and Adolescent Injuries Related to Sports, Driving, and Work

Along with Substance Abuse Information about Nicotine, Alcohol, and Drug Use, a Glossary, and Directory of Additional Resources

Edited by Joyce Brennfleck Shannon. 683 pages. 2006. 978-0-7808-0943-7.

"It is written in clear, nontechnical language aimed at general readers. . . . Recommended for public libraries, community colleges, and other agencies serving health care consumers."
— *American Reference Books Annual, 2003*

"Recommended for school and public libraries. Parents and professionals dealing with teens will appreciate the easy-to-follow format and the clearly written text. This could become a 'must have' for every high school teacher." — *E-Streams, Jan '03*

"A good starting point for information related to common medical, mental, and emotional concerns of adolescents." — *School Library Journal, Nov '02*

"This book provides accurate information in an easy to access format. It addresses topics that parents and caregivers might not be aware of and provides practical, useable information."
— *Doody's Health Sciences Book Review Journal, Sep-Oct '02*

"Recommended reference source."
— *Booklist, American Library Association, Sep '02*

▪

AIDS Sourcebook, 3rd Edition

Basic Consumer Health Information about Acquired Immune Deficiency Syndrome (AIDS) and Human Immunodeficiency Virus (HIV) Infection, Including Facts about Transmission, Prevention, Diagnosis, Treatment, Opportunistic Infections, and Other Complications, with a Section for Women and Children, Including Details about Associated Gynecological Concerns, Pregnancy, and Pediatric Care

Along with Updated Statistical Information, Reports on Current Research Initiatives, a Glossary, and Directories of Internet, Hotline, and Other Resources

Edited by Dawn D. Matthews. 664 pages. 2003. 978-0-7808-0631-3.

"The 3rd edition of the *AIDS Sourcebook*, part of Omnigraphics' *Health Reference Series*, is a welcome update. . . . This resource is highly recommended for academic and public libraries."
— *American Reference Books Annual, 2004*

"Excellent sourcebook. This continues to be a highly recommended book. There is no other book that provides as much information as this book provides."
— *AIDS Book Review Journal, Dec-Jan '00*

"Recommended reference source."
— *Booklist, American Library Association, Dec '99*

▪

Alcoholism Sourcebook, 2nd Edition

Basic Consumer Health Information about Alcohol Use, Abuse, and Dependence, Featuring Facts about the Physical, Mental, and Social Health Effects of Alcohol Addiction, Including Alcoholic Liver Disease, Pancreatic Disease, Cardiovascular Disease, Neurological Disorders, and the Effects of Drinking during Pregnancy

Along with Information about Alcohol Treatment, Medications, and Recovery Programs, in Addition to Tips for Reducing the Prevalence of Underage Drinking, Statistics about Alcohol Use, a Glossary of Related Terms, and Directories of Resources for More Help and Information

Edited by Amy L. Sutton. 653 pages. 2006. 978-0-7808-0942-0.

"This title is one of the few reference works on alcoholism for general readers. For some readers this will be a welcome complement to the many self-help books on the market. Recommended for collections serving general readers and consumer health collections."
— *E-Streams, Mar '01*

"This book is an excellent choice for public and academic libraries."
— *American Reference Books Annual, 2001*

"Recommended reference source."
— *Booklist, American Library Association, Dec '00*

"Presents a wealth of information on alcohol use and abuse and its effects on the body and mind, treatment, and prevention." — *SciTech Book News, Dec '00*

"Important new health guide which packs in the latest consumer information about the problems of alcoholism." — *Reviewer's Bookwatch, Nov '00*

SEE ALSO *Drug Abuse Sourcebook*

Allergies Sourcebook, 3rd Edition

Basic Consumer Health Information about Allergic Disorders, Such as Anaphylaxis, Hives, Eczema, Rhinitis, Sinusitis, and Conjunctivitis, and Their Triggers, Including Pollen, Mold, Dust Mites, Animal Dander, Insects, Chemicals, Food, Food Additives, and Medications;

Along with Advice about the Diagnosis and Treatment of Allergy Symptoms, a Glossary of Related Terms, a Directory of Resources for Help and Information, and Suggestions for Additional Reading

Edited by Amy L. Sutton. 598 pages. 2007. 978-0-7808-0950-5.

"This book brings a great deal of useful material together. . . . This is an excellent addition to public and consumer health library collections."

—*American Reference Books Annual, 2003*

"This second edition would be useful to laypersons with little or advanced knowledge of the subject matter. This book would also serve as a resource for nursing and other health care professions students. It would be useful in public, academic, and hospital libraries with consumer health collections." —*E-Streams, Jul '02*

◼

Alternative Medicine Sourcebook

SEE Complementary & Alternative Medicine Sourcebook

◼

Alzheimer's Disease Sourcebook, 3rd Edition

Basic Consumer Health Information about Alzheimer's Disease, Other Dementias, and Related Disorders, Including Multi-Infarct Dementia, AIDS Dementia Complex, Dementia with Lewy Bodies, Huntington's Disease, Wernicke-Korsakoff Syndrome (Alcohol-Related Dementia), Delirium, and Confusional States

Along with Information for People Newly Diagnosed with Alzheimer's Disease and Caregivers, Reports Detailing Current Research Efforts in Prevention, Diagnosis, and Treatment, Facts about Long-Term Care Issues, and Listings of Sources for Additional Information

Edited by Karen Bellenir. 645 pages. 2003. 978-0-7808-0666-5.

"This very informative and valuable tool will be a great addition to any library serving consumers, students and health care workers."

—*American Reference Books Annual, 2004*

"This is a valuable resource for people affected by dementias such as Alzheimer's. It is easy to navigate and includes important information and resources."

—*Doody's Review Service, Feb '04*

"Recommended reference source."
—*Booklist, American Library Association, Oct '99*

SEE ALSO *Brain Disorders Sourcebook*

Arthritis Sourcebook, 2nd Edition

Basic Consumer Health Information about Osteoarthritis, Rheumatoid Arthritis, Other Rheumatic Disorders, Infectious Forms of Arthritis, and Diseases with Symptoms Linked to Arthritis, Featuring Facts about Diagnosis, Pain Management, and Surgical Therapies

Along with Coping Strategies, Research Updates, a Glossary, and Resources for Additional Help and Information

Edited by Amy L. Sutton. 593 pages. 2004. 978-0-7808-0667-2.

"This easy-to-read volume is recommended for consumer health collections within public or academic libraries." —*E-Streams, May '05*

"As expected, this updated edition continues the excellent reputation of this series in providing sound, usable health information. . . . Highly recommended."

—*American Reference Books Annual, 2005*

"Excellent reference." —*The Bookwatch, Jan '05*

◼

Asthma Sourcebook, 2nd Edition

Basic Consumer Health Information about the Causes, Symptoms, Diagnosis, and Treatment of Asthma in Infants, Children, Teenagers, and Adults, Including Facts about Different Types of Asthma, Common Co-Occurring Conditions, Asthma Management Plans, Triggers, Medications, and Medication Delivery Devices

Along with Asthma Statistics, Research Updates, a Glossary, a Directory of Asthma-Related Resources, and More

Edited by Karen Bellenir. 609 pages. 2006. 978-0-7808-0866-9.

"A worthwhile reference acquisition for public libraries and academic medical libraries whose readers desire a quick introduction to the wide range of asthma information." —*Choice, Association of College & Research Libraries, Jun '01*

"Recommended reference source."
—*Booklist, American Library Association, Feb '01*

"Highly recommended." —*The Bookwatch, Jan '01*

"There is much good information for patients and their families who deal with asthma daily."
—*American Medical Writers Association Journal, Winter '01*

"This informative text is recommended for consumer health collections in public, secondary school, and community college libraries and the libraries of universities with a large undergraduate population."
—*American Reference Books Annual, 2001*

◼

Attention Deficit Disorder Sourcebook

Basic Consumer Health Information about Attention Deficit/Hyperactivity Disorder in Children and Adults,

Including Facts about Causes, Symptoms, Diagnostic Criteria, and Treatment Options Such as Medications, Behavior Therapy, Coaching, and Homeopathy

Along with Reports on Current Research Initiatives, Legal Issues, and Government Regulations, and Featuring a Glossary of Related Terms, Internet Resources, and a List of Additional Reading Material

Edited by Dawn D. Matthews. 470 pages. 2002. 978-0-7808-0624-5.

"Recommended reference source."
— Booklist, American Library Association, Jan '03

"This book is recommended for all school libraries and the reference or consumer health sections of public libraries." — American Reference Books Annual, 2003

■

Back & Neck Sourcebook, 2nd Edition

Basic Consumer Health Information about Spinal Pain, Spinal Cord Injuries, and Related Disorders, Such as Degenerative Disk Disease, Osteoarthritis, Scoliosis, Sciatica, Spina Bifida, and Spinal Stenosis, and Featuring Facts about Maintaining Spinal Health, Self-Care, Pain Management, Rehabilitative Care, Chiropractic Care, Spinal Surgeries, and Complementary Therapies

Along with Suggestions for Preventing Back and Neck Pain, a Glossary of Related Terms, and a Directory of Resources

Edited by Amy L. Sutton. 633 pages. 2004. 978-0-7808-0738-9.

"Recommended . . . an easy to use, comprehensive medical reference book." — E-Streams, Sep '05

"The strength of this work is its basic, easy-to-read format. Recommended." — Reference and User Services Quarterly, American Library Association, Winter '97

■

Blood & Circulatory Disorders Sourcebook, 2nd Edition

Basic Consumer Health Information about the Blood and Circulatory System and Related Disorders, Such as Anemia and Other Hemoglobin Diseases, Cancer of the Blood and Associated Bone Marrow Disorders, Clotting and Bleeding Problems, and Conditions That Affect the Veins, Blood Vessels, and Arteries, Including Facts about the Donation and Transplantation of Bone Marrow, Stem Cells, and Blood and Tips for Keeping the Blood and Circulatory System Healthy

Along with a Glossary of Related Terms and Resources for Additional Help and Information

Edited by Amy L. Sutton. 659 pages. 2005. 978-0-7808-0746-4.

"Highly recommended pick for basic consumer health reference holdings at all levels."
— The Bookwatch, Aug '05

"Recommended reference source."
— Booklist, American Library Association, Feb '99

"An important reference sourcebook written in simple language for everyday, non-technical users. "
— Reviewer's Bookwatch, Jan '99

■

Brain Disorders Sourcebook, 2nd Edition

Basic Consumer Health Information about Acquired and Traumatic Brain Injuries, Infections of the Brain, Epilepsy and Seizure Disorders, Cerebral Palsy, and Degenerative Neurological Disorders, Including Amyotrophic Lateral Sclerosis (ALS), Dementias, Multiple Sclerosis, and More

Along with Information on the Brain's Structure and Function, Treatment and Rehabilitation Options, Reports on Current Research Initiatives, a Glossary of Terms Related to Brain Disorders and Injuries, and a Directory of Sources for Further Help and Information

Edited by Sandra J. Judd. 625 pages. 2005. 978-0-7808-0744-0.

"Highly recommended pick for basic consumer health reference holdings at all levels."
— The Bookwatch, Aug '05

"Belongs on the shelves of any library with a consumer health collection." — E-Streams, Mar '00

"Recommended reference source."
— Booklist, American Library Association, Oct '99

SEE ALSO Alzheimer's Disease Sourcebook

■

Breast Cancer Sourcebook, 2nd Edition

Basic Consumer Health Information about Breast Cancer, Including Facts about Risk Factors, Prevention, Screening and Diagnostic Methods, Treatment Options, Complementary and Alternative Therapies, Post-Treatment Concerns, Clinical Trials, Special Risk Populations, and New Developments in Breast Cancer Research

Along with Breast Cancer Statistics, a Glossary of Related Terms, and a Directory of Resources for Additional Help and Information

Edited by Sandra J. Judd. 595 pages. 2004. 978-0-7808-0668-9.

"This book will be an excellent addition to public, community college, medical, and academic libraries."
— American Reference Books Annual, 2006

"It would be a useful reference book in a library or on loan to women in a support group."
— Cancer Forum, Mar '03

"Recommended reference source."
— Booklist, American Library Association, Jan '02

"This reference source is highly recommended. It is quite informative, comprehensive and detailed in nature, and yet it offers practical advice in easy-to-read language. It could be thought of as the 'bible' of breast cancer for the consumer." —*E-Streams, Jan '02*

"From the pros and cons of different screening methods and results to treatment options, *Breast Cancer Sourcebook* provides the latest information on the subject." —*Library Bookwatch, Dec '01*

"This thoroughgoing, very readable reference covers all aspects of breast health and cancer.... Readers will find much to consider here. Recommended for all public and patient health collections." —*Library Journal, Sep '01*

SEE ALSO Cancer Sourcebook for Women, Women's Health Concerns Sourcebook

■

Breastfeeding Sourcebook

Basic Consumer Health Information about the Benefits of Breastmilk, Preparing to Breastfeed, Breastfeeding as a Baby Grows, Nutrition, and More, Including Information on Special Situations and Concerns Such as Mastitis, Illness, Medications, Allergies, Multiple Births, Prematurity, Special Needs, and Adoption

Along with a Glossary and Resources for Additional Help and Information

Edited by Jenni Lynn Colson. 388 pages. 2002. 978-0-7808-0332-9.

"Particularly useful is the information about professional lactation services and chapters on breastfeeding when returning to work.... *Breastfeeding Sourcebook* will be useful for public libraries, consumer health libraries, and technical schools offering nurse assistant training, especially in areas where Internet access is problematic." —*American Reference Books Annual, 2003*

SEE ALSO Pregnancy & Birth Sourcebook

■

Burns Sourcebook

Basic Consumer Health Information about Various Types of Burns and Scalds, Including Flame, Heat, Cold, Electrical, Chemical, and Sun Burns

Along with Information on Short-Term and Long-Term Treatments, Tissue Reconstruction, Plastic Surgery, Prevention Suggestions, and First Aid

Edited by Allan R. Cook. 604 pages. 1999. 978-0-7808-0204-9.

"This is an exceptional addition to the series and is highly recommended for all consumer health collections, hospital libraries, and academic medical centers." —*E-Streams, Mar '00*

"This key reference guide is an invaluable addition to all health care and public libraries in confronting this ongoing health issue." —*American Reference Books Annual, 2000*

"Recommended reference source." —*Booklist, American Library Association, Dec '99*

SEE ALSO Dermatological Disorders Sourcebook

Cancer Sourcebook, 5th Edition

Basic Consumer Health Information about Major Forms and Stages of Cancer, Featuring Facts about Head and Neck Cancers, Lung Cancers, Gastrointestinal Cancers, Genitourinary Cancers, Lymphomas, Blood Cell Cancers, Endocrine Cancers, Skin Cancers, Bone Cancers, Metastatic Cancers, and More

Along with Facts about Cancer Treatments, Cancer Risks and Prevention, a Glossary of Related Terms, Statistical Data, and a Directory of Resources for Additional Information

Edited by Karen Bellenir. 1,133 pages. 2007. 978-0-7808-0947-5.

"With cancer being the second leading cause of death for Americans, a prodigious work such as this one, which locates centrally so much cancer-related information, is clearly an asset to this nation's citizens and others." —*Journal of the National Medical Association, 2004*

"This title is recommended for health sciences and public libraries with consumer health collections." —*E-Streams, Feb '01*

"... can be effectively used by cancer patients and their families who are looking for answers in a language they can understand. Public and hospital libraries should have it on their shelves." —*American Reference Books Annual, 2001*

"Recommended reference source." —*Booklist, American Library Association, Dec '00*

SEE ALSO Breast Cancer Sourcebook, Cancer Sourcebook for Women, Pediatric Cancer Sourcebook, Prostate Cancer Sourcebook

■

Cancer Sourcebook for Women, 3rd Edition

Basic Consumer Health Information about Leading Causes of Cancer in Women, Featuring Facts about Gynecologic Cancers and Related Concerns, Such as Breast Cancer, Cervical Cancer, Endometrial Cancer, Uterine Sarcoma, Vaginal Cancer, Vulvar Cancer, and Common Non-Cancerous Gynecologic Conditions, in Addition to Facts about Lung Cancer, Colorectal Cancer, and Thyroid Cancer in Women

Along with Information about Cancer Risk Factors, Screening and Prevention, Treatment Options, and Tips on Coping with Life after Cancer Treatment, a Glossary of Cancer Terms, and a Directory of Resources for Additional Help and Information

Edited by Amy L. Sutton. 715 pages. 2006. 978-0-7808-0867-6.

"An excellent addition to collections in public, consumer health, and women's health libraries." —*American Reference Books Annual, 2003*

"Overall, the information is excellent, and complex topics are clearly explained. As a reference book for the consumer it is a valuable resource to assist them to make informed decisions about cancer and its treatments." —*Cancer Forum, Nov '02*

SEE ALSO Breast Cancer Sourcebook, Women's Health Concerns Sourcebook

Cancer Survivorship Sourcebook

Basic Consumer Health Information about the Physical, Educational, Emotional, Social, and Financial Needs of Cancer Patients from Diagnosis, through Cancer Treatment, and Beyond, Including Facts about Researching Specific Types of Cancer and Learning about Clinical Trials and Treatment Options, and Featuring Tips for Coping with the Side Effects of Cancer Treatments and Adjusting to Life after Cancer Treatment Concludes

Along with Suggestions for Caregivers, Friends, and Family Members of Cancer Patients, a Glossary of Cancer Care Terms, and Directories of Related Resources

Edited by Karen Bellenir. 6561 pages. 2007. 978-0-7808-0985-7.

Cardiovascular Diseases & Disorders Sourcebook, 3rd Edition

Basic Consumer Health Information about Heart and Vascular Diseases and Disorders, Such as Angina, Heart Attacks, Arrhythmias, Cardiomyopathy, Valve Disease, Atherosclerosis, and Aneurysms, with Information about Managing Cardiovascular Risk Factors and Maintaining Heart Health, Medications and Procedures Used to Treat Cardiovascular Disorders, and Concerns of Special Significance to Women

Along with Reports on Current Research Initiatives, a Glossary of Related Medical Terms, and a Directory of Sources for Further Help and Information

Edited by Sandra J. Judd. 713 pages. 2005. 978-0-7808-0739-6.

Caregiving Sourcebook

Basic Consumer Health Information for Caregivers, Including a Profile of Caregivers, Caregiving Responsibilities and Concerns, Tips for Specific Conditions, Care Environments, and the Effects of Caregiving

Along with Facts about Legal Issues, Financial Information, and Future Planning, a Glossary, and a Listing of Additional Resources

Edited by Joyce Brennfleck Shannon. 600 pages. 2001. 978-0-7808-0331-2.

Child Abuse Sourcebook

Basic Consumer Health Information about the Physical, Sexual, and Emotional Abuse of Children, with Additional Facts about Neglect, Munchausen Syndrome by Proxy (MSBP), Shaken Baby Syndrome, and Controversial Issues Related to Child Abuse, Such as Withholding Medical Care, Corporal Punishment, and Child Maltreatment in Youth Sports, and Featuring Facts about Child Protective Services, Foster Care, Adoption, Parenting Challenges, and Other Abuse Prevention Efforts

Along with a Glossary of Related Terms and Resources for Additional Help and Information

Edited by Dawn D. Matthews. 620 pages. 2004. 978-0-7808-0705-1.

SEE ALSO: Domestic Violence Sourcebook

Childhood Diseases & Disorders Sourcebook

Basic Consumer Health Information about Medical Problems Often Encountered in Pre-Adolescent Children, Including Respiratory Tract Ailments, Ear Infections, Sore Throats, Disorders of the Skin and Scalp, Digestive and Genitourinary Diseases, Infectious Diseases, Inflammatory Disorders, Chronic Physical and Developmental Disorders, Allergies, and More

Along with Information about Diagnostic Tests, Common Childhood Surgeries, and Frequently Used Medications, with a Glossary of Important Terms and Resource Directory

Edited by Chad T. Kimball. 662 pages. 2003. 978-0-7808-0458-6.

"This is an excellent book for new parents and should be included in all health care and public libraries."
—*American Reference Books Annual, 2004*

SEE ALSO: Healthy Children Sourcebook

■

Colds, Flu & Other Common Ailments Sourcebook

Basic Consumer Health Information about Common Ailments and Injuries, Including Colds, Coughs, the Flu, Sinus Problems, Headaches, Fever, Nausea and Vomiting, Menstrual Cramps, Diarrhea, Constipation, Hemorrhoids, Back Pain, Dandruff, Dry and Itchy Skin, Cuts, Scrapes, Sprains, Bruises, and More

Along with Information about Prevention, Self-Care, Choosing a Doctor, Over-the-Counter Medications, Folk Remedies, and Alternative Therapies, and Including a Glossary of Important Terms and a Directory of Resources for Further Help and Information

Edited by Chad T. Kimball. 638 pages. 2001. 978-0-7808-0435-7.

"A good starting point for research on common illnesses. It will be a useful addition to public and consumer health library collections."
—*American Reference Books Annual, 2002*

"Will prove valuable to any library seeking to maintain a current, comprehensive reference collection of health resources. . . . Excellent reference."
—*The Bookwatch, Aug '01*

"Recommended reference source."
—*Booklist, American Library Association, Jul '01*

■

Communication Disorders Sourcebook

Basic Information about Deafness and Hearing Loss, Speech and Language Disorders, Voice Disorders, Balance and Vestibular Disorders, and Disorders of Smell, Taste, and Touch

Edited by Linda M. Ross. 533 pages. 1996. 978-0-7808-0077-9.

"This is skillfully edited and is a welcome resource for the layperson. It should be found in every public and medical library." —*Booklist Health Sciences Supplement, American Library Association, Oct '97*

■

Complementary & Alternative Medicine Sourcebook, 3rd Edition

Basic Consumer Health Information about Complementary and Alternative Medical Therapies, Including Acupuncture, Ayurveda, Traditional Chinese Medicine, Herbal Medicine, Homeopathy, Naturopathy, Biofeedback, Hypnotherapy, Yoga, Art Therapy, Aromatherapy, Clinical Nutrition, Vitamin and Mineral Supplements, Chiropractic, Massage, Reflexology, Crystal Therapy, Therapeutic Touch, and More

Along with Facts about Alternative and Complementary Treatments for Specific Conditions Such as Cancer, Diabetes, Osteoarthritis, Chronic Pain, Menopause, Gastrointestinal Disorders, Headaches, and Mental Illness, a Glossary, and a Resource List for Additional Help and Information

Edited by Sandra J. Judd. 657 pages. 2006. 978-0-7808-0864-5.

"Recommended for public, high school, and academic libraries that have consumer health collections. Hospital libraries that also serve the public will find this to be a useful resource." —*E-Streams, Feb '03*

"Recommended reference source."
—*Booklist, American Library Association, Jan '03*

"An important alternate health reference."
—*MBR Bookwatch, Oct '02*

"A great addition to the reference collection of every type of library." —*American Reference Books Annual, 2000*

■

Congenital Disorders Sourcebook, 2nd Edition

Basic Consumer Health Information about Nonhereditary Birth Defects and Disorders Related to Prematurity, Gestational Injuries, Congenital Infections, and Birth Complications, Including Heart Defects, Hydrocephalus, Spina Bifida, Cleft Lip and Palate, Cerebral Palsy, and More

Along with Facts about the Prevention of Birth Defects, Fetal Surgery and Other Treatment Options, Research Initiatives, a Glossary of Related Terms, and Resources for Additional Information and Support

Edited by Sandra J. Judd. 647 pages. 2006. 978-0-7808-0945-1.

"Recommended reference source."
—*Booklist, American Library Association, Oct '97*

SEE ALSO Pregnancy & Birth Sourcebook

■

Contagious Diseases Sourcebook

Basic Consumer Health Information about Infectious Diseases Spread by Person-to-Person Contact through

Direct Touch, Airborne Transmission, Sexual Contact, or Contact with Blood or Other Body Fluids, Including Hepatitis, Herpes, Influenza, Lice, Measles, Mumps, Pinworm, Ringworm, Severe Acute Respiratory Syndrome (SARS), Streptococcal Infections, Tuberculosis, and Others

Along with Facts about Disease Transmission, Antimicrobial Resistance, and Vaccines, with a Glossary and Directories of Resources for More Information

Edited by Karen Bellenir. 643 pages. 2004. 978-0-7808-0736-5.

"This easy-to-read volume is recommended for consumer health collections within public or academic libraries."
— E-Streams, May '05

"This informative book is highly recommended for public libraries, consumer health collections, and secondary schools and undergraduate libraries."
— American Reference Books Annual, 2005

"Excellent reference."
— The Bookwatch, Jan '05

■

Death & Dying Sourcebook, 2nd Edition

Basic Consumer Health Information about End-of-Life Care and Related Perspectives and Ethical Issues, Including End-of-Life Symptoms and Treatments, Pain Management, Quality-of-Life Concerns, the Use of Life Support, Patients' Rights and Privacy Issues, Advance Directives, Physician-Assisted Suicide, Caregiving, Organ and Tissue Donation, Autopsies, Funeral Arrangements, and Grief

Along with Statistical Data, Information about the Leading Causes of Death, a Glossary, and Directories of Support Groups and Other Resources

Edited by Joyce Brennfleck Shannon. 653 pages. 2006. 978-0-7808-0871-3.

"Public libraries, medical libraries, and academic libraries will all find this sourcebook a useful addition to their collections."
— American Reference Books Annual, 2001

"An extremely useful resource for those concerned with death and dying in the United States."
— Respiratory Care, Nov '00

"Recommended reference source."
— Booklist, American Library Association, Aug '00

"This book is a definite must for all those involved in end-of-life care."
— Doody's Review Service, 2000

■

Dental Care & Oral Health Sourcebook, 2nd Edition

Basic Consumer Health Information about Dental Care, Including Oral Hygiene, Dental Visits, Pain Management, Cavities, Crowns, Bridges, Dental Implants, and Fillings, and Other Oral Health Concerns, Such as Gum Disease, Bad Breath, Dry Mouth, Genetic and Developmental Abnormalities, Oral Cancers, Orthodontics, and Temporomandibular Disorders

Along with Updates on Current Research in Oral Health, a Glossary, a Directory of Dental and Oral Health Organizations, and Resources for People with Dental and Oral Health Disorders

Edited by Amy L. Sutton. 609 pages. 2003. 978-0-7808-0634-4.

"This book could serve as a turning point in the battle to educate consumers in issues concerning oral health."
— American Reference Books Annual, 2004

"Unique source which will fill a gap in dental sources for patients and the lay public. A valuable reference tool even in a library with thousands of books on dentistry. Comprehensive, clear, inexpensive, and easy to read and use. It fills an enormous gap in the health care literature."
— Reference & User Services Quarterly, American Library Association, Summer '98

"Recommended reference source."
— Booklist, American Library Association, Dec '97

■

Depression Sourcebook

Basic Consumer Health Information about Unipolar Depression, Bipolar Disorder, Postpartum Depression, Seasonal Affective Disorder, and Other Types of Depression in Children, Adolescents, Women, Men, the Elderly, and Other Selected Populations

Along with Facts about Causes, Risk Factors, Diagnostic Criteria, Treatment Options, Coping Strategies, Suicide Prevention, a Glossary, and a Directory of Sources for Additional Help and Information

Edited by Karen Bellenir. 602 pages. 2002. 978-0-7808-0611-5.

"Depression Sourcebook is of a very high standard. Its purpose, which is to serve as a reference source to the lay reader, is very well served."
— Journal of the National Medical Association, 2004

"Invaluable reference for public and school library collections alike."
— Library Bookwatch, Apr '03

"Recommended for purchase."
— American Reference Books Annual, 2003

■

Dermatological Disorders Sourcebook, 2nd Edition

Basic Consumer Health Information about Conditions and Disorders Affecting the Skin, Hair, and Nails, Such as Acne, Rosacea, Rashes, Dermatitis, Pigmentation Disorders, Birthmarks, Skin Cancer, Skin Injuries, Psoriasis, Scleroderma, and Hair Loss, Including Facts about Medications and Treatments for Dermatological Disorders and Tips for Maintaining Healthy Skin, Hair, and Nails

Along with Information about How Aging Affects the Skin, a Glossary of Related Terms, and a Directory of Resources for Additional Help and Information

Edited by Amy L. Sutton. 645 pages. 2005. 978-0-7808-0795-2.

"... comprehensive, easily read reference book."
— *Doody's Health Sciences Book Reviews, Oct '97*

SEE ALSO *Burns Sourcebook*

■

Diabetes Sourcebook, 3rd Edition

Basic Consumer Health Information about Type 1 Diabetes (Insulin-Dependent or Juvenile-Onset Diabetes), Type 2 Diabetes (Noninsulin-Dependent or Adult-Onset Diabetes), Gestational Diabetes, Impaired Glucose Tolerance (IGT), and Related Complications, Such as Amputation, Eye Disease, Gum Disease, Nerve Damage, and End-Stage Renal Disease, Including Facts about Insulin, Oral Diabetes Medications, Blood Sugar Testing, and the Role of Exercise and Nutrition in the Control of Diabetes

Along with a Glossary and Resources for Further Help and Information

Edited by Dawn D. Matthews. 622 pages. 2003. 978-0-7808-0629-0.

"This edition is even more helpful than earlier versions. . . . It is a truly valuable tool for anyone seeking readable and authoritative information on diabetes."
— *American Reference Books Annual, 2004*

"An invaluable reference." — *Library Journal, May '00*

Selected as one of the 250 "Best Health Sciences Books of 1999." — *Doody's Rating Service, Mar-Apr '00*

"Provides useful information for the general public."
— *Healthlines, University of Michigan Health Management Research Center, Sep/Oct '99*

". . . provides reliable mainstream medical information . . . belongs on the shelves of any library with a consumer health collection." — *E-Streams, Sep '99*

"Recommended reference source."
— *Booklist, American Library Association, Feb '99*

■

Diet & Nutrition Sourcebook, 3rd Edition

Basic Consumer Health Information about Dietary Guidelines and the Food Guidance System, Recommended Daily Nutrient Intakes, Serving Proportions, Weight Control, Vitamins and Supplements, Nutrition Issues for Different Life Stages and Lifestyles, and the Needs of People with Specific Medical Concerns, Including Cancer, Celiac Disease, Diabetes, Eating Disorders, Food Allergies, and Cardiovascular Disease

Along with Facts about Federal Nutrition Support Programs, a Glossary of Nutrition and Dietary Terms, and Directories of Additional Resources for More Information about Nutrition

Edited by Joyce Brennfleck Shannon. 633 pages. 2006. 978-0-7808-0800-3.

"This book is an excellent source of basic diet and nutrition information." — *Booklist Health Sciences Supplement, American Library Association, Dec '00*

"This reference document should be in any public library, but it would be a very good guide for beginning students in the health sciences. If the other books in this publisher's series are as good as this, they should all be in the health sciences collections."
— *American Reference Books Annual, 2000*

"This book is an excellent general nutrition reference for consumers who desire to take an active role in their health care for prevention. Consumers of all ages who select this book can feel confident they are receiving current and accurate information." — *Journal of Nutrition for the Elderly, Vol. 19, No. 4, 2000*

SEE ALSO *Digestive Diseases & Disorders Sourcebook, Eating Disorders Sourcebook, Gastrointestinal Diseases & Disorders Sourcebook, Vegetarian Sourcebook*

■

Digestive Diseases & Disorders Sourcebook

Basic Consumer Health Information about Diseases and Disorders that Impact the Upper and Lower Digestive System, Including Celiac Disease, Constipation, Crohn's Disease, Cyclic Vomiting Syndrome, Diarrhea, Diverticulosis and Diverticulitis, Gallstones, Heartburn, Hemorrhoids, Hernias, Indigestion (Dyspepsia), Irritable Bowel Syndrome, Lactose Intolerance, Ulcers, and More

Along with Information about Medications and Other Treatments, Tips for Maintaining a Healthy Digestive Tract, a Glossary, and Directory of Digestive Diseases Organizations

Edited by Karen Bellenir. 335 pages. 2000. 978-0-7808-0327-5.

"This title would be an excellent addition to all public or patient-research libraries."
— *American Reference Books Annual, 2001*

"This title is recommended for public, hospital, and health sciences libraries with consumer health collections." — *E-Streams, Jul-Aug '00*

"Recommended reference source."
— *Booklist, American Library Association, May '00*

SEE ALSO *Eating Disorders Sourcebook, Gastrointestinal Diseases & Disorders Sourcebook*

■

Disabilities Sourcebook

Basic Consumer Health Information about Physical and Psychiatric Disabilities, Including Descriptions of Major Causes of Disability, Assistive and Adaptive Aids, Workplace Issues, and Accessibility Concerns

Along with Information about the Americans with Disabilities Act, a Glossary, and Resources for Additional Help and Information

Edited by Dawn D. Matthews. 616 pages. 2000. 978-0-7808-0389-3.

"It is a must for libraries with a consumer health section." — *American Reference Books Annual, 2002*

"A much needed addition to the Omnigraphics *Health Reference Series*. A current reference work to provide people with disabilities, their families, caregivers or those who work with them, a broad range of information in one volume, has not been available until now. . . . It is recommended for all public and academic library reference collections." —*E-Streams, May '01*

"An excellent source book in easy-to-read format covering many current topics; highly recommended for all libraries." —*Choice, Association of College & Research Libraries, Jan '01*

"Recommended reference source."
—*Booklist, American Library Association, Jul '00*

■

Domestic Violence Sourcebook, 2nd Edition

Basic Consumer Health Information about the Causes and Consequences of Abusive Relationships, Including Physical Violence, Sexual Assault, Battery, Stalking, and Emotional Abuse, and Facts about the Effects of Violence on Women, Men, Young Adults, and the Elderly, with Reports about Domestic Violence in Selected Populations, and Featuring Facts about Medical Care, Victim Assistance and Protection, Prevention Strategies, Mental Health Services, and Legal Issues

Along with a Glossary of Related Terms and Resources for Additional Help and Information

Edited by Dawn D. Matthews. 628 pages. 2004. 978-0-7808-0669-6.

"Educators, clergy, medical professionals, police, and victims and their families will benefit from this realistic and easy-to-understand resource."
—*American Reference Books Annual, 2005*

"Recommended for all collections supporting consumer health information. It should also be considered for any collection needing general, readable information on domestic violence." —*E-Streams, Jan '05*

"This sourcebook complements other books in its field, providing a one-stop resource . . . Recommended."
—*Choice, Association of College & Research Libraries, Jan '05*

"Interested lay persons should find the book extremely beneficial. . . . A copy of *Domestic Violence and Child Abuse Sourcebook* should be in every public library in the United States."
—*Social Science & Medicine, No. 56, 2003*

"This is important information. The Web has many resources but this sourcebook fills an important societal need. I am not aware of any other resources of this type." —*Doody's Review Service, Sep '01*

"Recommended reference source."
—*Booklist, American Library Association, Apr '01*

"Important pick for college-level health reference libraries." —*The Bookwatch, Mar '01*

"Because this problem is so widespread and because this book includes a lot of issues within one volume, this work is recommended for all public libraries."
—*American Reference Books Annual, 2001*

SEE ALSO *Child Abuse Sourcebook*

■

Drug Abuse Sourcebook, 2nd Edition

Basic Consumer Health Information about Illicit Substances of Abuse and the Misuse of Prescription and Over-the-Counter Medications, Including Depressants, Hallucinogens, Inhalants, Marijuana, Stimulants, and Anabolic Steroids

Along with Facts about Related Health Risks, Treatment Programs, Prevention Programs, a Glossary of Abuse and Addiction Terms, a Glossary of Drug-Related Street Terms, and a Directory of Resources for More Information

Edited by Catherine Ginther. 607 pages. 2004. 978-0-7808-0740-2.

"Commendable for organizing useful, normally scattered government and association-produced data into a logical sequence."
—*American Reference Books Annual, 2006*

"This easy-to-read volume is recommended for consumer health collections within public or academic libraries." —*E-Streams, Sep '05*

"An excellent library reference."
—*The Bookwatch, May '05*

"Containing a wealth of information, this book will be useful to the college student just beginning to explore the topic of substance abuse. This resource belongs in libraries that serve a lower-division undergraduate or community college clientele as well as the general public." —*Choice, Association of College & Research Libraries, Jun '01*

"Recommended reference source."
—*Booklist, American Library Association, Feb '01*

SEE ALSO *Alcoholism Sourcebook*

■

Ear, Nose & Throat Disorders Sourcebook, 2nd Edition

Basic Consumer Health Information about Disorders of the Ears, Hearing Loss, Vestibular Disorders, Nasal and Sinus Problems, Throat and Vocal Cord Disorders, and Otolaryngologic Cancers, Including Facts about Ear Infections and Injuries, Genetic and Congenital Deafness, Sensorineural Hearing Disorders, Tinnitus, Vertigo, Ménière Disease, Rhinitis, Sinusitis, Snoring, Sore Throats, Hoarseness, and More

Along with Reports on Current Research Initiatives, a Glossary of Related Medical Terms, and a Directory of Sources for Further Help and Information

Edited by Sandra J. Judd. 659 pages. 2006. 978-0-7808-0872-0.

"Overall, this sourcebook is helpful for the consumer seeking information on ENT issues. It is recommended for public libraries."
— *American Reference Books Annual, 1999*

"Recommended reference source."
— *Booklist, American Library Association, Dec '98*

■

Eating Disorders Sourcebook, 2nd Edition

Basic Consumer Health Information about Anorexia Nervosa, Bulimia Nervosa, Binge Eating, Compulsive Exercise, Female Athlete Triad, and Other Eating Disorders, Including Facts about Body Image and Other Cultural and Age-Related Risk Factors, Prevention Efforts, Adverse Health Effects, Treatment Options, and the Recovery Process

Along with Guidelines for Healthy Weight Control, a Glossary, and Directories of Additional Resources

Edited by Joyce Brennfleck Shannon. 585 pages. 2007. 978-0-7808-0948-2.

"Recommended for health science libraries that are open to the public, as well as hospital libraries. This book is a good resource for the consumer who is concerned about eating disorders." — *E-Streams, Mar '02*

"This volume is another convenient collection of excerpted articles. Recommended for school and public library patrons; lower-division undergraduates; and two-year technical program students."
— *Choice, Association of College & Research Libraries, Jan '02*

"Recommended reference source."
— *Booklist, American Library Association, Oct '01*

SEE ALSO *Diet & Nutrition Sourcebook, Digestive Diseases & Disorders Sourcebook, Gastrointestinal Diseases & Disorders Sourcebook*

■

Emergency Medical Services Sourcebook

Basic Consumer Health Information about Preventing, Preparing for, and Managing Emergency Situations, When and Who to Call for Help, What to Expect in the Emergency Room, the Emergency Medical Team, Patient Issues, and Current Topics in Emergency Medicine

Along with Statistical Data, a Glossary, and Sources of Additional Help and Information

Edited by Jenni Lynn Colson. 494 pages. 2002. 978-0-7808-0420-3.

"Handy and convenient for home, public, school, and college libraries. Recommended."
— *Choice, Association of College & Research Libraries, Apr '03*

"This reference can provide the consumer with answers to most questions about emergency care in the United States, or it will direct them to a resource where the answer can be found."
— *American Reference Books Annual, 2003*

"Recommended reference source."
— *Booklist, American Library Association, Feb '03*

■

Endocrine & Metabolic Disorders Sourcebook

Basic Information for the Layperson about Pancreatic and Insulin-Related Disorders Such as Pancreatitis, Diabetes, and Hypoglycemia; Adrenal Gland Disorders Such as Cushing's Syndrome, Addison's Disease, and Congenital Adrenal Hyperplasia; Pituitary Gland Disorders Such as Growth Hormone Deficiency, Acromegaly, and Pituitary Tumors; Thyroid Disorders Such as Hypothyroidism, Graves' Disease, Hashimoto's Disease, and Goiter; Hyperparathyroidism; and Other Diseases and Syndromes of Hormone Imbalance or Metabolic Dysfunction

Along with Reports on Current Research Initiatives

Edited by Linda M. Shin. 574 pages. 1998. 978-0-7808-0207-0.

"Omnigraphics has produced another needed resource for health information consumers."
— *American Reference Books Annual, 2000*

"Recommended reference source."
— *Booklist, American Library Association, Dec '98*

■

Environmental Health Sourcebook, 2nd Edition

Basic Consumer Health Information about the Environment and Its Effect on Human Health, Including the Effects of Air Pollution, Water Pollution, Hazardous Chemicals, Food Hazards, Radiation Hazards, Biological Agents, Household Hazards, Such as Radon, Asbestos, Carbon Monoxide, and Mold, and Information about Associated Diseases and Disorders, Including Cancer, Allergies, Respiratory Problems, and Skin Disorders

Along with Information about Environmental Concerns for Specific Populations, a Glossary of Related Terms, and Resources for Further Help and Information

Edited by Dawn D. Matthews. 673 pages. 2003. 978-0-7808-0632-0.

"This recently updated edition continues the level of quality and the reputation of the numerous other volumes in Omnigraphics' *Health Reference Series*."
— *American Reference Books Annual, 2004*

"An excellent updated edition."
— *The Bookwatch, Oct '03*

"Recommended reference source."
— *Booklist, American Library Association, Sep '98*

"This book will be a useful addition to anyone's library." — *Choice Health Sciences Supplement, Association of College & Research Libraries, May '98*

". . . a good survey of numerous environmentally induced physical disorders . . . a useful addition to anyone's library."
— *Doody's Health Sciences Book Reviews, Jan '98*

Ethnic Diseases Sourcebook

Basic Consumer Health Information for Ethnic and Racial Minority Groups in the United States, Including General Health Indicators and Behaviors, Ethnic Diseases, Genetic Testing, the Impact of Chronic Diseases, Women's Health, Mental Health Issues, and Preventive Health Care Services

Along with a Glossary and a Listing of Additional Resources

Edited by Joyce Brennfleck Shannon. 664 pages. 2001. 978-0-7808-0336-7.

"Recommended for health sciences libraries where public health programs are a priority."
— E-Streams, Jan '02

"Not many books have been written on this topic to date, and the *Ethnic Diseases Sourcebook* is a strong addition to the list. It will be an important introductory resource for health consumers, students, health care personnel, and social scientists. It is recommended for public, academic, and large hospital libraries."
— American Reference Books Annual, 2002

"Recommended reference source."
— Booklist, American Library Association, Oct '01

"Will prove valuable to any library seeking to maintain a current, comprehensive reference collection of health resources. . . . An excellent source of health information about genetic disorders which affect particular ethnic and racial minorities in the U.S."
— The Bookwatch, Aug '01

■

Eye Care Sourcebook, 2nd Edition

Basic Consumer Health Information about Eye Care and Eye Disorders, Including Facts about the Diagnosis, Prevention, and Treatment of Common Refractive Problems Such as Myopia, Hyperopia, Astigmatism, and Presbyopia, and Eye Diseases, Including Glaucoma, Cataract, Age-Related Macular Degeneration, and Diabetic Retinopathy

Along with a Section on Vision Correction and Refractive Surgeries, Including LASIK and LASEK, a Glossary, and Directories of Resources for Additional Help and Information

Edited by Amy L. Sutton. 543 pages. 2003. 978-0-7808-0635-1.

". . . a solid reference tool for eye care and a valuable addition to a collection."
— American Reference Books Annual, 2004

■

Family Planning Sourcebook

Basic Consumer Health Information about Planning for Pregnancy and Contraception, Including Traditional Methods, Barrier Methods, Hormonal Methods, Permanent Methods, Future Methods, Emergency Contraception, and Birth Control Choices for Women at Each Stage of Life

Along with Statistics, a Glossary, and Sources of Additional Information

Edited by Amy Marcaccio Keyzer. 520 pages. 2001. 978-0-7808-0379-4.

"Recommended for public, health, and undergraduate libraries as part of the circulating collection."
— E-Streams, Mar '02

"Information is presented in an unbiased, readable manner, and the sourcebook will certainly be a necessary addition to those public and high school libraries where Internet access is restricted or otherwise problematic." — American Reference Books Annual, 2002

"Recommended reference source."
— Booklist, American Library Association, Oct '01

"Will prove valuable to any library seeking to maintain a current, comprehensive reference collection of health resources. . . . Excellent reference."
— The Bookwatch, Aug '01

SEE ALSO Pregnancy & Birth Sourcebook

■

Fitness & Exercise Sourcebook, 3rd Edition

Basic Consumer Health Information about the Physical and Mental Benefits of Fitness, Including Cardiorespiratory Endurance, Muscular Strength, Muscular Endurance, and Flexibility, with Facts about Sports Nutrition and Exercise-Related Injuries and Tips about Physical Activity and Exercises for People of All Ages and for People with Health Concerns

Along with Advice on Selecting and Using Exercise Equipment, Maintaining Exercise Motivation, a Glossary of Related Terms, and a Directory of Resources for More Help and Information

Edited by Amy L. Sutton. 663 pages. 2007. 978-0-7808-0946-8.

"This work is recommended for all general reference collections."
— American Reference Books Annual, 2002

"Highly recommended for public, consumer, and school grades fourth through college." — E-Streams, Nov '01

"Recommended reference source."
— Booklist, American Library Association, Oct '01

"The information appears quite comprehensive and is considered reliable. . . . This second edition is a welcomed addition to the series."
— Doody's Review Service, Sep '01

■

Food Safety Sourcebook

Basic Consumer Health Information about the Safe Handling of Meat, Poultry, Seafood, Eggs, Fruit Juices, and Other Food Items, and Facts about Pesticides, Drinking Water, Food Safety Overseas, and the Onset, Duration, and Symptoms of Foodborne Illnesses, Including Types of Pathogenic Bacteria, Parasitic Protozoa, Worms, Viruses, and Natural Toxins

*Along with the Role of the Consumer, the Food Hand-
ler, and the Government in Food Safety; a Glossary,
and Resources for Additional Help and Information*

Edited by Dawn D. Matthews. 339 pages. 1999. 978-0-
7808-0326-8.

"This book is recommended for public libraries and
universities with home economic and food science programs." — *E-Streams, Nov '00*

"Recommended reference source."
— *Booklist, American Library Association, May '00*

"This book takes the complex issues of food safety and
foodborne pathogens and presents them in an easily
understood manner. [It does] an excellent job of covering a large and often confusing topic."
— *American Reference Books Annual, 2000*

■

Forensic Medicine Sourcebook

*Basic Consumer Information for the Layperson about
Forensic Medicine, Including Crime Scene Investigation, Evidence Collection and Analysis, Expert Testi-
mony, Computer-Aided Criminal Identification, Digital Imaging in the Courtroom, DNA Profiling, Accident Reconstruction, Autopsies, Ballistics, Drugs and
Explosives Detection, Latent Fingerprints, Product
Tampering, and Questioned Document Examination*

*Along with Statistical Data, a Glossary of Forensics
Terminology, and Listings of Sources for Further Help
and Information*

Edited by Annemarie S. Muth. 574 pages. 1999. 978-0-
7808-0232-2.

"Given the expected widespread interest in its content
and its easy to read style, this book is recommended for
most public and all college and university libraries."
— *E-Streams, Feb '01*

"Recommended for public libraries."
— *Reference & User Services Quarterly, American
Library Association, Spring 2000*

"Recommended reference source."
— *Booklist, American Library Association, Feb '00*

"A wealth of information, useful statistics, references
are up-to-date and extremely complete. This wonderful
collection of data will help students who are interested
in a career in any type of forensic field. It is a great
resource for attorneys who need information about
types of expert witnesses needed in a particular case. It
also offers useful information for fiction and nonfiction
writers whose work involves a crime. A fascinating
compilation. All levels."
— *Choice, Association of College
& Research Libraries, Jan '00*

"There are several items that make this book attractive
to consumers who are seeking certain forensic data. . . .
This is a useful current source for those seeking general forensic medical answers."
— *American Reference Books Annual, 2000*

Gastrointestinal Diseases
& Disorders Sourcebook,
2nd Edition

*Basic Consumer Health Information about the Upper
and Lower Gastrointestinal (GI) Tract, Including the
Esophagus, Stomach, Intestines, Rectum, Liver, and
Pancreas, with Facts about Gastroesophageal Reflux
Disease, Gastritis, Hernias, Ulcers, Celiac Disease,
Diverticulitis, Irritable Bowel Syndrome, Hemorrhoids,
Gastrointestinal Cancers, and Other Diseases and Dis-
orders Related to the Digestive Process*

*Along with Information about Commonly Used
Diagnostic and Surgical Procedures, Statistics, Reports
on Current Research Initiatives and Clinical Trials, a
Glossary, and Resources for Additional Help and
Information*

Edited by Sandra J. Judd. 681 pages. 2006. 978-0-7808-
0798-3.

". . . very readable form. The successful editorial work
that brought this material together into a useful and
understandable reference makes accessible to all readers
information that can help them more effectively understand and obtain help for digestive tract problems."
— *Choice, Association of College &
Research Libraries, Feb '97*

SEE ALSO Diet & Nutrition Sourcebook, Digestive
Diseases & Disorders Sourcebook, Eating Disorders
Sourcebook

■

Genetic Disorders Sourcebook,
3rd Edition

*Basic Consumer Health Information about Hereditary
Diseases and Disorders, Including Facts about the Hu-
man Genome, Genetic Inheritance Patterns, Disorders
Associated with Specific Genes, Such as Sickle Cell
Disease, Hemophilia, and Cystic Fibrosis, Chromo-
some Disorders, Such as Down Syndrome, Fragile X
Syndrome, and Turner Syndrome, and Complex Dis-
eases and Disorders Resulting from the Interaction of
Environmental and Genetic Factors, Such as Allergies,
Cancer, and Obesity*

*Along with Facts about Genetic Testing, Suggestions for
Parents of Children with Special Needs, Reports on
Current Research Initiatives, a Glossary of Genetic
Terminology, and Resources for Additional Help and
Information*

Edited by Karen Bellenir. 777 pages. 2004. 978-0-7808-
0742-6.

"This text is recommended for any library with an
interest in providing consumer health resources."
— *E-Streams, Aug '05*

"This is a valuable resource for anyone wishing to have
an understandable description of any of the topics or
disorders included. The editor succeeds in making complex genetic issues understandable."
— *Doody's Book Review Service, May '05*

"A good acquisition for public libraries."
— *American Reference Books Annual, 2005*

Head Trauma Sourcebook

Basic Information for the Layperson about Open-Head and Closed-Head Injuries, Treatment Advances, Recovery, and Rehabilitation

Along with Reports on Current Research Initiatives

Edited by Karen Bellenir. 414 pages. 1997. 978-0-7808-0208-7.

Headache Sourcebook

Basic Consumer Health Information about Migraine, Tension, Cluster, Rebound and Other Types of Headaches, with Facts about the Cause and Prevention of Headaches, the Effects of Stress and the Environment, Headaches during Pregnancy and Menopause, and Childhood Headaches

Along with a Glossary and Other Resources for Additional Help and Information

Edited by Dawn D. Matthews. 362 pages. 2002. 978-0-7808-0337-4.

"Highly recommended for academic and medical reference collections." — *Library Bookwatch, Sep '02*

Healthy Aging Sourcebook

Basic Consumer Health Information about Maintaining Health through the Aging Process, Including Advice on Nutrition, Exercise, and Sleep, Help in Making Decisions about Midlife Issues and Retirement, and Guidance Concerning Practical and Informed Choices in Health Consumerism

Along with Data Concerning the Theories of Aging, Different Experiences in Aging by Minority Groups, and Facts about Aging Now and Aging in the Future; and Featuring a Glossary, a Guide to Consumer Help, Additional Suggested Reading, and Practical Resource Directory

Edited by Jenifer Swanson. 536 pages. 1999. 978-0-7808-0390-9.

"Recommended reference source."
— *Booklist, American Library Association, Feb '00*

SEE ALSO *Physical & Mental Issues in Aging Sourcebook*

Healthy Children Sourcebook

Basic Consumer Health Information about the Physical and Mental Development of Children between the Ages of 3 and 12, Including Routine Health Care, Preventative Health Services, Safety and First Aid,

Healthy Sleep, Dental Care, Nutrition, and Fitness, and Featuring Parenting Tips on Such Topics as Bedwetting, Choosing Day Care, Monitoring TV and Other Media, and Establishing a Foundation for Substance Abuse Prevention

Along with a Glossary of Commonly Used Pediatric Terms and Resources for Additional Help and Information.

Edited by Chad T. Kimball. 647 pages. 2003. 978-0-7808-0247-6.

"It is hard to imagine that any other single resource exists that would provide such a comprehensive guide of timely information on health promotion and disease prevention for children aged 3 to 12."
— *American Reference Books Annual, 2004*

"The strengths of this book are many. It is clearly written, presented and structured."
— *Journal of the National Medical Association, 2004*

SEE ALSO *Childhood Diseases & Disorders Sourcebook*

Healthy Heart Sourcebook for Women

Basic Consumer Health Information about Cardiac Issues Specific to Women, Including Facts about Major Risk Factors and Prevention, Treatment and Control Strategies, and Important Dietary Issues

Along with a Special Section Regarding the Pros and Cons of Hormone Replacement Therapy and Its Impact on Heart Health, and Additional Help, Including Recipes, a Glossary, and a Directory of Resources

Edited by Dawn D. Matthews. 336 pages. 2000. 978-0-7808-0329-9.

"A good reference source and recommended for all public, academic, medical, and hospital libraries."
— *Medical Reference Services Quarterly, Summer '01*

"Because of the lack of information specific to women on this topic, this book is recommended for public libraries and consumer libraries."
— *American Reference Books Annual, 2001*

"Contains very important information about coronary artery disease that all women should know. The information is current and presented in an easy-to-read format. The book will make a good addition to any library." — *American Medical Writers Association Journal, Summer '00*

"Important, basic reference."
— *Reviewer's Bookwatch, Jul '00*

SEE ALSO *Cardiovascular Diseases & Disorders Sourcebook, Women's Health Concerns Sourcebook*

Hepatitis Sourcebook

Basic Consumer Health Information about Hepatitis A, Hepatitis B, Hepatitis C, and Other Forms of Hepatitis, Including Autoimmune Hepatitis, Alcoholic Hepatitis, Nonalcoholic Steatohepatitis, and Toxic Hepatitis, with

657

Facts about Risk Factors, Screening Methods, Diagnostic Tests, and Treatment Options

Along with Information on Liver Health, Tips for People Living with Chronic Hepatitis, Reports on Current Research Initiatives, a Glossary of Terms Related to Hepatitis, and a Directory of Sources for Further Help and Information

Edited by Sandra J. Judd. 597 pages. 2005. 978-0-7808-0749-5.

"Highly recommended."
— American Reference Books Annual, 2006

■

Household Safety Sourcebook

Basic Consumer Health Information about Household Safety, Including Information about Poisons, Chemicals, Fire, and Water Hazards in the Home

Along with Advice about the Safe Use of Home Maintenance Equipment, Choosing Toys and Nursery Furniture, Holiday and Recreation Safety, a Glossary, and Resources for Further Help and Information

Edited by Dawn D. Matthews. 606 pages. 2002. 978-0-7808-0338-1.

"This work will be useful in public libraries with large consumer health and wellness departments."
— American Reference Books Annual, 2003

"As a sourcebook on household safety this book meets its mark. It is encyclopedic in scope and covers a wide range of safety issues that are commonly seen in the home." — E-Streams, Jul '02

■

Hypertension Sourcebook

Basic Consumer Health Information about the Causes, Diagnosis, and Treatment of High Blood Pressure, with Facts about Consequences, Complications, and Co-Occurring Disorders, Such as Coronary Heart Disease, Diabetes, Stroke, Kidney Disease, and Hypertensive Retinopathy, and Issues in Blood Pressure Control, Including Dietary Choices, Stress Management, and Medications

Along with Reports on Current Research Initiatives and Clinical Trials, a Glossary, and Resources for Additional Help and Information

Edited by Dawn D. Matthews and Karen Bellenir. 613 pages. 2004. 978-0-7808-0674-0.

"Academic, public, and medical libraries will want to add the Hypertension Sourcebook to their collections."
— E-Streams, Aug '05

"The strength of this source is the wide range of information given about hypertension."
— American Reference Books Annual, 2005

■

Immune System Disorders Sourcebook, 2nd Edition

Basic Consumer Health Information about Disorders of the Immune System, Including Immune System Function and Response, Diagnosis of Immune Disorders, Information about Inherited Immune Disease, Acquired Immune Disease, and Autoimmune Diseases, Including Primary Immune Deficiency, Acquired Immunodeficiency Syndrome (AIDS), Lupus, Multiple Sclerosis, Type 1 Diabetes, Rheumatoid Arthritis, and Graves' Disease

Along with Treatments, Tips for Coping with Immune Disorders, a Glossary, and a Directory of Additional Resources.

Edited by Joyce Brennfleck Shannon. 671 pages. 2005. 978-0-7808-0748-8.

"Highly recommended for academic and public libraries." — American Reference Books Annual, 2006

"The updated second edition is a 'must' for any consumer health library seeking a solid resource covering the treatments, symptoms, and options for immune disorder sufferers. . . . An excellent guide."
— MBR Bookwatch, Jan '06

■

Infant & Toddler Health Sourcebook

Basic Consumer Health Information about the Physical and Mental Development of Newborns, Infants, and Toddlers, Including Neonatal Concerns, Nutrition Recommendations, Immunization Schedules, Common Pediatric Disorders, Assessments and Milestones, Safety Tips, and Advice for Parents and Other Caregivers

Along with a Glossary of Terms and Resource Listings for Additional Help

Edited by Jenifer Swanson. 585 pages. 2000. 978-0-7808-0246-9.

"As a reference for the general public, this would be useful in any library." — E-Streams, May '01

"Recommended reference source."
— Booklist, American Library Association, Feb '01

"This is a good source for general use."
— American Reference Books Annual, 2001

■

Infectious Diseases Sourcebook

Basic Consumer Health Information about Non-Contagious Bacterial, Viral, Prion, Fungal, and Parasitic Diseases Spread by Food and Water, Insects and Animals, or Environmental Contact, Including Botulism, E. Coli, Encephalitis, Legionnaires' Disease, Lyme Disease, Malaria, Plague, Rabies, Salmonella, Tetanus, and Others, and Facts about Newly Emerging Diseases, Such as Hantavirus, Mad Cow Disease, Monkeypox, and West Nile Virus

Along with Information about Preventing Disease Transmission, the Threat of Bioterrorism, and Current Research Initiatives, with a Glossary and Directory of Resources for More Information

Edited by Karen Bellenir. 634 pages. 2004. 978-0-7808-0675-7.

"This reference continues the excellent tradition of the *Health Reference Series* in consolidating a wealth of information on a selected topic into a format that is easy to use and accessible to the general public."
— *American Reference Books Annual, 2005*

"Recommended for public and academic libraries."
— *E-Streams, Jan '05*

◼

Injury & Trauma Sourcebook

Basic Consumer Health Information about the Impact of Injury, the Diagnosis and Treatment of Common and Traumatic Injuries, Emergency Care, and Specific Injuries Related to Home, Community, Workplace, Transportation, and Recreation

Along with Guidelines for Injury Prevention, a Glossary, and a Directory of Additional Resources

Edited by Joyce Brennfleck Shannon. 696 pages. 2002. 978-0-7808-0421-0.

"This publication is the most comprehensive work of its kind about injury and trauma."
— *American Reference Books Annual, 2003*

"This sourcebook provides concise, easily readable, basic health information about injuries. . . . This book is well organized and an easy to use reference resource suitable for hospital, health sciences and public libraries with consumer health collections."
— *E-Streams, Nov '02*

"Practitioners should be aware of guides such as this in order to facilitate their use by patients and their families."
— *Doody's Health Sciences Book Review Journal, Sep-Oct '02*

"Recommended reference source."
— *Booklist, American Library Association, Sep '02*

"Highly recommended for academic and medical reference collections."
— *Library Bookwatch, Sep '02*

◼

Kidney & Urinary Tract Diseases & Disorders Sourcebook

SEE *Urinary Tract & Kidney Diseases & Disorders Sourcebook*

◼

Learning Disabilities Sourcebook, 2nd Edition

Basic Consumer Health Information about Learning Disabilities, Including Dyslexia, Developmental Speech and Language Disabilities, Non-Verbal Learning Disorders, Developmental Arithmetic Disorder, Developmental Writing Disorder, and Other Conditions That Impede Learning Such as Attention Deficit/Hyperactivity Disorder, Brain Injury, Hearing Impairment, Klinefelter Syndrome, Dyspraxia, and Tourette's Syndrome

Along with Facts about Educational Issues and Assistive Technology, Coping Strategies, a Glossary of Related Terms, and Resources for Further Help and Information

Edited by Dawn D. Matthews. 621 pages. 2003. 978-0-7808-0626-9.

"The second edition of Learning Disabilities Sourcebook far surpasses the earlier edition in that it is more focused on information that will be useful as a consumer health resource."
— *American Reference Books Annual, 2004*

"Teachers as well as consumers will find this an essential guide to understanding various syndromes and their latest treatments. [An] invaluable reference for public and school library collections alike."
— *Library Bookwatch, Apr '03*

Named "Outstanding Reference Book of 1999."
— *New York Public Library, Feb '00*

"An excellent candidate for inclusion in a public library reference section. It's a great source of information. Teachers will also find the book useful. Definitely worth reading."
— *Journal of Adolescent & Adult Literacy, Feb 2000*

"Readable . . . provides a solid base of information regarding successful techniques used with individuals who have learning disabilities, as well as practical suggestions for educators and family members. Clear language, concise descriptions, and pertinent information for contacting multiple resources add to the strength of this book as a useful tool."
— *Choice, Association of College & Research Libraries, Feb '99*

"Recommended reference source."
— *Booklist, American Library Association, Sep '98*

"A useful resource for libraries and for those who don't have the time to identify and locate the individual publications."
— *Disability Resources Monthly, Sep '98*

◼

Leukemia Sourcebook

Basic Consumer Health Information about Adult and Childhood Leukemias, Including Acute Lymphocytic Leukemia (ALL), Chronic Lymphocytic Leukemia (CLL), Acute Myelogenous Leukemia (AML), Chronic Myelogenous Leukemia (CML), and Hairy Cell Leukemia, and Treatments Such as Chemotherapy, Radiation Therapy, Peripheral Blood Stem Cell and Marrow Transplantation, and Immunotherapy

Along with Tips for Life During and After Treatment, a Glossary, and Directories of Additional Resources

Edited by Joyce Brennfleck Shannon. 587 pages. 2003. 978-0-7808-0627-6.

"Unlike other medical books for the layperson, . . . the language does not talk down to the reader. . . . This volume is highly recommended for all libraries."
— *American Reference Books Annual, 2004*

". . . a fine title which ranges from diagnosis to alternative treatments, staging, and tips for life during and after diagnosis."
— *The Bookwatch, Dec '03*

Liver Disorders Sourcebook

Basic Consumer Health Information about the Liver and How It Works; Liver Diseases, Including Cancer, Cirrhosis, Hepatitis, and Toxic and Drug Related Diseases; Tips for Maintaining a Healthy Liver; Laboratory Tests, Radiology Tests, and Facts about Liver Transplantation

Along with a Section on Support Groups, a Glossary, and Resource Listings

Edited by Joyce Brennfleck Shannon. 591 pages. 2000. 978-0-7808-0383-1.

"A valuable resource."
—American Reference Books Annual, 2001

"This title is recommended for health sciences and public libraries with consumer health collections."
—E-Streams, Oct '00

"Recommended reference source."
—Booklist, American Library Association, Jun '00

■

Lung Disorders Sourcebook

Basic Consumer Health Information about Emphysema, Pneumonia, Tuberculosis, Asthma, Cystic Fibrosis, and Other Lung Disorders, Including Facts about Diagnostic Procedures, Treatment Strategies, Disease Prevention Efforts, and Such Risk Factors as Smoking, Air Pollution, and Exposure to Asbestos, Radon, and Other Agents

Along with a Glossary and Resources for Additional Help and Information

Edited by Dawn D. Matthews. 678 pages. 2002. 978-0-7808-0339-8.

"This title is a great addition for public and school libraries because it provides concise health information on the lungs."
—American Reference Books Annual, 2003

"Highly recommended for academic and medical reference collections." *—Library Bookwatch, Sep '02*

SEE ALSO *Respiratory Diseases & Disorders Sourcebook*

■

Medical Tests Sourcebook, 2nd Edition

Basic Consumer Health Information about Medical Tests, Including Age-Specific Health Tests, Important Health Screenings and Exams, Home-Use Tests, Blood and Specimen Tests, Electrical Tests, Scope Tests, Genetic Testing, and Imaging Tests, Such as X-Rays, Ultrasound, Computed Tomography, Magnetic Resonance Imaging, Angiography, and Nuclear Medicine

Along with a Glossary and Directory of Additional Resources

Edited by Joyce Brennfleck Shannon. 654 pages. 2004. 978-0-7808-0670-2.

"Recommended for hospital and health sciences

libraries with consumer health collections."
—E-Streams, Mar '00

"This is an overall excellent reference with a wealth of general knowledge that may aid those who are reluctant to get vital tests performed."
—Today's Librarian, Jan '00

"A valuable reference guide."
—American Reference Books Annual, 2000

■

Men's Health Concerns Sourcebook, 2nd Edition

Basic Consumer Health Information about the Medical and Mental Concerns of Men, Including Theories about the Shorter Male Lifespan, the Leading Causes of Death and Disability, Physical Concerns of Special Significance to Men, Reproductive and Sexual Concerns, Sexually Transmitted Diseases, Men's Mental and Emotional Health, and Lifestyle Choices That Affect Wellness, Such as Nutrition, Fitness, and Substance Use

Along with a Glossary of Related Terms and a Directory of Organizational Resources in Men's Health

Edited by Robert Aquinas McNally. 644 pages. 2004. 978-0-7808-0671-9.

"A very accessible reference for non-specialist general readers and consumers." *—The Bookwatch, Jun '04*

"This comprehensive resource and the series are highly recommended."
—American Reference Books Annual, 2000

"Recommended reference source."
—Booklist, American Library Association, Dec '98

■

Mental Health Disorders Sourcebook, 3rd Edition

Basic Consumer Health Information about Mental and Emotional Health and Mental Illness, Including Facts about Depression, Bipolar Disorder, and Other Mood Disorders, Phobias, Post-Traumatic Stress Disorder (PTSD), Obsessive-Compulsive Disorder, and Other Anxiety Disorders, Impulse Control Disorders, Eating Disorders, Personality Disorders, and Psychotic Disorders, Including Schizophrenia and Dissociative Disorders

Along with Statistical Information, a Special Section Concerning Mental Health Issues in Children and Adolescents, a Glossary, and Directories of Resources for Additional Help and Information

Edited by Karen Bellenir. 661 pages. 2005. 978-0-7808-0747-1.

"Recommended for public libraries and academic libraries with an undergraduate program in psychology."
—American Reference Books Annual, 2006

"Recommended reference source."
—Booklist, American Library Association, Jun '00

Mental Retardation Sourcebook

Basic Consumer Health Information about Mental Retardation and Its Causes, Including Down Syndrome, Fetal Alcohol Syndrome, Fragile X Syndrome, Genetic Conditions, Injury, and Environmental Sources

Along with Preventive Strategies, Parenting Issues, Educational Implications, Health Care Needs, Employment and Economic Matters, Legal Issues, a Glossary, and a Resource Listing for Additional Help and Information

Edited by Joyce Brennfleck Shannon. 642 pages. 2000. 978-0-7808-0377-0.

"Public libraries will find the book useful for reference and as a beginning research point for students, parents, and caregivers."
— American Reference Books Annual, 2001

"The strength of this work is that it compiles many basic fact sheets and addresses for further information in one volume. It is intended and suitable for the general public. This sourcebook is relevant to any collection providing health information to the general public."
— E-Streams, Nov '00

"From preventing retardation to parenting and family challenges, this covers health, social and legal issues and will prove an invaluable overview."
— Reviewer's Bookwatch, Jul '00

Movement Disorders Sourcebook

Basic Consumer Health Information about Neurological Movement Disorders, Including Essential Tremor, Parkinson's Disease, Dystonia, Cerebral Palsy, Huntington's Disease, Myasthenia Gravis, Multiple Sclerosis, and Other Early-Onset and Adult-Onset Movement Disorders, Their Symptoms and Causes, Diagnostic Tests, and Treatments

Along with Mobility and Assistive Technology Information, a Glossary, and a Directory of Additional Resources

Edited by Joyce Brennfleck Shannon. 655 pages. 2003. 978-0-7808-0628-3.

". . . a good resource for consumers and recommended for public, community college and undergraduate libraries." *— American Reference Books Annual, 2004*

Muscular Dystrophy Sourcebook

Basic Consumer Health Information about Congenital, Childhood-Onset, and Adult-Onset Forms of Muscular Dystrophy, Such as Duchenne, Becker, Emery-Dreifuss, Distal, Limb-Girdle, Facioscapulohumeral (FSHD), Myotonic, and Ophthalmoplegic Muscular Dystrophies, Including Facts about Diagnostic Tests, Medical and Physical Therapies, Management of Co-Occurring Conditions, and Parenting Guidelines

Along with Practical Tips for Home Care, a Glossary, and Directories of Additional Resources

Edited by Joyce Brennfleck Shannon. 577 pages. 2004. 978-0-7808-0676-4.

"This book is highly recommended for public and academic libraries as well as health care offices that support the information needs of patients and their families."
— E-Streams, Apr '05

"Excellent reference." *— The Bookwatch, Jan '05*

Obesity Sourcebook

Basic Consumer Health Information about Diseases and Other Problems Associated with Obesity, and Including Facts about Risk Factors, Prevention Issues, and Management Approaches

Along with Statistical and Demographic Data, Information about Special Populations, Research Updates, a Glossary, and Source Listings for Further Help and Information

Edited by Wilma Caldwell and Chad T. Kimball. 376 pages. 2001. 978-0-7808-0333-6.

"The book synthesizes the reliable medical literature on obesity into one easy-to-read and useful resource for the general public."
— American Reference Books Annual, 2002

"This is a very useful resource book for the lay public."
— Doody's Review Service, Nov '01

"Well suited for the health reference collection of a public library or an academic health science library that serves the general population." *— E-Streams, Sep '01*

"Recommended reference source."
— Booklist, American Library Association, Apr '01

"Recommended pick both for specialty health library collections and any general consumer health reference collection." *— The Bookwatch, Apr '01*

Oral Health Sourcebook

SEE *Dental Care & Oral Health Sourcebook*

Osteoporosis Sourcebook

Basic Consumer Health Information about Primary and Secondary Osteoporosis and Juvenile Osteoporosis and Related Conditions, Including Fibrous Dysplasia, Gaucher Disease, Hyperthyroidism, Hypophosphatasia, Myeloma, Osteopetrosis, Osteogenesis Imperfecta, and Paget's Disease

Along with Information about Risk Factors, Treatments, Traditional and Non-Traditional Pain Management, a Glossary of Related Terms, and a Directory of Resources

Edited by Allan R. Cook. 584 pages. 2001. 978-0-7808-0239-1.

"This would be a book to be kept in a staff or patient library. The targeted audience is the layperson, but the therapist who needs a quick bit of information on a particular topic will also find the book useful."
— Physical Therapy, Jan '02

661

"This resource is recommended as a great reference source for public, health, and academic libraries, and is another triumph for the editors of Omnigraphics."
— *American Reference Books Annual, 2002*

"Recommended for all public libraries and general health collections, especially those supporting patient education or consumer health programs."
— *E-Streams, Nov '01*

"Will prove valuable to any library seeking to maintain a current, comprehensive reference collection of health resources. . . . From prevention to treatment and associated conditions, this provides an excellent survey."
— *The Bookwatch, Aug '01*

"Recommended reference source."
— *Booklist, American Library Association, Jul '01*

SEE ALSO *Healthy Aging Sourcebook, Physical & Mental Issues in Aging Sourcebook, Women's Health Concerns Sourcebook*

■

Pain Sourcebook, 2nd Edition

Basic Consumer Health Information about Specific Forms of Acute and Chronic Pain, Including Muscle and Skeletal Pain, Nerve Pain, Cancer Pain, and Disorders Characterized by Pain, Such as Fibromyalgia, Shingles, Angina, Arthritis, and Headaches

Along with Information about Pain Medications and Management Techniques, Complementary and Alternative Pain Relief Options, Tips for People Living with Chronic Pain, a Glossary, and a Directory of Sources for Further Information

Edited by Karen Bellenir. 670 pages. 2002. 978-0-7808-0612-2.

"A source of valuable information. . . . This book offers help to nonmedical people who need information about pain and pain management. It is also an excellent reference for those who participate in patient education."
— *Doody's Review Service, Sep '02*

"Highly recommended for academic and medical reference collections." — *Library Bookwatch, Sep '02*

"The text is readable, easily understood, and well indexed. This excellent volume belongs in all patient education libraries, consumer health sections of public libraries, and many personal collections."
— *American Reference Books Annual, 1999*

"The information is basic in terms of scholarship and is appropriate for general readers. Written in journalistic style . . . intended for non-professionals. Quite thorough in its coverage of different pain conditions and summarizes the latest clinical information regarding pain treatment." — *Choice, Association of College and Research Libraries, Jun '98*

"Recommended reference source."
— *Booklist, American Library Association, Mar '98*

■

Pediatric Cancer Sourcebook

Basic Consumer Health Information about Leukemias, Brain Tumors, Sarcomas, Lymphomas, and Other Cancers in Infants, Children, and Adolescents, Including Descriptions of Cancers, Treatments, and Coping Strategies

Along with Suggestions for Parents, Caregivers, and Concerned Relatives, a Glossary of Cancer Terms, and Resource Listings

Edited by Edward J. Prucha. 587 pages. 1999. 978-0-7808-0245-2.

"An excellent source of information. Recommended for public, hospital, and health science libraries with consumer health collections." — *E-Streams, Jun '00*

"Recommended reference source."
— *Booklist, American Library Association, Feb '00*

"A valuable addition to all libraries specializing in health services and many public libraries."
— *American Reference Books Annual, 2000*

SEE ALSO *Childhood Diseases & Disorders Sourcebook, Healthy Children Sourcebook*

■

Physical & Mental Issues in Aging Sourcebook

Basic Consumer Health Information on Physical and Mental Disorders Associated with the Aging Process, Including Concerns about Cardiovascular Disease, Pulmonary Disease, Oral Health, Digestive Disorders, Musculoskeletal and Skin Disorders, Metabolic Changes, Sexual and Reproductive Issues, and Changes in Vision, Hearing, and Other Senses

Along with Data about Longevity and Causes of Death, Information on Acute and Chronic Pain, Descriptions of Mental Concerns, a Glossary of Terms, and Resource Listings for Additional Help

Edited by Jenifer Swanson. 660 pages. 1999. 978-0-7808-0233-9.

"This is a treasure of health information for the layperson." — *Choice Health Sciences Supplement, Association of College & Research Libraries, May '00*

"Recommended for public libraries."
— *American Reference Books Annual, 2000*

"Recommended reference source."
— *Booklist, American Library Association, Oct '99*

SEE ALSO *Healthy Aging Sourcebook*

■

Podiatry Sourcebook, 2nd Edition

Basic Consumer Health Information about Disorders, Diseases, Deformities, and Injuries that Affect the Foot and Ankle, Including Sprains, Corns, Calluses, Bunions, Plantar Warts, Plantar Fasciitis, Neuromas, Clubfoot, Flat Feet, Achilles Tendonitis, and Much More

Along with Information about Selecting a Foot Care Specialist, Foot Fitness, Shoes and Socks, Diagnostic Tests and Corrective Procedures, Financial Assistance for Corrective Devices, a Glossary of Related Terms, and a Directory of Resources for Additional Help and Information

Edited by Ivy L. Alexander. 543 pages. 2007. 978-0-7808-0944-4.

"Recommended reference source."
— *Booklist, American Library Association, Feb '02*

"There is a lot of information presented here on a topic that is usually only covered sparingly in most larger comprehensive medical encyclopedias."
— *American Reference Books Annual, 2002*

Pregnancy & Birth Sourcebook, 2nd Edition

Basic Consumer Health Information about Conception and Pregnancy, Including Facts about Fertility, Infertility, Pregnancy Symptoms and Complications, Fetal Growth and Development, Labor, Delivery, and the Postpartum Period, as Well as Information about Maintaining Health and Wellness during Pregnancy and Caring for a Newborn

Along with Information about Public Health Assistance for Low-Income Pregnant Women, a Glossary, and Directories of Agencies and Organizations Providing Help and Support

Edited by Amy L. Sutton. 626 pages. 2004. 978-0-7808-0672-6.

"Will appeal to public and school reference collections strong in medicine and women's health. . . . Deserves a spot on any medical reference shelf."
— *The Bookwatch, Jul '04*

"A well-organized handbook. Recommended."
— *Choice, Association of College & Research Libraries, Apr '98*

"Recommended reference source."
— *Booklist, American Library Association, Mar '98*

"Recommended for public libraries."
— *American Reference Books Annual, 1998*

SEE ALSO *Breastfeeding Sourcebook, Congenital Disorders Sourcebook, Family Planning Sourcebook*

Prostate & Urological Disorders Sourcebook

Basic Consumer Health Information about Urogenital and Sexual Disorders in Men, Including Prostate and Other Andrological Cancers, Prostatitis, Benign Prostatic Hyperplasia, Testicular and Penile Trauma, Cryptorchidism, Peyronie Disease, Erectile Dysfunction, and Male Factor Infertility, and Facts about Commonly Used Tests and Procedures, Such as Prostatectomy, Vasectomy, Vasectomy Reversal, Penile Implants, and Semen Analysis

Along with a Glossary of Andrological Terms and a Directory of Resources for Additional Information

Edited by Karen Bellenir. 631 pages. 2005. 978-0-7808-0797-6.

Prostate Cancer Sourcebook

Basic Consumer Health Information about Prostate Cancer, Including Information about the Associated Risk Factors, Detection, Diagnosis, and Treatment of Prostate Cancer

Along with Information on Non-Malignant Prostate Conditions, and Featuring a Section Listing Support and Treatment Centers and a Glossary of Related Terms

Edited by Dawn D. Matthews. 358 pages. 2001. 978-0-7808-0324-4.

"Recommended reference source."
— *Booklist, American Library Association, Jan '02*

"A valuable resource for health care consumers seeking information on the subject. . . . All text is written in a clear, easy-to-understand language that avoids technical jargon. Any library that collects consumer health resources would strengthen their collection with the addition of the *Prostate Cancer Sourcebook*."
— *American Reference Books Annual, 2002*

SEE ALSO *Men's Health Concerns Sourcebook*

Reconstructive & Cosmetic Surgery Sourcebook

Basic Consumer Health Information on Cosmetic and Reconstructive Plastic Surgery, Including Statistical Information about Different Surgical Procedures, Things to Consider Prior to Surgery, Plastic Surgery Techniques and Tools, Emotional and Psychological Considerations, and Procedure-Specific Information

Along with a Glossary of Terms and a Listing of Resources for Additional Help and Information

Edited by M. Lisa Weatherford. 374 pages. 2001. 978-0-7808-0214-8.

"An excellent reference that addresses cosmetic and medically necessary reconstructive surgeries. . . . The style of the prose is calm and reassuring, discussing the many positive outcomes now available due to advances in surgical techniques."
— *American Reference Books Annual, 2002*

"Recommended for health science libraries that are open to the public, as well as hospital libraries that are open to the patients. This book is a good resource for the consumer interested in plastic surgery."
— *E-Streams, Dec '01*

"Recommended reference source."
— *Booklist, American Library Association, Jul '01*

Rehabilitation Sourcebook

Basic Consumer Health Information about Rehabilitation for People Recovering from Heart Surgery, Spinal Cord Injury, Stroke, Orthopedic Impairments, Amputation, Pulmonary Impairments, Traumatic Injury, and More, Including Physical Therapy, Occupational Therapy, Speech/Language Therapy, Massage Therapy, Dance Therapy, Art Therapy, and Recreational Therapy

Along with Information on Assistive and Adaptive Devices, a Glossary, and Resources for Additional Help and Information

Edited by Dawn D. Matthews. 531 pages. 1999. 978-0-7808-0236-0.

"This is an excellent resource for public library reference and health collections."
— American Reference Books Annual, 2001

"Recommended reference source."
— Booklist, American Library Association, May '00

Respiratory Diseases & Disorders Sourcebook

Basic Information about Respiratory Diseases and Disorders, Including Asthma, Cystic Fibrosis, Pneumonia, the Common Cold, Influenza, and Others, Featuring Facts about the Respiratory System, Statistical and Demographic Data, Treatments, Self-Help Management Suggestions, and Current Research Initiatives

Edited by Allan R. Cook and Peter D. Dresser. 771 pages. 1995. 978-0-7808-0037-3.

"Designed for the layperson and for patients and their families coping with respiratory illness. . . . an extensive array of information on diagnosis, treatment, management, and prevention of respiratory illnesses for the general reader." — Choice, Association of College & Research Libraries, Jun '96

"A highly recommended text for all collections. It is a comforting reminder of the power of knowledge that good books carry between their covers."
— Academic Library Book Review, Spring '96

"A comprehensive collection of authoritative information presented in a nontechnical, humanitarian style for patients, families, and caregivers."
— Association of Operating Room Nurses, Sep/Oct '95

SEE ALSO Lung Disorders Sourcebook

Sexually Transmitted Diseases Sourcebook, 3rd Edition

Basic Consumer Health Information about Chlamydial Infections, Gonorrhea, Hepatitis, Herpes, HIV/AIDS, Human Papillomavirus, Pubic Lice, Scabies, Syphilis, Trichomoniasis, Vaginal Infections, and Other Sexually Transmitted Diseases, Including Facts about Risk Factors, Symptoms, Diagnosis, Treatment, and the Prevention of Sexually Transmitted Infections

Along with Updates on Current Research Initiatives, a Glossary of Related Terms, and Resources for Additional Help and Information

Edited by Amy L. Sutton. 629 pages. 2006. 978-0-7808-0824-9.

"Recommended for consumer health collections in public libraries, and secondary school and community college libraries."
— American Reference Books Annual, 2002

"Every school and public library should have a copy of this comprehensive and user-friendly reference book."
— Choice, Association of College & Research Libraries, Sep '01

"This is a highly recommended book. This is an especially important book for all school and public libraries."
— AIDS Book Review Journal, Jul-Aug '01

"Recommended reference source."
— Booklist, American Library Association, Apr '01

Sleep Disorders Sourcebook, 2nd Edition

Basic Consumer Health Information about Sleep and Sleep Disorders, Including Insomnia, Sleep Apnea, Restless Legs Syndrome, Narcolepsy, Parasomnias, and Other Health Problems That Affect Sleep, Plus Facts about Diagnostic Procedures, Treatment Strategies, Sleep Medications, and Tips for Improving Sleep Quality

Along with a Glossary of Related Terms and Resources for Additional Help and Information

Edited by Amy L. Sutton. 567 pages. 2005. 978-0-7808-0743-3.

"This book will be useful for just about everybody, especially the 40 million Americans with sleep disorders."
— American Reference Books Annual, 2006

"Recommended for public libraries and libraries supporting health care professionals." — E-Streams, Sep '05

". . . key medical library acquisition."
— The Bookwatch, Jun '05

Smoking Concerns Sourcebook

Basic Consumer Health Information about Nicotine Addiction and Smoking Cessation, Featuring Facts about the Health Effects of Tobacco Use, Including Lung and Other Cancers, Heart Disease, Stroke, and Respiratory Disorders, Such as Emphysema and Chronic Bronchitis

Along with Information about Smoking Prevention Programs, Suggestions for Achieving and Maintaining a Smoke-Free Lifestyle, Statistics about Tobacco Use, Reports on Current Research Initiatives, a Glossary of Related Terms, and Directories of Resources for Additional Help and Information

Edited by Karen Bellenir. 621 pages. 2004. 978-0-7808-0323-7.

"Provides everything needed for the student or general reader seeking practical details on the effects of tobacco use." — The Bookwatch, Mar '05

"Public libraries and consumer health care libraries will find this work useful."
— American Reference Books Annual, 2005

Sports Injuries Sourcebook, 3rd Edition

Basic Consumer Health Information about Sprains and Strains, Fractures, Growth Plate Injuries, Overtraining Injuries, and Injuries to the Head, Face, Shoulders, Elbows, Hands, Spinal Column, Knees, Ankles, and Feet, and with Facts about Heat-Related Illness, Steroids and Sport Supplements, Protective Equipment, Diagnostic Procedures, Treatment Options, and Rehabilitation

Along with a Glossary of Related Terms and a Directory of Resources for Additional Help and Information

Edited by Sandra J. Judd. 651 pages. 2007. 978-0-7808-0949-9.

"This is an excellent reference for consumers and it is recommended for public, community college, and undergraduate libraries."
— *American Reference Books Annual, 2003*

"Recommended reference source."
— *Booklist, American Library Association, Feb '03*

■

Stress-Related Disorders Sourcebook

Basic Consumer Health Information about Stress and Stress-Related Disorders, Including Stress Origins and Signals, Environmental Stress at Work and Home, Mental and Emotional Stress Associated with Depression, Post-Traumatic Stress Disorder, Panic Disorder, Suicide, and the Physical Effects of Stress on the Cardiovascular, Immune, and Nervous Systems

Along with Stress Management Techniques, a Glossary, and a Listing of Additional Resources

Edited by Joyce Brennfleck Shannon. 610 pages. 2002. 978-0-7808-0560-6.

"Well written for a general readership, the *Stress-Related Disorders Sourcebook* is a useful addition to the health reference literature."
— *American Reference Books Annual, 2003*

"I am impressed by the amount of information. It offers a thorough overview of the causes and consequences of stress for the layperson. . . . A well-done and thorough reference guide for professionals and nonprofessionals alike." — *Doody's Review Service, Dec '02*

■

Stroke Sourcebook

Basic Consumer Health Information about Stroke, Including Ischemic, Hemorrhagic, Transient Ischemic Attack (TIA), and Pediatric Stroke, Stroke Triggers and Risks, Diagnostic Tests, Treatments, and Rehabilitation Information

Along with Stroke Prevention Guidelines, Legal and Financial Information, a Glossary, and a Directory of Additional Resources

Edited by Joyce Brennfleck Shannon. 606 pages. 2003. 978-0-7808-0630-6.

"This volume is highly recommended and should be in every medical, hospital, and public library."
— *American Reference Books Annual, 2004*

"Highly recommended for the amount and variety of topics and information covered." — *Choice, Nov '03*

■

Surgery Sourcebook

Basic Consumer Health Information about Inpatient and Outpatient Surgeries, Including Cardiac, Vascular, Orthopedic, Ocular, Reconstructive, Cosmetic, Gynecologic, and Ear, Nose, and Throat Procedures and More

Along with Information about Operating Room Policies and Instruments, Laser Surgery Techniques, Hospital Errors, Statistical Data, a Glossary, and Listings of Sources for Further Help and Information

Edited by Annemarie S. Muth and Karen Bellenir. 596 pages. 2002. 978-0-7808-0380-0.

"Large public libraries and medical libraries would benefit from this material in their reference collections."
— *American Reference Books Annual, 2004*

"Invaluable reference for public and school library collections alike." — *Library Bookwatch, Apr '03*

■

Thyroid Disorders Sourcebook

Basic Consumer Health Information about Disorders of the Thyroid and Parathyroid Glands, Including Hypothyroidism, Hyperthyroidism, Graves Disease, Hashimoto Thyroiditis, Thyroid Cancer, and Parathyroid Disorders, Featuring Facts about Symptoms, Risk Factors, Tests, and Treatments

Along with Information about the Effects of Thyroid Imbalance on Other Body Systems, Environmental Factors That Affect the Thyroid Gland, a Glossary, and a Directory of Additional Resources

Edited by Joyce Brennfleck Shannon. 599 pages. 2005. 978-0-7808-0745-7.

"Recommended for consumer health collections."
— *American Reference Books Annual, 2006*

"Highly recommended pick for basic consumer health reference holdings at all levels."
— *The Bookwatch, Aug '05*

■

Transplantation Sourcebook

Basic Consumer Health Information about Organ and Tissue Transplantation, Including Physical and Financial Preparations, Procedures and Issues Relating to Specific Solid Organ and Tissue Transplants, Rehabilitation, Pediatric Transplant Information, the Future of Transplantation, and Organ and Tissue Donation

Along with a Glossary and Listings of Additional Resources

Edited by Joyce Brennfleck Shannon. 628 pages. 2002. 978-0-7808-0322-0.

"Along with these advances [in transplantation technology] have come a number of daunting questions for potential transplant patients, their families, and their health care providers. This reference text is the best single tool to address many of these questions. . . . It will be a much-needed addition to the reference collections in health care, academic, and large public libraries."
— American Reference Books Annual, 2003

"Recommended for libraries with an interest in offering consumer health information." — E-Streams, Jul '02

"This is a unique and valuable resource for patients facing transplantation and their families."
— Doody's Review Service, Jun '02

■

Traveler's Health Sourcebook

Basic Consumer Health Information for Travelers, Including Physical and Medical Preparations, Transportation Health and Safety, Essential Information about Food and Water, Sun Exposure, Insect and Snake Bites, Camping and Wilderness Medicine, and Travel with Physical or Medical Disabilities

Along with International Travel Tips, Vaccination Recommendations, Geographical Health Issues, Disease Risks, a Glossary, and a Listing of Additional Resources

Edited by Joyce Brennfleck Shannon. 613 pages. 2000. 978-0-7808-0384-8.

"Recommended reference source."
— Booklist, American Library Association, Feb '01

"This book is recommended for any public library, any travel collection, and especially any collection for the physically disabled."
— American Reference Books Annual, 2001

SEE ALSO Worldwide Health Sourcebook

■

Urinary Tract & Kidney Diseases & Disorders Sourcebook, 2nd Edition

Basic Consumer Health Information about the Urinary System, Including the Bladder, Urethra, Ureters, and Kidneys, with Facts about Urinary Tract Infections, Incontinence, Congenital Disorders, Kidney Stones, Cancers of the Urinary Tract and Kidneys, Kidney Failure, Dialysis, and Kidney Transplantation

Along with Statistical and Demographic Information, Reports on Current Research in Kidney and Urologic Health, a Summary of Commonly Used Diagnostic Tests, a Glossary of Related Terms, and a Directory of Resources for Additional Help and Information

Edited by Ivy L. Alexander. 649 pages. 2005. 978-0-7808-0750-1.

"A good choice for a consumer health information library or for a medical library needing information to refer to their patients."
— American Reference Books Annual, 2006

Vegetarian Sourcebook

Basic Consumer Health Information about Vegetarian Diets, Lifestyle, and Philosophy, Including Definitions of Vegetarianism and Veganism, Tips about Adopting Vegetarianism, Creating a Vegetarian Pantry, and Meeting Nutritional Needs of Vegetarians, with Facts Regarding Vegetarianism's Effect on Pregnant and Lactating Women, Children, Athletes, and Senior Citizens

Along with a Glossary of Commonly Used Vegetarian Terms and Resources for Additional Help and Information

Edited by Chad T. Kimball. 360 pages. 2002. 978-0-7808-0439-5.

"Organizes into one concise volume the answers to the most common questions concerning vegetarian diets and lifestyles. This title is recommended for public and secondary school libraries." — E-Streams, Apr '03

"Invaluable reference for public and school library collections alike." — Library Bookwatch, Apr '03

"The articles in this volume are easy to read and come from authoritative sources. The book does not necessarily support the vegetarian diet but instead provides the pros and cons of this important decision. The Vegetarian Sourcebook is recommended for public libraries and consumer health libraries."
— American Reference Books Annual, 2003

SEE ALSO Diet & Nutrition Sourcebook

■

Women's Health Concerns Sourcebook, 2nd Edition

Basic Consumer Health Information about the Medical and Mental Concerns of Women, Including Maintaining Health and Wellness, Gynecological Concerns, Breast Health, Sexuality and Reproductive Issues, Menopause, Cancer in Women, Leading Causes of Death and Disability among Women, Physical Concerns of Special Significance to Women, and Women's Mental and Emotional Health

Along with a Glossary of Related Terms and Directories of Resources for Additional Help and Information

Edited by Amy L. Sutton. 746 pages. 2004. 978-0-7808-0673-3.

"This is a useful reference book, which makes the reader knowledgeable about several issues that concern women's health. It is recommended for public libraries and home library collections." — E-Streams, May '05

"A useful addition to public and consumer health library collections."
— American Reference Books Annual, 2005

"A highly recommended title."
— The Bookwatch, May '04

"Handy compilation. There is an impressive range of diseases, devices, disorders, procedures, and other physical and emotional issues covered . . . well organized, illustrated, and indexed." — Choice, Association of College & Research Libraries, Jan '98

SEE ALSO *Breast Cancer Sourcebook, Cancer Sourcebook for Women, Healthy Heart Sourcebook for Women, Osteoporosis Sourcebook*

■

Workplace Health & Safety Sourcebook

Basic Consumer Health Information about Workplace Health and Safety, Including the Effect of Workplace Hazards on the Lungs, Skin, Heart, Ears, Eyes, Brain, Reproductive Organs, Musculoskeletal System, and Other Organs and Body Parts

Along with Information about Occupational Cancer, Personal Protective Equipment, Toxic and Hazardous Chemicals, Child Labor, Stress, and Workplace Violence

Edited by Chad T. Kimball. 626 pages. 2000. 978-0-7808-0231-5.

"As a reference for the general public, this would be useful in any library." — *E-Streams, Jun '01*

"Provides helpful information for primary care physicians and other caregivers interested in occupational medicine. . . . General readers; professionals."
— *Choice, Association of College & Research Libraries, May '01*

"Recommended reference source."
— *Booklist, American Library Association, Feb '01*

"Highly recommended." — *The Bookwatch, Jan '01*

■

Worldwide Health Sourcebook

Basic Information about Global Health Issues, Including Malnutrition, Reproductive Health, Disease Dispersion and Prevention, Emerging Diseases, Risky Health Behaviors, and the Leading Causes of Death

Along with Global Health Concerns for Children, Women, and the Elderly, Mental Health Issues, Research and Technology Advancements, and Economic, Environmental, and Political Health Implications, a Glossary, and a Resource Listing for Additional Help and Information

Edited by Joyce Brennfleck Shannon. 614 pages. 2001. 978-0-7808-0330-5.

"Named an Outstanding Academic Title."
— *Choice, Association of College & Research Libraries, Jan '02*

"Yet another handy but also unique compilation in the extensive *Health Reference Series*, this is a useful work because many of the international publications reprinted or excerpted are not readily available. Highly recommended." — *Choice, Association of College & Research Libraries, Nov '01*

"Recommended reference source."
— *Booklist, American Library Association, Oct '01*

SEE ALSO *Traveler's Health Sourcebook*

667

Teen Health Series
Helping Young Adults Understand, Manage, and Avoid Serious Illness

List price $65 per volume. **School and library price $58 per volume.**

Alcohol Information for Teens
Health Tips about Alcohol and Alcoholism

Including Facts about Underage Drinking, Preventing Teen Alcohol Use, Alcohol's Effects on the Brain and the Body, Alcohol Abuse Treatment, Help for Children of Alcoholics, and More

Edited by Joyce Brennfleck Shannon. 370 pages. 2005. 978-0-7808-0741-9.

"Boxed facts and tips add visual interest to the well-researched and clearly written text."
— *Curriculum Connection, Apr '06*

Allergy Information for Teens
Health Tips about Allergic Reactions Such as Anaphylaxis, Respiratory Problems, and Rashes

Including Facts about Identifying and Managing Allergies to Food, Pollen, Mold, Animals, Chemicals, Drugs, and Other Substances

Edited by Karen Bellenir. 410 pages. 2006. 978-0-7808-0799-0.

Asthma Information for Teens
Health Tips about Managing Asthma and Related Concerns

Including Facts about Asthma Causes, Triggers, Symptoms, Diagnosis, and Treatment

Edited by Karen Bellenir. 386 pages. 2005. 978-0-7808-0770-9.

"Highly recommended for medical libraries, public school libraries, and public libraries."
— *American Reference Books Annual, 2006*

"It is so clearly written and well organized that even hesitant readers will be able to find the facts they need, whether for reports or personal information. . . . A succinct but complete resource."
— *School Library Journal, Sep '05*

Body Information for Teens
Health Tips about Maintaining Well-Being for a Lifetime

Including Facts about the Development and Functioning of the Body's Systems, Organs, and Structures and the Health Impact of Lifestyle Choices

Edited by Sandra Augustyn Lawton. 458 pages. 2007. 978-0-7808-0443-2.

Cancer Information for Teens
Health Tips about Cancer Awareness, Prevention, Diagnosis, and Treatment

Including Facts about Frequently Occurring Cancers, Cancer Risk Factors, and Coping Strategies for Teens Fighting Cancer or Dealing with Cancer in Friends or Family Members

Edited by Wilma R. Caldwell. 428 pages. 2004. 978-0-7808-0678-8.

"Recommended for school libraries, or consumer libraries that see a lot of use by teens."
— *E-Streams, May '05*

"A valuable educational tool."
— *American Reference Books Annual, 2005*

"Young adults and their parents alike will find this new addition to the *Teen Health Series* an important reference to cancer in teens."
— *Children's Bookwatch, Feb '05*

Complementary and Alternative Medicine Information for Teens
Health Tips about Non-Traditional and Non-Western Medical Practices

Including Information about Acupuncture, Chiropractic Medicine, Dietary and Herbal Supplements, Hypnosis, Massage Therapy, Prayer and Spirituality, Reflexology, Yoga, and More

Edited by Sandra Augustyn Lawton. 405 pages. 2006. 978-0-7808-0966-6.

Diabetes Information for Teens
Health Tips about Managing Diabetes and Preventing Related Complications

Including Information about Insulin, Glucose Control, Healthy Eating, Physical Activity, and Learning to Live with Diabetes

Edited by Sandra Augustyn Lawton. 410 pages. 2006. 978-0-7808-0811-9.

Diet Information for Teens, 2nd Edition

Health Tips about Diet and Nutrition

Including Facts about Dietary Guidelines, Food Groups, Nutrients, Healthy Meals, Snacks, Weight Control, Medical Concerns Related to Diet, and More

Edited by Karen Bellenir. 432 pages. 2006. 978-0-7808-0820-1.

"Full of helpful insights and facts throughout the book. . . . An excellent resource to be placed in public libraries or even in personal collections."
— *American Reference Books Annual, 2002*

"Recommended for middle and high school libraries and media centers as well as academic libraries that educate future teachers of teenagers. It is also a suitable addition to health science libraries that serve patrons who are interested in teen health promotion and education." — *E-Streams, Oct '01*

"This comprehensive book would be beneficial to collections that need information about nutrition, dietary guidelines, meal planning, and weight control. . . . This reference is so easy to use that its purchase is recommended." — *The Book Report, Sep-Oct '01*

"This book is written in an easy to understand format describing issues that many teens face every day, and then provides thoughtful explanations so that teens can make informed decisions. This is an interesting book that provides important facts and information for today's teens." — *Doody's Health Sciences Book Review Journal, Jul-Aug '01*

"A comprehensive compendium of diet and nutrition. The information is presented in a straightforward, plain-spoken manner. This title will be useful to those working on reports on a variety of topics, as well as to general readers concerned about their dietary health." — *School Library Journal, Jun '01*

Drug Information for Teens, 2nd Edition

Health Tips about the Physical and Mental Effects of Substance Abuse

Including Information about Marijuana, Inhalants, Club Drugs, Stimulants, Hallucinogens, Opiates, Prescription and Over-the-Counter Drugs, Herbal Products, Tobacco, Alcohol, and More

Edited by Sandra Augustyn Lawton. 468 pages. 2006. 978-0-7808-0862-1.

"A clearly written resource for general readers and researchers alike." — *School Library Journal*

"This book is well-balanced. . . . a must for public and school libraries."
— *VOYA: Voice of Youth Advocates, Dec '03*

"The chapters are quick to make a connection to their teenage reading audience. The prose is straightforward and the book lends itself to spot reading. It should be useful both for practical information and for research, and it is suitable for public and school libraries."
— *American Reference Books Annual, 2003*

"Recommended reference source."
— *Booklist, American Library Association, Feb '03*

"This is an excellent resource for teens and their parents. Education about drugs and substances is key to discouraging teen drug abuse and this book provides this much needed information in a way that is interesting and factual." — *Doody's Review Service, Dec '02*

Eating Disorders Information for Teens

Health Tips about Anorexia, Bulimia, Binge Eating, and Other Eating Disorders

Including Information on the Causes, Prevention, and Treatment of Eating Disorders, and Such Other Issues as Maintaining Healthy Eating and Exercise Habits

Edited by Sandra Augustyn Lawton. 337 pages. 2005. 978-0-7808-0783-9.

"An excellent resource for teens and those who work with them."
— *VOYA: Voice of Youth Advocates, Apr '06*

"A welcome addition to high school and undergraduate libraries." — *American Reference Books Annual, 2006*

"This book covers the topic in a lucid manner but delves deeper into every aspect of an eating disorder. A solid addition for any nonfiction or reference collection." — *School Library Journal, Dec '05*

Fitness Information for Teens

Health Tips about Exercise, Physical Well-Being, and Health Maintenance

Including Facts about Aerobic and Anaerobic Conditioning, Stretching, Body Shape and Body Image, Sports Training, Nutrition, and Activities for Non-Athletes

Edited by Karen Bellenir. 425 pages. 2004. 978-0-7808-0679-5.

"Another excellent offering from Omnigraphics in their *Teen Health Series*. . . . This book will be a great addition to any public, junior high, senior high, or secondary school library."
— *American Reference Books Annual, 2005*

Learning Disabilities Information for Teens

Health Tips about Academic Skills Disorders and Other Disabilities That Affect Learning

Including Information about Common Signs of Learning Disabilities, School Issues, Learning to Live with a Learning Disability, and Other Related Issues

Edited by Sandra Augustyn Lawton. 337 pages. 2005. 978-0-7808-0796-9.

"This book provides a wealth of information for any reader interested in the signs, causes, and consequences

of learning disabilities, as well as related legal rights and educational interventions.... Public and academic libraries should want this title for both students and general readers."
— *American Reference Books Annual, 2006*

■

Mental Health Information for Teens, 2nd Edition
Health Tips about Mental Wellness and Mental Illness

Including Facts about Mental and Emotional Health, Depression and Other Mood Disorders, Anxiety Disorders, Behavior Disorders, Self-Injury, Psychosis, Schizophrenia, and More

Edited by Karen Bellenir. 400 pages. 2006. 978-0-7808-0863-8.

"In both language and approach, this user-friendly entry in the *Teen Health Series* is on target for teens needing information on mental health concerns."
— *Booklist, American Library Association, Jan '02*

"Readers will find the material accessible and informative, with the shaded notes, facts, and embedded glossary insets adding appropriately to the already interesting and succinct presentation."
— *School Library Journal, Jan '02*

"This title is highly recommended for any library that serves adolescents and parents/caregivers of adolescents."
— *E-Streams, Jan '02*

"Recommended for high school libraries and young adult collections in public libraries. Both health professionals and teenagers will find this book useful."
— *American Reference Books Annual, 2002*

"This is a nice book written to enlighten the society, primarily teenagers, about common teen mental health issues. It is highly recommended to teachers and parents as well as adolescents."
— *Doody's Review Service, Dec '01*

■

Sexual Health Information for Teens
Health Tips about Sexual Development, Human Reproduction, and Sexually Transmitted Diseases

Including Facts about Puberty, Reproductive Health, Chlamydia, Human Papillomavirus, Pelvic Inflammatory Disease, Herpes, AIDS, Contraception, Pregnancy, and More

Edited by Deborah A. Stanley. 391 pages. 2003. 978-0-7808-0445-6.

"This work should be included in all high school libraries and many larger public libraries.... highly recommended."
— *American Reference Books Annual, 2004*

"*Sexual Health* approaches its subject with appropriate seriousness and offers easily accessible advice and information."
— *School Library Journal, Feb '04*

Skin Health Information for Teens
Health Tips about Dermatological Concerns and Skin Cancer Risks

Including Facts about Acne, Warts, Hives, and Other Conditions and Lifestyle Choices, Such as Tanning, Tattooing, and Piercing, That Affect the Skin, Nails, Scalp, and Hair

Edited by Robert Aquinas McNally. 429 pages. 2003. 978-0-7808-0446-3.

"This volume, as with others in the series, will be a useful addition to school and public library collections." — *American Reference Books Annual, 2004*

"There is no doubt that this reference tool is valuable."
— *VOYA: Voice of Youth Advocates, Feb '04*

"This volume serves as a one-stop source and should be a necessity for any health collection."
— *Library Media Connection*

■

Sports Injuries Information for Teens
Health Tips about Sports Injuries and Injury Protection

Including Facts about Specific Injuries, Emergency Treatment, Rehabilitation, Sports Safety, Competition Stress, Fitness, Sports Nutrition, Steroid Risks, and More

Edited by Joyce Brennfleck Shannon. 405 pages. 2003. 978-0-7808-0447-0.

"This work will be useful in the young adult collections of public libraries as well as high school libraries."
— *American Reference Books Annual, 2004*

■

Suicide Information for Teens
Health Tips about Suicide Causes and Prevention

Including Facts about Depression, Risk Factors, Getting Help, Survivor Support, and More

Edited by Joyce Brennfleck Shannon. 368 pages. 2005. 978-0-7808-0737-2.

■

Tobacco Information for Teens
Health Tips about the Hazards of Using Cigarettes, Smokeless Tobacco, and Other Nicotine Products

Including Facts about Nicotine Addiction, Immediate and Long-Term Health Effects of Tobacco Use, Related Cancers, Smoking Cessation, Tobacco Use Prevention, and Tobacco Use Statistics

Edited by Karen Bellenir. 440 pages. 2007. 978-0-7808-0976-5.

Health Reference Series